LIVING WITH DISFIGUREMENT

This book is the seventh in a series published in association with CEDR

Series Editor: *Robin Lovelock*

Already published:

CHANGING PATTERNS OF MENTAL HEALTH CARE
A case study in the development of local services
Jackie Powell and Robin Lovelock

PARTNERSHIP IN PRACTICE
The Children Act 1989
Edited by Ann Buchanan

DISABILITY: BRITAIN IN EUROPE
An evaluation of UK participation in the HELIOS
programme (1988-1991)
Robin Lovelock and Jackie Powell

THE PROBATION SERVICE AND INFORMATION TECHNOLOGY
David Colombi

VISUAL IMPAIRMENT; SOCIAL SUPPORT
Recent research in context
Robin Lovelock

WORKLOADS
Measurement and management
Joan Orme

Forthcoming titles:

EDUCATING FOR SOCIAL WORK: ARGUMENTS FOR OPTIMISM
Edited by Peter Ford and Patrick Hayes

DEMENTIA CARE: KEEPING INTACT AND IN TOUCH
A search for occupational therapy interventions
Cathy Conroy

Living With Disfigurement:

Psychosocial implications of being born with a cleft lip and palate

POPPY NASH

Avebury

Aldershot • Brookfield USA • Hong Kong • Singapore • Sydney

Published by
Avebury
Ashgate Publishing Limited
Gower House
Croft Road
Aldershot
Hants GU11 3HR
England

Ashgate Publishing Company
Old Post Road
Brookfield
Vermont 05036
USA

British Library Cataloguing in Publication Data

Nash, Poppy
Living with Disfigurement: Psychosocial
Implications of Being Born with a Cleft Lip
and Palate. - (CEDR Series)
I. Title   II. Series
362.1975225

ISBN 1 85628 967 2

Library of Congress Catalog Card Number: 95-80355

Printed and bound by Athenaeum Press, Ltd.,
Gateshead, Tyne & Wear.

Contents

List of tables

List of figures

Acknowledgements

I would like to take this opportunity to remember those without whose involvement the study could not have taken place. This not only includes the participants, but also Mrs. Beryl Hammond herself, for affording me the chance to pursue such an enjoyable and stimulating area of study.

Alongside these acknowledgements, I wish to my express gratitude for the advice and encouragement which I have received from Professor Bryan Glastonbury, Hazel Osborne and Robin Lovelock at the University of Southampton; in addition, to Mr. Robert McDowall (Consultant Plastic Surgeon), Shirley Smith (my former Speech and Language Therapy Manager), and my colleagues in the Speech and Language Therapy Department and on the Cleft Palate Team at Odstock Hospital (now Salisbury District Hospital). Without their support the research could not have been undertaken. I wish also to acknowledge the generous financial assistance given to me by the Wessex Regional Research Committee, and funds from the Wessex Centre for Plastic and Maxillo-facial Surgery, Odstock Hospital, which enabled the development of the study.

My thanks is extended to those who have lived and breathed the research with me from the outset, especially Robin, Alison, my parents and family. Their support and understanding have been integral to the completion of the study.

1 Introduction

General introduction

> From the beginning, the life experiences of the baby with cleft lip and cleft palate are different from those of normal infants. (Tisza and Gumpertz, 1962, p.87)

The neonatal diagnosis of cleft lip and/or palate, can be a devastating psychological shock to the infant's parents and family. This may be particularly so if there is no prior knowledge of the cleft deformity, since the anticipation of producing a 'perfect baby' is obliterated.

Whilst the newborn baby receives immediate care from a variety of professionals, the need for adequate attention to be paid to the parents at this stage cannot be underestimated. Indeed, there appears to be a direct relationship between the parents' (especially the mother's) psychological well-being during the child's early life, and the subsequent effects of the cleft upon the developing child (for example, Brantley and Clifford, 1980). Therefore, the birth of an infant with a cleft necessitates a concerted effort by both professionals and parents, to work together in minimizing the potentially adverse implications of the condition.

According to Pigott (1986), in the United Kingdom approximately 900 infants a year are born with one form of cleft lip and/or palate. About half of this population will require the advice of specialists comprising the Cleft Palate Team, into late adolescence. Thus, about 15,000 cleft-impaired patients will be receiving professional help at any given time.

1

The majority of patients with a cleft are treated under the National Health Service in a district general hospital. However, the services offered in this country are very diverse. For example, some regions place much emphasis upon joint clinics, in which all those involved in treating the patient are present. In other areas, members of the Cleft Palate Team attend clinics only if, and when their particular expertise is required. In a small minority of situations, a Cleft Palate Team does not exist at all, leaving the managing clinician to call upon the relevant specialists at his/her discretion, or at the request of the patient.

Before addressing the particular problems encountered by the cleft population and their families, and the treatment offered by the Cleft Palate Team, the nature of the cleft deformity itself will be examined.

The nature of cleft lip and/or palate

As cleft of the lip and/or palate is a congenital malformation, examination of foetal development can intimate how such a deformity takes place. Berkovitz (1986, p.1) states that facial development evolves during the fourth week of gestation. Clefting of the lip and/or palate is believed to occur in early pregnancy during the first trimester. Having reviewed various research findings relating to the aetiology of clefts, Noar (1988, p.11) concludes: 'What seems apparent is that there is a 'critical time and a critical dose' for the induction of a cleft in a foetus by environmental agents (DePaola, 1975).'

Classification of clefts

Clefts can take various forms, differing in both type and severity from the lip to the soft palate. A variety of classifications exist, some of which are morphological (such as Davis and Ritchie, 1922; Veau, 1931). Others emphasize embryological development (for example, Fogh-Anderson, 1942; Kernahan and Stark, 1958). The practice these days, however, is to describe the deformity in detail, as and when it is presented clinically, since categorizing the defect too specifically can be misleading.

In acknowledging the complex nature of cleft lip and palate, Hathorn (1986, p.17) has put forward a descriptive categorization of clefts, which can be compared with the most frequently cited classification of Kernahan and Stark (1958) below. Before considering these taxonomies, the location of the different anatomical features to which they refer will be identified.

If the lips are thought of as the most anterior part of the oral cavity, with that cavity extending posteriorly to the uvula (free edge of the soft palate), the position of the various features which may be associated with cleft impairment is described below (some definitions derive from Albery et al., 1986, p.84-87).

Upper Lip   (soft tissue)
|
Alveolus   (gum ridge and bone incorporating teeth)
|
Premaxilla   (bone between two parts of upper jaw holding incisors)
|
Hard Palate   (bony structure partially forming the roof of mouth)
|
Soft Palate   (incisive foramen divides soft tissue from hard palate)
↓
Uvula   (muscular structure hanging from free edge of soft palate)

Figure 1.1   Anatomical features potentially implicated in cleft lip and/or palate

Table 1.1
An outline of Hathorn's (1986) classification of clefts

i) *Cleft Lip*
   Right or left sided (unilateral) or both sides (bilateral).
   With or without the involvement of the alveolus.

ii) *Unilateral Cleft lip and Palate*
   Right or left sided.
   With involvement of the upper lip, premaxilla, hard and soft palate.

iii) *Bilateral Cleft Lip and Palate*
   Right and left sides.
   With involvement of the upper lip, premaxilla, hard and soft palate.

iv) *Cleft Palate*
   No lip involvement.
   Cleft of the hard and soft palate, or soft palate only.
   Submucous cleft is included in this category.

Hathorn's delineation of the different presentations of clefts as preented in Table 1.1, can be contrasted with the earlier, and more widely documented description proposed by Kernahan and Stark (1958). The latter authors speak in terms of the 'primary' and 'secondary' palate (taken from Stengelhofen, 1989, p.4), as indicated in their classification of clefts in Table 1.2. In clarifying the terminology used, the 'incisive foramen' refers to small orifices within the hard palate, occurring at the junction in the midline between the premaxilla and posterior palatal segments (Albery et al., 1986, p.85).

3

Table 1.2
Kernahan and Stark's (1958) classification of clefts

i) *Clefts of the Primary Palate*
Lies anterior to (in front of) the incisive foramen.
May involve both lip and alveolus.
1. Unilateral (right or left)
2. Median
3. Bilateral

ii) *Clefts of the Secondary Palate*
Cleft of the palate only.
Lies posterior to (behind) the incisive foramen.
Ranges from bifid uvula to complete hard and soft palate.
1. Total (or complete)
2. Sub-Total (or incomplete)
3. Sub-Mucous

iii) *Clefts of the Primary and Secondary Palate*
Affects both primary and secondary palate.
Wide range of manifestations and degrees of severity.
1. Unilateral (right or left)
2. Median
3. Bilateral

Incidence and prevalence of clefts

The accurate estimation of the incidence and prevalence of cleft lip and/or palate is fraught with difficulties, since a central register for cleft births is still being compiled in this country. More precisely, the Craniofacial Anomalies Register (CARE) was launched in January 1989 by the Craniofacial Society of Great Britain, as a national register for all forms of craniofacial anomaly including cleft lip and/or palate. Prior to this, epidemiological data have been collected without reference to standard and universally accepted criteria. For example, reports including still and live births, and abortions in their statistics, contrast with those excluding one or two of these groups.

Goodman and Gorlin (1983, p.56) report that cleft lip and palate is more common in males than females (about 2:1). Stengelhofen (1989) notes that isolated cleft of the palate is the only instance of cleft, which occurs more frequently in females.

Hathorn (1986, p.17) has calculated the proportion of each type of cleft occurring as a percentage of the overall incidence of clefts, in accordance with his classification of clefts (Table 1.3). It should be pointed out that Hathorn states the overall incidence of clefts (of all types), as approximately 1 in 600. This is contrary to the incidence cited by Pigott (1986) referred to earlier, who posits a 1 in 900 incidence. A further discrepancy arises with Blenkinsop's (1989) estimated incidence of 1 in 800 births.

Table 1.3
Incidence of clefts according to type of cleft

Type of cleft	Percentage incidence of total clefts
Cleft lip only	25.0
Unilateral cleft lip and palate	40.0
Bilateral cleft lip and palate	10.0
Cleft palate only (including submucous cleft)	25.0
Total	100.0

The incidence and prevalence of clefts in this country appears to follow a distinct geographical pattern of distribution, according to Richards and Lowe (1971). The lowest incidence of the deformity is found in south-east England. There is then a gradual increase in incidence over the west and north of the United Kingdom. This is evident in Wales for example, where the incidence of clefts is reported to be over 2.00 per 1000. The pattern of distribution appears to correspond to the nationwide division of social and economic affluence. That is, the incidence of clefts seems to be greater in the regions associated with less affluence in social and economic terms.

In describing the differential diagnosis of clefts in infants, Goodman and Gorlin (1983, p.56), stress the necessary exclusion of the 200 facial cleft syndromes in doing so, as genetic counselling may differ greatly in each case. The majority of individuals presenting with cleft lip and palate, however, do not have additional congenital anomalies.

Cleft of the lip

In embryological terms, the face develops with the fusion of specific features. In the case of cleft lip, the fusion between the maxillary process and the median nasal process (the primary palate) fails to take place (Goodman and Gorlin, 1983). The mildest manifestation of cleft lip involves a slight notching, or natural scarring of the vermilion border of the upper lip. Surgery may not be required if there is no open cleft to repair. In contrast, the most severe form of cleft lip presents as a complete bilateral cleft of the lip and the alveolus behind it. Between these two extremes there are varying degrees of clefting, which may be either unilateral (left or right side only), or bilateral (both left and right sides).

Regarding the severity of clefting, the cleft may be evident at the fleshy border of the upper lip, and extend through the soft tissue of the prolabium towards the nostril on the affected side. Sometimes, the nostril is also affected by the cleft, giving a characteristic flat nose profile. In the more severe cases, the cleft continues through the maxillary arch, with further clefting of the alveolus. Clefts of the lip may occur with or without additional cleft palate.

Cleft of the palate

Cleft palate is reported to be: 'the most common malformation in human babies' (Blenkinsop, 1989, p.D11). The malformation is due to the failed fusion of the secondary palate. That is, the midline fusion of the two palatine processes which is critical to normal development, has not occurred. A more extensive form of clefting involves the hard and soft palate. The hard palate lies beyond the alveolus, with the soft palate extending behind it. It presents in both unilateral and bilateral forms. The degree of clefting again varies, depending upon how incomplete or complete the deformity appears to be. Although cleft palate may be accompanied by additional cleft lip, isolated cleft palate (no cleft lip) is considered to be a genetically different disorder from cleft of the lip and palate (for example, Goodman and Gorlin, 1983).

Submucous cleft

A submucous cleft may not be diagnosed at birth since it occurs below the mucous membrane of the soft palate, and the visible surface of the palate may appear to be unblemished and intact. As the effects of the deformity may not be recognized until the emergence of speech (Stengelhofen, 1989), diagnosis of submucous cleft may be made much later during childhood. In view of the generally later pattern of diagnosis and treatment, it will not be discussed further in this study.

Genetic counselling

Osborne (1986, p.76) advocates that since most cleft lip or palate disorders arise from multifactorial inheritance, the precise prescription of genetic inheritance is unclear. He presents statistics pertinent to genetic counselling.

• Where there is one child with cleft lip with or without cleft palate, the probability of the defect recurring in subsequent children is approximately 1 in 25.

• Where the child has cleft of the palate only, the probability of recurrence in subsequent children is approximately 1 in 50.

• Where a parent has a cleft, the probability of the defect recurring in his/her children, is approximately 1 in 25 for cleft lip with or without cleft palate, and 1 in 16 for cleft palate only.

Genetic counselling can be an essential part of the overall treatment programme, involving the patient and also his/her parents and family.
The two types of cleft under investigation in the current study are cleft

palate and cleft lip and palate, with no instances of cleft lip only. With the exception of Pierre Robin syndrome, the participants did not evidence any cleft-related syndromes.

Potential problems associated with a cleft

Cleft impairment signals a diversity of potential problems or anomalies affecting development and physical growth. The extent to which these additional 'handicaps' are experienced varies from person to person. Thus, the notion that the child can be discharged to live a 'normal' and carefree life, once the cleft has been surgically repaired is usually unrealistic. Indeed, some individuals continue to receive intermittent cleft-related treatment over a period of twenty or more years. The following table indicates predominant cleft-related problems, according to the age and stage of treatment at which they generally occur.

Table 1.4
The nature of cleft management over a twenty year period:
the identification of potential cleft-related problems and their implications
for the patient's maturation at various ages

In utero (occurring approximately 9-12 weeks gestation)

Potential cleft-related problems	Implications for development
Congenital cleft deformity exists. Severe clefts of lip can now be detected by ultrasound scanning. Clefts of the palate cannot yet be accurately identified in utero.	Diagnosis made.

Infancy (0-2 years old)

Potential cleft-related problems	Implications for development
Repair surgery for cleft lip and/ or palate.	Hazards associated with general anaesthetic necessary for surgery.
Cleft lip: diffculties obtaining adequate lip seal for sucking. Cleft palate: regurgitation of food and/or liquid through the nasal cavity. Inability to gain adequate intra-oral pressure necessary for effective feeding. Tongue may adopt a deviant position.	Feeding lengthy and fraught, therefore creating unrewarding interaction between infant and parent (especially mother), and disrupting routine. Inadequate nutrition obtained by infant on account of feeding complications.

Potential cleft-related problems	Implications for development
Psychosocial and language development.	Interaction and bonding between infant and parents, may be adversely affected by impaired communication skills, feeding, parental attitude towards infant and requisite hospitalization.
Speech development.	Deviant patterns of articulation from defective articulators may become established, such as compensatory tongue positions due to cleft palate. Resonatory and phonatory features may be apparent where velopharyngeal insufficiency (VPI) occurs.
Hearing impairment.	Conductive hearing loss with middle ear problems, which may adversely affect interaction and speech acquisition. Grommets (or drainage tubes) may be surgically inserted to counter impaired hearing, at the time of repair surgery or later on. Frequent upper respiratory tract infections (URTI) associated with cleft palate may impede hearing.

Childhood (approximately 3-12 years old)

Potential cleft-related problems	Implications for development
Revision surgery to the lip and/or palate, and/or closure of fistula(e). Cosmetic surgery may be offered to improve the appearance of the nose.	Trauma of hospitalization, and absence from school. Peers may mark child out as 'different' since he/she requires treatment.
Dental anomalies.	Orthodontic treatment may be lengthy and obvious (e.g. if child is required to wear an appliance, such as a brace).
Psychosocial development.	A problematic parental attitude towards child may hamper his/ her self-esteem and functioning. Adverse effects of sibling rivalry and victimization by peers (such as teasing) upon socialization.

Language development.	Language delay can impede effective communication and interaction with other people.
Speech development.	Impaired articulation and/or nasality may affect the intelligibility of speech, disrupt communication and invite ridicule by peers.
Hearing impairment.	As for Infancy above. Education may be also hampered by inadequate hearing in the classroom.
Education and intellectual development.	Language delay can exert a deleterious effect upon learning. Possible special educational needs which may necessitate special schooling. Victimization by school peers may influence child's perception of school and his/her school performance. Cleft defect may adversely affect school teacher's expectations of child's academic capabilities. Disrupted schooling due to attendance at requisite out-patient follow-up clinics and/or hospitalization. Frequent upper respiratory tract infections may mean further absence from school.

Adolescence (13-17 years old)

Potential cleft-related problems

Implications for development

As for Childhood above.
On leaving school various options are available to the individual, such as pursuing Further or Higher Education, or seeking some form of employment or remaining unemployed. Marriage and/or parenthood is also a possibility.

Problems of childhood now divide individiduals into four distinct groups as follows, depending upon their personal circumstances.

1. Few or no problems are encountered.
2. Problems identified by the professionals have now been resolved or diminish with intervention.
3. Problems identified by the professionals persist despite intervention.
4. Problems remain unidentified by the professionals, and persist with no intervention

9

Potential cleft-related problems	Implications for development
As for Adolescence above.	By now, various operational strategies have been adopted in response to the various problems encountered (where applicable).
	These strategies will largely determine how effectively, in psychosocial terms, the person will function in adulthood.

Although the same diagnosis may be given to two different infants (for instance, cleft palate), their treatment and life experience of living with that diagnosis may vary enormously. Whilst Table 1.4 above identifies the most common cleft-related problems, each individual's response to those difficulties may differ. There is, therefore, no such concept as the 'typical' cleft patient. This notion is misleading and undermines the heterogeneity of the cleft population. The extent to which the physical problems (such as the anatomical cleft defect, the disruption of dentition and middle ear complications), exacerbate the less tangible psychosocial impairment, largely depends upon the interaction of several factors.

Professional domain   the appropriate timing and type of hospital treatment, and professional attitude shown towards those receiving it.

Parental domain   parental attitude towards not only the cleft-impaired child, but also towards the cleft-related treatment offered to him/her.

Patient domain   the personality (including self-esteem) of the individual born with a cleft.

Where the equation denotes the positive and optimal aspects of the three domains listed, it is anticipated that the individual's life experiences will not be significantly marred by the cleft impairment. Where, however, the equation breaks down in even one of the three factors, the likelihood of negative repercussions of having a cleft increases.

To take an extreme example, an infant who receives hospital treatment which, with hindsight, did not adequately address his/her needs for various reasons, is reared by parents who are deeply disappointed that they have not produced a 'perfect' baby. This disappointment may be realised by an indifferent attitude towards their child, and towards all those offering cleft-related intervention. In that the youngster's temperament may be critical to his/her psychological survival, the vulnerable child may be less resilient to the effects of parental indifference than the naturally ebullient child.

Alongside a child's personality disposition, develops self-esteem. Although some personality traits appear to be strongly genetically determined, self-

10

esteem is largely shaped by environmental influences, such as parenting style. Further discussion of the complex interaction of the three domains, and their implications for the management of the cleft population will be pursued in chapter two (literature on disfigurement).

The Cleft Palate Team (CPT)

The diversity of the potential problems facing the cleft-impaired (Table 1.4), requires the expertise of an equally diverse range of specialists to address the problems. As suggested earlier, the composition of the Cleft Palate Team and its method of delivering the necessary services to the patient, tends to differ across hospital units. Since cleft lip and/or palate repair is usually undertaken by a plastic or maxillo-facial surgeon, the infant is generally referred to the nearest plastic or maxillo-facial surgery unit. These take the form of units run on a regional basis, which are fed by a number of hospitals within the region which do not provide the requisite service. Some Cleft Palate Teams visit the peripheral hospitals for out-patient follow-up clinics, enabling patients to be seen at their local hospital. However, when specific surgery, and/or intensive speech therapy are indicated, patients are invited to the unit run on a regional basis.

The frequency of the follow-up clinics also varies depending upon the needs and the number of patients in the locality. For example, clinics may be held on a monthly basis at one hospital, but on a six monthly basis at another hospital. Similarly, the patient may be requested to attend the clinic twice a year, or once every two years. Frequency of attendance is largely determined by the patient's age and stage of treatment and progress.

The precise timing and type of repair surgery continue to be widely debated, and as such provide a fine example of the variation between the services offered by Cleft Palate Teams. For instance, whilst some surgeons favour lip repair within the first forty-eight hours of birth, others prefer to wait until the infant is about three months old, when the he/she is considered to be less vulnerable. The differing viewpoints have fundamental implications regarding parental bonding and interaction with the infant, which will be addressed in due course.

Table 1.5 below indicates the professionals and carers who represent the 'extended' Cleft Palate Team, in that they could conceivably be involved in the management of cleft-impaired individuals. However, it is usually only the hospital-based specialists who officially comprise the team. Since the organization of provision may differ between units, the sources of help cited below are not ordered according to their degree of involvement. Rather, the sequence follows a broadly developmental framework with those most involved during the patient's infancy appearing first. The particular responsibilities of those most frequently involved in cleft management will be subsequently delineated.

Table 1.5
The potential sources of help and advice available to the patient

Community-based	Hospital-based
Parents	Obstetrician
Relatives	Paediatrician
Friends	Nursing Staff
Health Visitor	Obstetric Social Worker
General Practitioner	Plastic/Maxillo-Facial Surgeon
Speech Therapist	Speech Therapist
Pre-School Staff	ENT Surgeon
Peer Group	Anaesthetist
CLAPA Support Group	CLAPA Support Group
Social Services	Paediatric Social Worker
School Staff	Audiologist
Dentist	Orthodontist
Educational Psychologist	Oral Surgeon
Clinical Psychologist	Clinical Psychologist
Psychiatrist	Psychiatrist
College Staff	Radiologist
Spouse/Partner	Dietitian
Employer(s)	

With respect to the hospital procedure generally adopted following the birth of an infant with a cleft, the paediatrician and nursing staff are first on the scene. Medical care during the initial weeks of the baby's life, may be crucial in allaying respiratory and feeding problems. The obstetric social worker may also be involved at this stage to assist the patient's family.

The orthodontist may wish to provide the infant with a feeding plate and/or an active pre-surgical orthodontic appliance. The former enables the infant to be fed whilst waiting for repair surgery. The latter, pre-surgical orthopaedic treatment tends to be favoured in some areas in preparation for repair surgery.

Further intervention by the orthodontist often occurs throughout childhood once surgery has been completed. The school-aged patient may be offered dental and/or orthodontic treatment, for dental and/or occlusal problems.

When the plastic or maxillo-facial surgeon is confident of the infant's satisfactory health, the cleft will be surgically repaired (primary surgery). Revision and cosmetic surgery may be offered at a later stage if necessary. Middle ear problems, which can cause conductive hearing loss, are often associated with a cleft defect. Where indicated, the ear, nose and throat (ENT) surgeon will undertake a myringotomy operation, with possible insertion of grommets (drainage tubes). This may be carried out during palatal repair surgery. Some children with cleft palate suffer extensive hearing and ear problems throughout their schooling. Therefore, close links are maintained with the ENT department including the audiologist, since frequent hearing tests are essential for these patients.

From birth, the speech therapist can advise the parents and nursing staff on appropriate feeding methods, depending upon the type and extent of the infant's cleft. In some hospitals, this responsibility may be additionally undertaken by the nursing staff.

The speech therapist also recommends ways in which parents can actively encourage communication, and lip and tongue mobility in the young cleft-impaired child. These areas of development are particularly vulnerable in infancy and early guidance can assuage future problems. In this sense the help given is primarily preventative, compared with the more curative treatment which may be required later on.

Since each child's needs vary, speech therapy may be indicated for one individual throughout childhood, but be contra-indicated for another child. In general, the infant with cleft lip only will see the speech therapist during the early stages of treatment, to ensure that the repair surgery has allowed sufficient lip mobility for speech acquisition.

With cleft palate, however, speech therapy may be required for a prolonged period, since attainment of satisfactory speech may be hampered by impaired hearing, deviant articulation and a nasal voice quality. Stengelhofen (1989) notes that approximately forty per cent of patients with cleft lip and palate experience long term problems affecting their communication skills. Indeed, in addition to cleft-related problems of articulation and nasality, the speech therapist may need to address the wider domain of poor communication skills.

A proportion of individuals with a cleft will require the assistance of the oral surgeon, who is responsible for treating anomalies of facial bone structure. Oral surgery is generally postponed until adolescence when the individual's bone structure is more stabilized.

In the United States of America, the inclusion of a psychologist in the Cleft Palate Team is considered essential. In this country, such practice is generally deemed inappropriate or unnecessary, possibly due to restricted financial resources. As will become clear in the subsequent chapters, the low priority which may be given to the psychological aspects associated with a cleft, may reflect a lack of awareness of the apparent trauma experienced by many individuals. Needless to say, by paying insufficient attention to the psychological needs of the cleft-impaired and their parents from birth, the repercussions of the unmet needs may emerge in the future. Psychological problems detected and addressed in adulthood, are generally much more resistant to treatment than they are in their infancy, when the individual is younger.

Having said this, the hospital-based social worker and the community-based health visitor, continue to play an invaluable role in detecting and attending to everyday problems faced by families of the cleft-impaired.

In recognizing that the cleft population is susceptible to multiple problems, the concept of the Cleft Palate Team's facility to offer appropriate treatment as and when necessary, is becoming increasingly attractive and universally accepted. In identifying the role of the Cleft Palate Team, Noar (1988, p.22) comments: 'The overall aim of the treatment for these patients is to foster the development of a child who speaks well, has a pleasing appearance and a reasonably satisfactory dentition (Mordecai, 1984).'

This widely held perception of the objectives of cleft management exemplifies the focus upon cleft-related treatment. That is, attention is paid to improving the auditory and visible (physical) features of cleft impairment, but no mention is made of the possible psychosocial problems requiring attention. Thus, emphasis is placed upon satisfactory 'treatment' outcomes rather than holistic 'management' of the patient.

An invaluable adjunct to the hospital-based services available to the cleft population, is the Cleft Lip and Palate Association (CLAPA). This self-support group was begun over ten years ago, in response to the perceived need for such a group. The Association is now a national network, with regional branches around the country. Regular meetings are held to which patients, their parents and professionals are invited.

The aims of the support group are to counsel and support the parents of cleft-impaired children. The group also seeks to increase public awareness of the defect, and to educate the providers of cleft-related treatment. Educational literature is published and distributed to parents and those working in the field. Research into congenital head and neck anomalies is encouraged by the high priority given to fund raising events. Forging links between professionals and parents is also esteemed (CLAPA literature).

Having outlined the nature of cleft lip and/or palate, potential cleft-related problem areas, and the specialists involved in cleft management, it is now possible to recount the main concerns of this study. Initially, this will take the form of a statement of the problem, in which the predominant themes of the study will be identified.

Statement of the problem

Since the research being presented has evolved in response to an earlier study undertaken over twenty years ago, a statement of the problem regarding this study is only valuable if sufficient background information has preceded it. It is for this reason, that a description of the previous, formative investigation is given prior to detailing the writer's research.

The research of Beryl N. Hammond (1950s-1980s)

The latter part of the notably distinguished speech therapy career of the late Mrs. Beryl N. Hammond (hereafter referred to as BNH), was spent as Consultant Speech Therapist at the Wessex Centre for Plastic and Maxillo-Facial Surgery, Odstock Hospital, Salisbury, Wiltshire. Up until her death in 1987, BNH pursued her particular interest in children with cleft lip and/or palate, by conducting detailed research on surgical and non-surgical factors influencing child development. The current research has sought to address and extend the implications of BNH's research findings. Attention is turned

14

first to outlining the most notable findings.

With the development of Salisbury District Hospital on the site of Odstock Hospital in the early 1990s, the Wessex Centre has been superseded by the Odstock Centre for Burns, Plastic and Maxillo-Facial Surgery. In reporting the current study, reference to the Wessex Centre at Odstock Hospital will be preserved, since this is where the study took place. Similarly, in the early 1990s the profession of speech therapy became formally recognized as that of speech and language therapy. As the former term was current in BNH's day, it has been maintained in writing this book.

The survey of 249 cleft-impaired children (1968-1972)

In examining the long term speech development of cleft-impaired patients, BNH advocated early assessment of the child's speech, and the importance of concurrent guidance to be given to the patient (and to his/her parents) when appropriate, by the speech therapist and surgeon. Whilst these practices are now commonplace in many plastic and maxillo-facial surgery units, they would have been regarded as entrepreneurial in BNH's time. Further details are given in Appendix 1.

Between the years 1968-1972, Hammond and O'Riain (Consultant plastic surgeon at Odstock Hospital) conducted a survey on the speech development of 249 cleft-impaired children, who were receiving treatment at the Wessex Centre for Plastic and Maxillo-Facial Surgery. The survey examined the nature and progress of the children's speech at the start of their schooling (aged five years). The participants were aged up to five years old. Data collection spanned over a sixteen year period, and was undertaken by the same speech therapist, team of surgeons and ward sister. The survey is reported in O'Riain and Hammond, 1972.

Conclusions drawn by O'Riain and Hammond (1972)

Whilst acknowledging the limitations of their retrospective study, O'Riain and Hammond offer some points for consideration.

- Relatively little is known about the contributory factors affecting the speech development of children with clefts. The survey identifies 32% of 5 year olds, with either 'unacceptable' or 'grossly defective' speech. Three factors showed marked statistical significance in the study; the nature of the cleft, the child's linguistic and general development, and parental influence during the formative years.

- The following point is perhaps the most significant finding for the current study (O'Riain and Hammond, 1972, p.386):

... having observed the influence on these children and their speech of the many variable surgical factors, such as types of operation, and non-surgical factors, such as parental influence and other environmental and psychological considerations, we would say that further research into the latter aspects is more likely to lead to progress in this field.

• The researchers stress the need for a team work approach to thetreatment of all clefts (p. 386): '... our findings emphasize the vital importance of the overall treatment of the child as an individual, rather than of his palatal condition alone.'

• BNH's concluding remarks set a challenge (Hammond, 1970, p.9):

Of course there are many surgical factors also at work but why should so many of these children be below average, not only in language development but in overall maturation? Why should nearly 1/3 of the parents be unable or unwilling to help their children and approximately 1/6 exert an influence which is definitely harmful to the child's speech progress? There is much work to be done on further investigation of these problems.

The survey produces a quantitative outcome to the original objective regarding the proportion of 'acceptable' speakers at school age (68%). However, this result also highlights the underlying complexities of the less tangible factors operating upon the 32% of children who failed to 'make the grade' by five years old.

Subsequent research undertaken by BNH (1976-1979)

The research outlined above served as a preliminary study for a larger scale investigation involving 561 cleft-impaired children (aged between 4.5 and 5.5 years) with hypernasality, which is a characteristic problem affecting the speech of some individuals with cleft palate. It is defined as the nasal quality of voice, perceived auditorily, and resulting from the excess or inappropriate coupling of the nasal and the oral cavities. As the effectiveness of the velopharyngeal valve, which controls the quantity of air flowing into the nose is reduced, the excess air entering the nasal cavity produces nasal resonance, or hypernasality (Stengelhofen, 1989).

The 561 patient participants in the investigation, which included the 249 children mentioned earlier (O'Riain and Hammond, 1972), were grouped according to the location and age at which primary palatal closure was undertaken. Three groupings emerged as outlined below.

Series I   Primary palatal closure undertaken at Odstock Hospital prior to patient being 30 months old (n=501)
Series II   Primary palatal closure undertaken elsewhere prior to patient being 30 months old (n=29).

Series III   Primary palatal closure undertaken at Odstock Hospital when patient aged between 30 and 60 months (n=31).

The period between the first and last patient assessed spanned over twenty years. Although the assessment team remained constant throughout this time, during the latter years of the survey additional staff comprised several junior speech therapists, a further consultant plastic surgeon, and an oral surgeon. The registrars undertook some palatal surgery. It should be noted that assessments were based upon clinical observations during the patients' visits to hospital, and that no home visits were undertaken according to BNH's documentation.

The findings of this study were presented by BNH in a paper entitled 'Hypernasality Among 561 Children With Cleft Palate' (Hammond, 1977). Correlations were clearly evident between articulatory defects, a 'detrimental' home environment and overall 'retarded' development (Hammond, 1976). Whilst the results proved valuable for detailed examination of patients' speech problems and consequent clinical treatment, on account of the current research objectives they will not be discussed further on this occasion. However, the data collected for the study on hypernasality, were integral to BNH's subsequent survey.

The survey of 561 cleft-impaired children (1979-1982)

Having obtained information on the extent of hypernasality in 561 children, BNH extended the survey by assembling data on 'all aspects' of the same 561 patients with cleft palate (with or without lip involvement), preserving the same deadline of 31st December 1975. Details were collected on the children's hearing acuity, intellectual capability, home background and parental influence amongst other aspects. The medical and social histories of those patients included in the hypernasality study, but not involved in the preceding study (n=312), were assessed according to the criteria adopted for the original 249 children (O'Riain and Hammond, 1972) as BNH explains in her unpublished notes p.2): 'Information is tabulated on 561 separate cards - No conclusions have been drawn and there is no text other than a brief description and a key to the interpretation of numbers recorded on the cards.'

Unfortunately, following the death of BNH's surgical colleague, and her own death in 1987, this additional data remained unanalysed and in its raw form. The existence of the extensive data base has instigated the development of the current study. In pursuing the investigation, the writer had the opportunity to interview two eminent colleagues of BNH, who recalled the original survey being undertaken. The colleagues concerned were both members of the same Cleft Palate Team as BNH. They, therefore, knew many of the children as in-patients when they were admitted to Odstock Hospital for cleft-related treatment.

Having transcribed the interviews with the two former members of the plastic surgery unit, mention can be made of their observations concerning

17

BNH and the work in which they were all involved. In the following excerpts the writer has edited out redundant filler speech (such as 'you know'), and diversions of conversation, and indicated these occurrences (...). Further reference is made to these interviews in Appendix 2. On asking the colleagues about BNH's research, the subsequent responses were elicited. Although the assessments were made jointly by the professionals concerned, BNH was very much regarded as the prime instigator of the survey, as implicated in the following extracts.

> *She (BNH) was always the sort of person that wanted to talk about it (the survey) ... after clinics, and that sort of thing. She was wonderful ... she used to stimulate everybody, ... this is all her own work ... no question about that.*

The intrinsic priority given to a team work approach to treatment is reflected in the folowing observations.

> *... in developing policy for a group of people like this, it was important ... it was the early days of palate surgery ... and she (BNH) always felt it was important for us to talk about ... principles and that sort of thing, which was very helpful to us.*

> *I think I was more interested in getting the parents to form a team with my lot, than I was in doing surgery on them ... because ... the differences are enormous in the years to come.*

> *... as soon as she (BNH) found a situation where the parental side or the home side wasn't up to scratch according to her, she would arrange special appointments to see them ... they used to come to the clinics, but she would have them in a different group ... she would try very hard ... with some of these parents ... trying to explain how the ultimate ... person that would end up ... who had a cleft was very largely dependent upon home influence ... I remember she was very interested in the parents.*

> *... if you take on cleft lip and palate work, you're not taking on just the child, you are very much taking on the parents.*

Summary of the implications of BNH's work for the present study

O'Riain and Hammond (1972) undertook a thorough assessment procedure. It is notable that given the range of areas covered, the authors specifically pin-point the non-surgical factors (such as parental influence or attitude), as warranting urgent further investigation. The importance of these factors is still unclear, since the bulk of research into the cleft defect, has been devoted to cleft-related treatment. The role of

18

non-surgical factors upon the developing cleft-impaired child has, therefore, remained comparatively untapped and sporadically documented.

BNH stresses throughout her research the need for a comprehensive approach to the treatment of patients with a cleft. Thus, adequate attention must be paid to all areas of need, and not exclusively to the obvious medical and paramedical problems presented by the child (such as those warranting surgery, orthodontics and speech therapy). If a truly holistic treatment programme is to be established, the child's parents should be regarded as co-workers, in helping to consolidate treatment objectives. In addition, it may benefit the cleft-impaired child if his/her parents are considered patients too, by being offered the appropriate advice and support where necessary.

A particularly poignant finding by O'Riain and Hammond (1972) with respect to parenting the child with a cleft, concerns the extent to which the defect is visible. Although the proportion having additional lip involvement in their study is relatively small (post-alveolar and lip group comprising 12% of the patients, n=30), this group showed the highest incidence of 'detrimental' parental influence. The implications of this result beg further consideration not only for the cleft population, but also for those with some form of facial disfigurement.

Bickel (1970) emphasizes the close association between parental attitude and acceptance of the child, and the child's personality. Thus, the impact of an indifferent parental attitude upon a resilient child, can contrast dramatically with that exerted upon a more vulnerable child. Unlike the largely inherited characteristics of one's personality, the development of self-esteem appears to be more directly determined by the environment. However, the complex network of contributory factors to personality (including self-esteem) continues to operate throughout the individual's life. Nevertheless, the significance of the influences exerted upon the child during the formative years, is generally deemed to be the most potent in developmental terms. These factors need to be borne in mind in discussing the nature and efficacy of cleft-related treatment. Indeed, failure to do so may undermine the most crucial aspects of the individual's psychological 'survival kit'.

The availability of the extensive, largely raw data base accumulated by BNH and her colleagues, offered the writer the opportunity to undertake a retrospective follow-up study of as many of the original participants as could be traced. By way of introducing the main issues to be examined, a distinction needs to be made at this stage between the potential 'overt' and 'covert' problems encountered by the cleft population. The 'overt' category refers to anomalies which are visibly and/or audibly detectible, for example, cleft lip and/or palate, impaired dentition and speech. The specialists responsible for treating these areas comprise the core members of the hospital-based Cleft Palate Team, and generally operate under the ideology of the medical model.

In contrast, 'covert' difficulties, are largely invisible and even disguised. For example, the stigma attached to facial disfigurement (however minor that disfigurement may seem to others), the humiliation of being teased about one's speech and/or appearance, the trauma of going to hospital yet again and so forth. Unlike 'overt' problems which are usually identified and treated, 'covert' problems may not be identified nor acknowledged, and therefore, remain unaddressed. In the most extreme cases, this neglect can lead to social maladjustment or social withdrawal. The cleft-impaired individual is expected to develop personal coping strategies at a super human speed, if he/she is to survive victimization, and other adverse cleft-related experiences. Since the development of these strategies is largely presumed, their discussion may not be considered a treatment priority.

On the basis that there is biased attention paid to the 'overt' problems of the cleft patient, compared with the 'covert' problem areas, the present study seeks to address the following hypotheses in relation to the participants involved in the study. These areas of interest reflect the theoretical infrastructure upon which the study is based. As will become apparent, the statements are termed 'hypotheses' in the broadest sense of the word, since they are not subjected to experimental methodology. Following a report of the investigation and findings, the implications for clinical practice and future research will be discussed, in addition to suggestions as to how they might be put into operation.

Hypotheses to be addressed

Factors relating to the participants' psychosocial development and functioning during the developmental years

Factors relating to the home environment

Hypothesis i The home environment of the cleft population implicated in the study, has distinguishable features which are attributable to the cleft defect.

Hypothesis ii A 'detrimental' parental attitude towards the cleft-impaired patient identified during the child's pre-school years, has an adverse effect upon his/her psychosocial development and later psychosocial functioning.

Factors relating to the school environment

Hypothesis iii The school environment of the cleft population implicated in the study, has distinguishable features which are attributable to the cleft defect.

Hypothesis iv The victims of teasing portray a particular personality 'type'.

Hypothesis v Negative experiences of interaction with peers during childhood and/or adolescence, exert an adverse influence upon his/her psychosocial development and later functioning.

Implications for clinical practice

Hypothesis vi Developmental trends amongst the participants in the study can be identified from information gleaned from independent data sets. Consequently, an 'at risk' group of individuals for psychosocial maldevelopment/malfunction can be detected during the developmental years, on the basis of their diagnosis, personal circumstances and/or social experiences.

The adult participants' retrospective perceptions of being born with a cleft and factors relating to their current psychosocial functioning

Factors relating to the type of cleft diagnosed

Hypothesis vii Participants born with a cleft lip and palate experience greater and more persistent psychosocial trauma, than participants born with cleft palate only.

Implications for clinical practice

Hypothesis viii An 'at risk' group of individuals for psychosocial maldevelopment/ malfunction can be identified during the adult years, on the basis of their diagnosis, personal circumstances and/or social experiences.

Factors determining the impact of circumstances and experiences encountered during the developmental years, upon the participants' psychosocial functioning in adulthood

Implications for clinical practice

Hypothesis ix Coping mechanisms are a function of innate and/or learned behavioural responses to environmental stimuli.

Hypothesis x The cleft-impaired are perceived as a 'normal' rather than a pathological population, by professionals involved in cleft-related treatment.

2 Literature on disfigurement

Introduction

> When someone stands in the library, he is, metaphorically speaking, surrounded by voices begging to be heard. Every book, every magazine article, represents at least one person's view. In these publications, people converse, announce positions, argue with a variety of eloquence, and describe events or scenes in different ways. The researcher needs only to discover the voices in the library to release them for his analytic use.
> (Glaser and Strauss, 1968)

The literature has been reviewed in such a way as to reflect the retrospective nature of the current investigation. By perusing the pertinent literature according to developmental stages (and the corresponding chronological ages), the natural progression of developmental processes can be more fully appreciated from a holistic perspective. In doing so, the particular influences and concerns of the different phases are highlighted, which are fundamental to the objectives of the follow-up study.

The literature review comprises four sections, namely, pre-school (0-approximately 5 years old, childhood (5-12 years old), adolescence (13-17 years old) and adulthood (18 years old and over). Each section represents a specific developmental stage, and examines the literature relevant to that stage. The relationship between the developmental stages and educational levels is indicated below (Figure 2.1).

Pre-school: 0-approximately 5 years old
Play group or nursery school may be attended.

Childhood: approximately 5-12 years old
By five years old children have generally entered primary school, and remain there until aged eleven when they tend to join secondary school.

Adolescence: 13-17 years old
Attendance at secondary school terminates at fifteen or sixteen years old, depending upon academic aspirations and achievements. On leaving school, the individual may continue his/her studies at college, begin a training scheme or start employment, amongst the most usual options available.

Adulthood: 18 years and over
At the age of eighteen, some young adults will pursue their studies at college, start a training scheme, or become employed. Others may have taken on the responsibilities of marriage and/or parenthood, or be unemployed.

Figure 2.1   Relationship between developmental stages and educational levels

The pre-school stage: 0-approximately 5 years old

> When a baby with a cleft is born, the parents face an immediate crisis, which they will handle in accordance with their own strengths and weaknesses, their previous backgrounds, their established mechanisms for coping with stress, and their personal philosophies of living. (McWilliams, 1982, p.317)

A baby's entrance into the world following birth signals a fundamental change in the parents' lives. How the parents react to, and handle their new charge will, to a certain extent shape the nature and quality of the baby's future life. It is appropriate, therefore, to begin by examining literature which focuses on the implications for parents in producing, and rearing a child with a cleft.

The psychosocial functioning of parents following the birth of a child with a cleft, and its implications for their parenting style

With respect to the parental reaction to the birth of a cleft-impaired child, it appears that only a minority of parents are aware that such a deformity is possible (for example, Biglund, 1990), or anticipate the deformity following antenatal scanning procedures. Since the majority of parents are ignorant of their unborn child's cleft lip and/or palate, the impact of the diagnosis following the birth of the presumed 'perfect' baby is all the more intense and distressing.

Tisza and Gumpertz's (1962) study of maternal reactions to the infant with cleft palate, relates the need for mothers to experience a grieving process, in order to work through the strong emotions of disappointment, resentment and failure as mothers in producing a damaged child. Once the immediate feelings of loss and rejection have been overcome, the more positive reaction of compassion and nurturance can gradually emerge. The essential mother-child bonding may be jeopardized, if the mother continues to be haunted by feelings of guilt, perceiving the child as visible proof of her maternal inadequacy (Tisza and Gumpertz, 1962). Lefebvre and Munro (1978, cited by Palkes et al., 1986) found that the attitudes displayed by friends and relatives played an influential role regarding the parents' ability to cope with having a deformed child.

In reviewing the literature, Brantley and Clifford (1980) refer to the documentation of negative parental affect displayed to defects which are not only immediately visible, but also to the delayed diagnosis of less detectable problems (for example, Burton, 1975). Other sources suggest the transience of such negative parental feelings (for example, Spriestersbach, 1973). Brantley and Clifford's (1980) own findings, however, suggest that parental attitudes, and socio-economic status (SES) may exert an adverse influence upon the child's psychological maturation, and jeopardize healthy family interaction. That is, they assessed the maternal attitudes towards the child's birth of 200 mothers of whom 97 had a child with a cleft lip/palate, and 103 had unaffected children. The children ranged from newborns to 18 years old. Whilst the mothers' responses were essentially retrospective they were considered to reflect the mothers' current projected feelings.

Brantley and Clifford (1980) report the consistently lower measures of mothers of children with cleft palate, which evidence greater parental anxiety, and less maternal and paternal positive affect.

> The lack of significant correlations between age of child and factor scores supports the idea of the continuing influence of parental perceptions of early childhood on present attitudes ... The interaction found between SES and subject type is reflective of our clinical experiences. Upper class mothers are more negatively affected by the birth of a child with a defect than lower class parents. On the other hand, lower SES mothers of normal children express fewer positive feelings about the birth than higher socioeconomic classes. (p.623)

According to Clifford and Brantley (1977), the degree to which parents harbour negative associations of the child's birth may reflect their current acceptance of the child. McWilliams (1982) proposes that the speed and effectiveness with which parents accept the cleft diagnosis, are determined by external factors, such as the severity of the infant's cleft, which supports other investigations (for example, Spriestersbach, 1973). Thus, the more extensive the cleft, the greater the parents' adjustment and their need for professional help, although some parents will be overwhelmed by a comparatively minor cleft deformity.

The influence of cleft type upon parental reactions is reported by Natsume et al. (1987), who noted the feelings of 300 mothers, according to their baby's cleft type. They found that 13.5% of mothers in the cleft lip and palate group denied the existence of their infants as human beings, which contrasts with the 6.2% of mothers in the cleft lip only group. Regarding the cleft palate only group, 23.1% of the mothers were not apparently distressed by the birth, although 45.8% of this group pitied their child.

The high incidence of mothers contemplating suicide following the birth of an infant with cleft lip (32.0%), or cleft lip and palate (36.0%), reflects the intensity of negative emotions. In view of no suicidal thoughts in the cleft palate only group, Natsume et al. (1987) conclude that the mothers' psychological state following delivery, was more adversely affected by a visible, than a non-visible cleft. Furthermore, mothers of children with visible defects feared for the child's social life, especially regarding his/her future employment and marriage prospects. The sole concern of the cleft palate only group, appeared to centre on the child's possible speech difficulties.

Cramer (1976) stresses that mother-child bonding may be particularly vulnerable following the unanticipated delivery of a premature and congenitally impaired baby, not least because maternal problems regarding self-esteem, guilt and separation are likely to be intensified. The mother's pre-crisis personality also shapes her response to a premature delivery and her subsequent coping capacity. Needless to say, the cleft-impaired baby may be premature.

Rosenberg's (1965) notable work on the self-esteem of non-affected children, suggests that parental indifference towards the child is not only associated with the child's low self-esteem, but appears to be more deleterious than the display of punitive reactions. Rosenberg qualifies his observations by stating that parental disinterest probably represents a variety of negative factors, such as lack of love, failure to regard the child with respect or give encouragement, an inclination to view him/her as a nuisance, all of which may be expressed in parental irritation, anger and impatience. Indeed, the development of a sense of self-worth may be directly related to the sense of being important to a 'significant other'.

Coopersmith's (1967) pioneering research on the antecedents of self-esteem explores the characteristics of 'low', 'medium' and 'high' parental (especially maternal) self-esteem, and documents their effects on the child's self-esteem. He surmises a close relationship between parental self-esteem and parental values, in that the former is generally reflected in the latter. Since the significance of positive self-esteem as a vital coping mechanism for the cleft population will become increasingly apparent, it is necessary to examine, at this stage how such self-esteem is cultivated (if at all).

On the basis of questionnaires given to both parents and their children, Coopersmith describes the likely characteristics and consequences of 'low', 'medium' and 'high' self-esteem represented by the respondents, and draws tentative cause and effect conclusions concerning the nature of parent-child interaction. For example, regarding the apparent differences in childrearing practices between the three levels of self-esteem assigned to the mothers, he reports on the greater self-reliance, and possibly ability of mothers of high self-esteem children to cope with and accept the responsibilities of parenthood. This contrasts sharply with the mothers of low self-esteem children who perceive themselves to be less able to manage the problems of birth and early child care. Concerning the tendency for children to both inherit and assimilate the values of their parents Coopersmith (1967, p.261) indicates:

> Children with high self-esteem appear to learn quite early that they must respond to the challenges and troublesome conditions they encounter. It may be the model of decisive parents and the clear demands that are enforced and thus provide solutions, or it may be that parental acceptance and respect makes them more responsive to themselves and more expressive and assertive in their actions. Whichever of these prevails in a given case, our study provides clear indications that the individual with high self-esteem feels capable of coping with adversity and competent enough to achieve success, and that the individual with low self-esteem feels helpless, vulnerable, and inadequate.

During the pre-school stage of development, therefore, the child with a cleft is learning (or conversely is failing to learn), how to cope with challenging situations. This learning is largely governed by whether or not the parents have the discernment of these fundamental life skills at their disposal to pass on to their child. If this has not taken place, on reaching school age the task will become increasingly difficult, since the 'golden opportunity' for acquiring a vital piece of psychological 'survival equipment' has been missed.

Having looked at the parental input to the child's development during the pre-school stage in psychosocial terms, it is now appropriate to consider what is taking place on the child's side of the equation. That is, the constituent parts of parent-child interaction must each be addressed, if the nature and complexity of the relationship itself is to be fully appreciated.

The psychosocial development and functioning of the pre-school child

The previous section alludes to the parent-child relationship as two parts of an equation. The contribution of the infant to the relationship is reinforced by Schaffer (1977, p.31).

> ... from the beginning the baby is active, not passive; his behaviour is organized, not 'absent'; and even to the earliest social interactions he brings certain characteristics which will affect the behaviour of other people towards him. A mother's task is thus not to create something out of nothing but rather to dovetail her behaviour to that of the infant's.

Coopersmith (1967) and Lowe (1972) similarly stress the increasing influence of the child's persona upon his/her own development and treatment by others. Whilst this is evident in the predominantly parent and family-orientated interaction of the pre-school child, on reaching school age, it is additionally prevalent in peer-orientated interaction.

The literature on the impact of clefting upon the pre-school child's psychosocial functioning, will be subsequently reviewed according to the four predominant areas of greatest psychosocial influence, namely, physical growth, personality development, cognitive development, and family dynamics.

Aspects of cleft-related physical growth having psychosocial implications

Although the medical model approach to the diagnosis and treatment of cleft lip and/or palate is well documented in literature focusing upon the child's physical growth, in the context of the present study, greater attention will be placed upon the psychosocial aspects of diagnosis and treatment. However, the literature on clefts is bestrewn with only fleeting references to the psychological implications of living with a cleft lip and/or palate. The emphasis upon the medical model seems particularly marked, when compared to the more psychosocially-orientated American literature on clefting. The areas of the pre-school child's physical growth most affected by a cleft, of particular psychosocial significance are feeding, hearing loss, and speech acquisition. Each of these areas will be now examined.

Feeding According to Campbell and Watson (1980, cited by Albery and Russell, 1990), feeding is often the first and most evident problem faced by the baby with a cleft lip and palate and one of the mother's first challenges. Inherent in the feeding process is the extent to which the mother satisfies, or fails to satisfy the baby's fundamental need for nutrition and security. The tendency to delay the surgical repair of cleft lip until approximately three months after birth, and cleft palate until at least six months old, implicates feeding problems. The situation is not helped by the fluctuating recommendation for breast-feeding (for example, Palmer, 1988), which may or may not be feasible for the cleft-deformed infant.

The mother may have to contend with her feelings of inadequacy and failure if she does not breast-feed her baby. At the same time, where there is cleft palate, the usual pleasures surrounding feeding the baby (whatever method is used), are often replaced by anguish and frustration since the cleft can mitigate against the swallowing of fluids and food, due to the lack of intra-oral pressure required, resulting in the possible nasal regurgitation of the feed. Problems may be heightened where babies have both cleft lip and palate, due to the impairment of reflex co-ordination which enables breathing whilst sucking (Hathorn, 1986). Stengelhofen (1989) indicates that feeding problems may be encountered by as much as 85% (Spriestersbach, 1973) of the cleft population. The lengthy and stressful feeding periods, sometimes taking two hours to complete, may jeopardize mother-child bonding (for example, Phillips and Stengelhofen, 1989).

The cleft deformity may also encourage abnormal tongue movement, which

28

may hamper feeding and later speech acquisition. That is, the cleft can effect impaired oro-sensory and oral motor development (Edwards, 1980), and deviant neuro-motor patterns because neuromotor encoding, and auditory decoding skills are mastered by the infant with a malfunctioning cleft palate (Bzoch, 1979).

Hearing Cleft palate deformity can affect the child's hearing abilities, especially malfunction of the Eustacian tube. The virtually universal incidence of otitis media (conductive hearing loss) in cleft palate from birth, is well documented (for example, Maw, 1986). Otitis media is characteristically intermittent, particularly in conjunction with the frequent cleft-related upper respiratory tract infections. It can seriously interfere with the infant's auditory acuity, thereby disrupting the course of speech and language development, and the nature and quality of parent-child interaction (Bamford and Saunders, 1985). The less common form of sensori-neural form of hearing loss may also be experienced by the child with cleft palate (Albery and Russell, 1990).

Since most of the treatment-oriented literature emanates from medical and speech therapy perspectives (for example, Fria et al., 1987), the researcher whose predominant interest lies in the psychosocial impact of hearing problems, needs to extrapolate the psychological implications from the essentially non-psychological documentation available. For example, reduced hearing can impede the reciprocal flow of communication if the mother's messages are not consistently received by the child. Moreover, the child's verbal contributions may be distorted by the unintelligible speech associated with hearing loss (Albery and Russell, 1990). Maw (1986, p.65) highlights that the hearing loss may not be detected until the child's learning difficulties at school (such as reading) are investigated by the teacher.

Speech In that speech production involves the mechanical co-ordination of anatomical structures in the vocal tract, it is incorporated under the present subheading of physical growth. However, in that the function of speech is to express language, the pertinent literature is addressed in the later section on cognitive development.

Various authorities describe the potentially adverse effect of the abnormal anatomy of cleft palate, or velopharyngeal malfunction and the consequent deviant neuromotor patterns upon phonetic (or articulation) development. That is, as clefting disrupts the regulation of air pressure by the vocal tract, the individual may be unable to acquire the necessary intra-oral pressure for the formation of oral consonants (for example, Albery and Russell, 1990).

Speech development can be disrupted or delayed prior to palatal repair surgery, during the 'babbling' phase as the nasal (rather than oral) emission of air, prevents adequate intra-oral pressure for the production of 'pressure' consonants (for example, Albery and Russell, 1990). This tendency explains the child's delayed speech acquisition and/or adoption of 'compensatory' articulation patterns (McWilliams et al., 1984), such as deviant humping of the tongue, or glottis constriction (Albery and Russell, 1990). Nasality due to velopharyngeal insufficiency also characterizes 'cleft palate speech' (Albery, 1986).

The commonly perceived effects of clefting upon articulation and/or nasality, is reduced intelligibility of speech, thereby adversely influencing communication and social interaction, especially if complicated by additional hearing loss (Stengelhofen, 1989). Speech intelligibility may also be compounded by dental malocclusion and/or oro-nasal fistula(e) (Stengelhofen, 1990). Dental malocclusion (especially Class III) is evident in a high proportion of the cleft lip and/or palate population, due to the grossly deformed dento-alveolar structures of the maxillary arch and palate (Foster, 1980).

The significance of palatal repair surgery undertaken before or after 12 months old for speech sound development has been investigated (for example, O'Gara and Logemann, 1988). These studies suggest that more normal phonetic characteristics were displayed by those undergoing earlier surgery, although still delayed compared to non-cleft children. Controversy prevails regarding the influence upon speech of oro-nasal fistulae (usually caused by surgical breakdown of the repair), which affects intra-oral air pressure as it communicates with the nasal cavity. Although fistula size was a contributory factor, Stengelhofen and Foster (1979) detected both phonetic problems and nasal emission in their study.

In addition to phonetic (speech sound) development, the degree to which clefting causes delayed and/or deviant phonological development (the way in which sounds signal meaning), is widely debated by speech therapists, since both are documented. The findings reflect the considerable variation within the heterogeneous cleft population (for example, Grunwell and Russell, 1988). Regarding the incidence of speech problems Albery (1986) indicates that approximately half of children with cleft palate naturally acquire acceptable articulation. However, Pannbacker (1988, p.406) documents:

> ...recent reports (Bardach, Morris, and Olin, 1984; Smith, Skef, Cohen, and Dorf, 1986; Van Demark and Olin, 1986) suggest a wide variation in reported success rates (20%-90%) following surgery for cleft palate.

Whilst therapeutic intervention is recommended as early as possible for both phonetic and phonological delay (Stengelhofen, 1990), in preventing later problems, some authorities evidence persisting speech impairment throughout childhood into adulthood (McWilliams et al., 1984).

Personality development

It should be pointed out at this stage, that where the literature refers to investigations with 'children' but does not specify the age range of the population, it will be reviewed in the subsequent section concerned with the childhood stage of development. This practice, similarly adopted for the literature on cognitive development, reflects the notable paucity of research devoted exclusively to the pre-school years of the cleft population.

Within the theoretical arena of personality development, the controversial 'nature/nurture' debate prevails concerning the extent to which personality is inherited (predetermined from birth), and/or acquired (learned from the environment). The debate has crucial implications regarding the child's response to untoward experiences. For example, if the child is born with a naturally resilient personality, the effect of threatening situations upon his or her development may be less potent than if the child has to learn to acquire such a personality disposition.

Concerning the 'nurture', or environmental influence upon human development, the once heralded significance of the irreversibility of influences and experiences during the child's first five or 'critical' years of life upon later development is in dispute. As Schaffer (1977, p.24) postulates, it may be more appropriate to speak of a 'sensitive' period, when the pre-school child is more sensitive to certain influences than at other times. He stipulates: 'One event may thus produce a multitude of effects that continue to reverberate for many years.' (p.25) This notion gathers credibility in reviewing the literature.

In delineating the course of personality development, Lowe (1972) emphasizes the particular psychosocial significance of the mother's (or primary care-giver's) attentiveness or indifference towards the infant. In learning to discriminate between mother and other people, the baby establishes his or her first human relationship. The detrimental impact of maternal separation upon mother (or 'significant other') and child bonding is also documented (Bowlby, e.g., 1973), especially upon the child's development of trust and subsequent separation from his/her primary caregiver (Bretherton, 1985). Periods of hospitalization are usually essential for surgical repair of the cleft. Although mothers are now usually encouraged to stay with their infants in hospital, this would not have been possible for the majority of parents of those involved in the current study, due to policy changes over time.

Family interaction

In describing the differential experiences which clefting can effect, Stengelhofen (1989) cites Spriestersbach (1973) in suggesting that a particular role is imposed upon the disfigured child. This role is largely learned and acquired from early experiences of family interaction.

> ... cleft palate children tend not to be treated in the same way as their potentially normal communicating peers. For example, they are given less encouragement to babble; given less chances to talk as much as they want; take less part in family conversations; talk less frequently than their peers; are less willing to talk to strangers and have less speaking parts in school. This list of factors gives clear indication that they may become poor communicators, less because of their specific speech problems, but more because they are given a role as a poor communicator and deprived of usual encouragement and opportunities. (Stengelhofen, 1989, p.27)

In view of the notably sparse literature relating to family interaction in the cleft population, attention is turned to the documentation of family life with a disabled child, since it offers a valuable contribution. The terminology used is clarified by Philp and Duckworth (1982, p.5):

> Impairments are the outward and visible signs of a pathological state; disabilities are what the child cannot do or does to excess in consequence of his or her impairments, while handicaps are the disadvantages and discordances in certain important dimensions of experience which stem from the presence of impairments and disabilities.

Regarding the application of these terms to the cleft population, it appears that the criteria of all three labels are met, which underlines the generally disadvantaged status of this population (however heterogeneous), and the relevance of the literature on disability. Following a review of the literature on families with a disabled child, Philp and Duckworth (1982) observe that whilst not collapsing, many families are not coping as well as might appear. The accumulation of secondary problems, rather than the disability itself, particularly jeopardizes family and social interaction (Jaehnig, 1974).

Various authors describe the strained relationships between siblings and the impaired child. Kew (1975) refers to the siblings' 'characteristic' jealousy, rivalry, fear, aggression and anxiety, whilst Podeanu-Czehofsky (1975) notes the hostility and cruelty of siblings. Schutt (1977) suggests that siblings may be embarrassed by the visibility of the child's impairment. Philp and Duckworth (1982) note that only a minority of siblings appear to experience social difficulties in the literature (Rutter et al., 1970b).

Based on research into the antecedents of self-esteem, Coopersmith (1967) postulates that although family size and self-esteem are unrelated, the child's ordinal position exerts a notable influence upon early social interaction. That is, the eldest children may benefit from not having to compete for affection, attention and status which may be required of later children. As with other contributory factors, the dynamics of family interaction within the cleft population appear to depend upon the particular circumstances of each family.

Cognitive development

At the pre-school stage, one of the most well-documented areas of cognitive development is that of language acquisition. However, the literature reflects a lack of universal agreement regarding the language development of the cleft population. According to some authorities, cleft palate is associated with very early evidence of delayed language comprehension and expression (for example, Bzoch, 1971), and later language delay when compared with unaffected children (for example, Nation and Wetherbee, 1985). This assertion, however, is contested by other investigators (such as McWilliams and Matthews, 1979).

Concerning the complex relationship between cognitive and language development, Stengelhofen (1990, p.23) refers to Heineman-de Boer's (1985) work, in suggesting:

Intellectual impairment is recognised as a cause of delayed language development, but it could also be a factor in relation to a child's ability to adapt to an inadequate mechanism. However, it should be noted that the suggestion that intellectual impairment has a high incidence in individuals with cleft palate is not supported by recent research evidence.

With respect to the cleft lip and palate population, Long and Dalston (1982) advocate that whilst language impairment may be apparent in later childhood, infant communication skills seem within the normal range (p < .189). The significance of age differences, may be attributed to the paucity of adequate pre-verbal communication assessments, which until recently, hampered research in this area. Investigations with non-cleft infants continue to provide valuable instrumentation (for example, Bates, 1976). However, Long and Dalston (1982) document that, excepting refusal behaviour, the cleft subjects (aged 12 to 13 months) employed fewer gestural behaviours compared with unaffected infants.

Differences in communication style were detected in Seidman et al.'s (1986) study of 2 year old subjects with oral-facial or orthopaedic deformities. The mean length of utterance (MLU) was shorter, and the vocabularies were smaller in these children, compared to unimpaired subjects.

Wasserman et al. (1988) studied maternal interaction and language development of infants (aged 23 to 29 months), with (cleft lip and/or palate, or with nasal obstruction) and without speech-related anomalies (with facial or different peripheral anomalies) and control subjects. Those with speech-related anomalies performed significantly poorer on standardized assessments than the controls. The mothers of the former group displayed significantly more 'Initiating' and 'Physical Teaching', and the mothers of both anomalous groups significantly more 'Attention Management', compared to controls in the observed play sessions.

In conclusion, the researchers postulate that, as expected subjects with speech-related anomalies evidence both below-average cognitive functioning and language delay. However, because the overlap between intelligence and language assessment is substantial at this stage, whether the results indicate a global, rather than a specific language delay is unclear. Maternal interactive behaviour appears to be determined by the child's particular disabilities and not a global response to disability, which endorses Wasserman et al. (1986).

Stengelhofen (1989, p.26; 1990, p.22) observes that whilst children with cleft palate are not members of a homogeneous group, they are particularly prone to language impairment for various reasons as outlined below.

- Where mother-baby bonding is under tension in the early days, the quality of the interaction between them may be compromised, giving the infant a disadvantageous start to life.

- Hearing loss may have an adverse effect upon the child's acquisition of language comprehension, thereby, also jeopardizing the development of expressive language.

- Hospitalization necessary during the pre-school period can interfere with the child's normal range of experiences essential for language stimulation.

- The association between low self-confidence and delayed language development is alluded to, especially as the young child may not wish to initiate or pursue interaction with others.

- Parents who are inclined to be overprotective of their congenitally deformed child, may actively discourage the child from expressing him/herself.

- At the same time, parents who are neglectful or indifferent, possibly in reaction to the cleft deformity, may not provide the young child with the appropriate and stimulating experiences which nurture language acquisition, thus making language delay more likely.

- In preserving intelligibility, those with impaired or deviant speech may reduce the length of words and sentences, and sentence complexity, which may impoverish communication.

In view of the vulnerable language and communication development of the cleft population, children with cleft palate are deemed to be 'at risk' according to some authorities (such as Russell, 1989). Pannbacker (1988) identifies the potential risk factors to include the many surgical interventions, parental separation and anxiety, early feeding complications and middle ear disease. This view supports Fox et al.'s (1978) contention that the deficits evidenced in older children and adults with cleft palate, can be detected during the initial three years of life.

Pannbacker (1988, p.403) provides a more optimistic view regarding language acquisition.

> Several early reports indicated significant differences between the language skills of cleft palate and noncleft children; however, more recent reports suggest that if these differences exist, they are minimal. Bradley (1977, p.326) attributed these decreasing differences to 'more emphasis in the early years on language stimulation in the home and early intervention'. Bzoch, Kemker, and Wood (1984, p.107) reported on the analysis of long term effects of early intervention on 50 infants with cleft palate. They stated 'early intervention results in a significant decrease in delayed language development in preschool children with cleft palate'.

Other literature, however, contributes to the controversial field. In the previously cited study, Nation (1970) investigated pre-school children with cleft palate (with or without additional cleft lip), and found notable differences between cleft palate subjects and siblings or other normal children. The former exhibited significantly reduced proficiency in the comprehension and usage of vocabulary. Although the subjects' comprehension and usage of vocabulary generally increased in accordance with chronological age, this outcome does not support the earlier finding of Philips and Harrison (1969), that pre-school cleft palate subjects showed consistent language retardation. Philips and Harrison report that in the areas of receptive and expressive language, those with cleft palate functioned below their unaffected contemporaries.

Fox et al. (1978) have examined the question of global developmental delay in children with cleft palate (some having additional cleft lip), aged 2 to 33 months. The linguistic and non-linguistic abilities of the 24 cleft subjects (12 female, 12 male) and the control subjects were assessed using developmental scales, and full medical histories. Regarding the results, the cleft group's performance paralleled that of their unaffected peers, but failed to reach the same standard on all behaviours assessed by screening tests. Therefore, the cleft group were found to function at a level ranging from one to three months below their peer group.

The results of Fox et al.'s study, appear to reinforce the findings of McWilliams and Musgrave (1972), that those with the most severe clefts are at greater risk for developmental problems, including language acquisition. Other variables investigated by Fox et al. namely, length of hospital stay, sex, body weight and middle ear problems were not statistically significant.

In conclusion, whilst the literature pertaining to the cognitive development of the cleft population is clearly controversial regarding the quality of early language skills, it is more united in describing evidence of impoverished cognitive functioning at a later stage. How this affects the child's schooling will be addressed in the subsequent section.

The childhood stage: approximately 5 - 12 years old

In addition to the start of schooling at the age of about five, the childhood stage reflects, and capitalizes upon that which was learned during the first five years of life. The emerging significance of peers during childhood is apparent in the literature's preoccupation with factors relating to the child's social and communicative skills, upon which much of his or her 'success' in psychosocial terms lies.

The impact of hospital treatment upon the school-aged child with a cleft

Throughout childhood, the impact of hospital treatment upon the child continues to be determined by individual circumstances, such as the severity of the cleft, social environment and psychological disposition. The implications of hospital treatment for the patient and the patient's family should not be underestimated. Admission to hospital for surgery can engender a whole range of emotions, including fear of the unknown and anticipation of improved functioning following surgery. Patients and their families may have unrealistically high expectations regarding the outcome of surgery. which can cause a negative reaction to the treatment (Pruzinsky and Edgerton (1990).

Personality (personal identity) In examining literature which focuses upon the child's personality development some studies characterize the 'cleft personality', and suggest that the cleft population is at risk for personality maladjustment and social isolation. For example, Freudian theorists attach significance to early feeding and sucking difficulties (Prugh, 1956). However, later investigations generally refute this advocation. Goodstein (1968) refers to the increased muscular rigidity, greater motor activity and postural tension, and distorted psychomotor performance of the cleft palate subjects compared to their unaffected peers (aged 5 to 8) in Tisza et al.'s (1958) study; however, questionable methodology was adopted on this occasion.

On reviewing a series of research reports Goodstein (1968) concludes that in view of the unconvincing evidence, children with cleft palate do not display serious psychological or emotional disturbance, although they may experience problems relating to social acceptance.

Self-concept appears to play a determining role in psychological adjustment to the defect, as Broder and Strauss (1989, p.114) suggest: '...perceptions, beliefs, feeling, attitudes, and values that the individual considers descriptive of him-or herself. Self-concept can affect school achievement (Piers-Harris, 1964), self-confidence (Richman, 1976), and social skills (Piers-Harris, 1964).' The relationship between self-concept and psychosocial adjustment has been highlighted by Kapp (1979), who administered the Piers-Harris Self-Concept Scale to 34 cleft lip and/or palate, and 34 control subjects (aged 11 to 13 years). The cleft group, especially female subjects obtained significantly lower scores on anxiety, intellectual and school status, in addition to happiness and satisfaction than control subjects. They also displayed lower scores pertaining to physical appearance.

More recently, Broder and Strauss' (1989) examination of the self-concept of 7 year olds with cleft lip (visible), cleft palate (non-visible) or cleft lip and palate (mixed) and control subjects, found significant differences between the cleft and control groups. The relationship between adjustment and type and severity of cleft is suggested by those with cleft lip and palate exhibiting the lowest self-concept measures. This contradicts Kapp-Simon's (1986) finding of no differences between cleft types. Broder and Strauss propound the likelihood that both visible (cleft lip) and invisible (cleft palate) impairments exert a compounding adverse influence upon self-concept. In accordance with earlier research, on measures regarding physical adequacy (Broder, 1982) and social acceptance (Sigelman et al., 1986), the scores of those with visible cleft were lower than those obtained by individuals with invisible or no deformity. Broder and Strauss (1989, p.116) conclude:

> ... the findings illustrate the negative impact and stigmatizing consequences of facial defects on the self-concept of children with clefts as early as 7 years ... the findings are consistent with person perception literature and the 'beauty-is-good' hypothesis. The findings suggest that future research should consider each cleft type

as a distinct and discreet group ... If adaptive behavior and school achievement are influenced by self concepts, early primary school age children with clefts appear to be at risk.

As Richman's (1989) commentary on Broder and Strauss' (1989) work suggests, cleft-impaired children are more prone than their unaffected peers, and at a younger than expected age to possess a low self-concept, social inhibition, and dissatisfaction with appearance. Moreover, the findings endorse the potential etiologic factors of low self-esteem in the cleft population advanced in other investigations, namely, discriminatory treatment and negative attitudes of parents, and negative teacher and peer perceptions. Thus, those with the most severe cleft defects appear to be at greatest risk for psychosocial problems.

Leonard et al. (1991) also highlight the particular vulnerability of the visible cleft population. Whilst noting that nutrition and communication problems pose the earliest primary challenges for the child with cleft lip and palate, low self-concept is identified as a secondary risk for this group, since it is usually confounded by visible facial disfigurement and expressive language deficits. Moreover, physical appearance is integral to the development of one's self-concept. Leahy and Shirk (1985) document the significance of appearance to children, as evidenced by the self-descriptions given at a stage of emerging self-concept.

With respect to the determinants of self-concept, Leonard et al. refer to the potentially influential role played by the child's parents. They cite the work of Harvey and Greenway (1982), who found that children with a low self-concept had parents who expressed more concern and felt hampered by the cleft deformity. In doing so, it is advocated that parents convey their anxiety to their children, who are profoundly sensitive to such messages.

In view of the literature which surmises that facial disfigurement negatively impacts self-concept, Leonard et al. (1991) question why the children with cleft lip and palate in their own investigation (aged between 8 and 11 years), tended to exhibit self-concepts that were average or above average. They posit that the children may have been denying or minimizing the import of their interpersonal world, in such a way as to preserve their self-concept. The researchers hypothesize that on this occasion, the self-concept characterizes a maladaptive response, which was perpetuated by:

> ... poor reality testing that compromises an accurate assessment of their functioning within a social context and undermines the formation of a healthier and more reality based social involvement. (p.351)

These findings contrast sharply with the suggestion that children with cleft lip and/or palate should be regarded as individuals with a chronic illness (Kapp-Simon et al., 1992). In their study of youngsters with craniofacial anomalies (including cleft lip and/or palate), the researchers explain that the potential stressors associated with chronic physical illness, are shared by the cleft population. For example, these stressors include the need for frequent hospital evaluations throughout childhood, repeated hospitalization and physical anomalies (Varni and Setoguchi, 1991). By conceptualizing cleft impairment as chronic illness, Kapp-Simon et al. (1992) propose that it is legitimate to consult the literature on children with chronic illness regarding psychological functioning.

In examining the self-perception of children with craniofacial anomalies (aged 10-16 years), Kapp-Simon et al. (1992) report similarities to those with chronic illness. That is, a significant proportion of the children are deemed to be at risk for psychological maladjustment, but not for poor self-concept. The authors' findings reinforce Leonard et al.'s (1991) suggestion that children with anomalies may preserve their self-concept by withdrawing from the social world. However, Kapp-Simon et al. (1992) comment that self-concept measures may not be accurate indicators of psychological functioning, and recommend that children at risk should be identified using a well-validated instrument of psychological adjustment.

Fishman and Fishman (1971) suggest that the self-concept of the disabled youngster is affected by the mother's understanding of the disability, her competence to seek information and to communicate openly to the child about it, and whether or not she holds a positive attitude towards her offspring and the future. Bickel (1970) emphasizes that as parental acceptance of the child is related directly to the child's personality, assistance must be offered to the family, especially the mother as early as possible.

In another study of self-concept, children whose appearance was impaired by skin depigmentation were examined by Hill-Beuf and Porter (1984). The authors observed that children can cope well with their disfigurement, if they are able to boost their self-concept by developing aptitude in other areas.

Stricker et al. (1979) looked at the psychological impact of dento-facial anomalies, often associated with clefts upon self-image, and note that body experience is intrinsic to early personality development. Body image can be fundamentally affected by damaged or lost body parts (Parkes, 1972).

> A poor self-image may not result from malocclusion or craniofacial malformation alone but also may be a function of our society which attaches a stigma to those who are different. The victim of any malformation may receive a negative social message, and the result may be self-devaluation. (Stricker et al., 1979)

The socialization of the child with a cleft (social identity) As the child becomes increasingly independent, the development of his/her social interactions (or social identity) is integral to healthy psychosocial maturation. Therefore, if a child has to contend with communication difficulties in addition to physical deformity, such as clefting, he/she may suffer detrimentally in social situations. The occurrence of social and psychological maladaptations may handicap the individual more than the initial diagnosis (Lencione, 1980). Variations in behavioural norms of children were examined by Spriestersbach (1973), who found that the parents of those with clefts perceived their children as less aggressive, less independent and less self-confident compared to their non-cleft contemporaries (as cited by Richman and Eliason, 1982).

38

The minimal data available advocating disability-specific personality types (for example, Schontz, 1975), suggests that the visibility, rather than the type of disability could be of greater significance to psychosocial development (Wright, 1964).

Steinhausen (1981) examined the impact of a visible deformity upon an individual's psychosocial adjustment, by comparing the responses of 104 children and adolescents (mean age 12.11 years), with various non-cleft physical impairments (such as cerebral palsy) with haemophilic, diabetic and control subjects. In comparing the groups, Steinhausen suggests that the visibility of the impairment plays a major part in determining how well the child copes with the deformity. The psychological significance of a visible impairment is also evidenced in the literature concerned with the psychosocial impact of face and hand burns (Chang and Herzog, 1974).

Richman and Harper (1979), studied the self-reported impact of different visible physical anomalies upon personality development and behaviour of 45 cleft lip and palate subjects and 45 orthopaedically and visibly impaired subjects (aged 8 and 9). Differences across and within the groups are evidenced by both male and female cleft lip and palate subjects displaying significantly higher measures regarding 'Maturity' and 'Inhibition'. The authors suggest that whilst both females and males with clefts exhibit similar social reserve during the elementary stage, adolescent females' greater concern over appearance may contribute to their increased self-doubt and dissatisfaction. The psychosocial implications of the results are indicated by Richman and Harper (1979, p.260): 'High scorers on Inhibition have been identified as displaying shyness, withdrawal, and social inhibition (Owen, 1970).'

Thus, although the visibly impaired may demonstrate similar modes of behaviour (for example, Wright, 1964), Richman and Harper (1979) propound that the type of visible disability may effect different personality traits, but significant psychopathology was not detected (Richman and Harper, 1978). Moreover, regarding the excessive inhibition of impulse of children with clefts reported by teachers in Richman's (1976) study, it is surmised these individuals may actually learn to avoid situations or behaviours which either attract attention to themselves, or provoke negative reactions from others. This finding is more likely to reflect socially adaptive behaviour, than maladjustment.

In response to attempts to investigate the psychosocial functioning of children with physical deformities, Clifford (1983) asks provocatively 'Why are they so normal?', and alludes to the growing evidence of the relative normality of the cleft population. Although applauding the efficiency of the professional management of clefts, he suggests that cleft-related problems may be over-exaggerated. Tobiasen (1984, p.131), propounds that Clifford's inference repudiates clinical experience (for example, Kapp-Simon, 1981): '...which suggests that individuals with visible facial anomalies and their families often experience painful social and personal adjustments which have long lasting psychosocial effects.'

Pursuing the question as to why (as opposed to what problems) those with a congenital cleft may experience psychosocial difficulties, Tobiasen (1984) consults the social psychological literature on the concept of facial attractiveness, and its influence upon self-concept. As she points out, the psychosocial difficulties of those with facial clefts may be associated with a negative or unattractive physical appearance, since two-thirds of this population have visible impairments. In identifying the relevance of 'person perception theory' Tobiasen cites Schneider et al. (1979).

> ... people go beyond the immediate information given to them about others to make inferences and conclusions about personality and behavior. Attractiveness is one of the cues that people use to make conclusions about others. This is one of the most consistent findings in contemporary social psychology (Berscheid and Walster, 1974; Kleinke, 1975; Patzer, 1984). (Tobiasen, 1984, p.102)

Tobiasen (1989) reports a fundamental finding emerging from the literature on dental and facial attractiveness. That is, the more socially prized facial characteristics are more likely to warrant significant psychosocial benefits (she cites Bell et al., 1985 amongst others). In addition, Adams (1977) and (Langlois and Stephan 1981) stress the impact
upon society's expectations that external beauty reflects internal goodness. Such expectations actively determine the ways in which 'beautiful' and 'ugly' individuals are treated by others, effectively discriminating against the less attractive members of society in favouring attractive people. Unattractive children are thus regarded by many to be antisocial and dishonest (Dion, 1972).

> Facially attractive people are assumed to possess many positive personality and behavioral traits, including friendliness, intelligence ... and kindness. Facially attractive individuals receive preferential treatment. For example, attractive children are punished less for behavior infractions than are their less attractive peers (Dion, 1972). (Tobiasen, 1989, p.103)

Concerning the cleft population, Tobiasen (1989) indicates that the findings are generally consistent with the social-psychological studies of global facial attractiveness, orthognathic appearance and malocclusion (Tobiasen, 1984). That is, facial appearance which is impaired by a cleft tends to be less acceptable to others than unimpaired facial appearance (she cites Schneidermann and Harding, 1984 amongst others). A study of the peer perceptions of cleft-related defects conducted by Tobiasen (1987), showed individuals (aged 8 to 16) photographs of children with either facial clefts, or with photographically corrected non-cleft appearance. Those with cleft impairments were rated as being less friendly, less popular, less intelligent and less likely to be selected as a potential friend.

Tobiasen and Hiebert (1988), found considerable consensus between children and adolescent judgements of the social acceptability of children with clefts, based on photographic slides showing varying degrees of cleft-related impairments and global facial attractiveness. The subjects discriminated the extent of impairment and facial attractiveness.

The 'beauty is good' stereotype described by Dion (1974), has been detected in three year old children (Adams, 1971), in addition to adult groups (Berscheid and Walster, 1974). The fact that disfigurement is observed from early childhood (Conant and Budoff, 1983), means that the adverse and accumulative effects of stigmatization may be experienced from this age. In view of this, Pillemer and Cook (1989) speak in terms of the craniofacially disfigured being 'at risk' for future psychosocial maladjustment, and caution: 'psychosocial problems appear rooted in years of prior negative experiences' (p.206).

Shaw et al.'s (1980) study of teasing amongst Welsh school children, suggests that victimization by peers may not be exclusive to the craniofacially disfigured population. Regarding features which provoked teasing, teeth emerged fourth out of fourteen physical features (after height, weight and hair). However, the researchers document that the most distress was elicited by teasing related to teeth

Other studies (for example, Rapoport and Quinn, 1975), suggest that as the number of minor physical impairments increase (such as widely separated eyes), there is a corresponding increase in the child's withdrawn, impulsive or aggressive behaviour, resulting in negative peer perception and less peer interaction. Regarding the psychological implications of dentofacial defects, Stricker et al. (1979, p.411) point out: '... the emotional impact of deformity on the individual does not always seem to be related directly to the degree of disfigurement (MacGregor, 1973).'

In this context, Reich (1969) surmises that severely impaired individuals may accurately predict a negative reaction from others, such as being teased, and therefore, resign themselves to the likelihood of receiving such treatment. Less severely deformed individuals may experience heightened anxiety and feelings of insecurity because of the unpredictability of other people's responses to their defect. Similarly, Lansdown et al. (1991) note that an inability to anticipate other peoples' reactions causes anxiety (Kelly, 1955).

There appears to be a notable discrepancy between the perceptions of the individual and society, as Stricker et al. (1979, p.412) postulate: 'It is expected that both society and the person are more accepting of relatively mild deviations in appearance or function.' Lansdown et al. (1991) hypothesize that severe facial defects may have less adverse psychological consequences than mild facial defects, which supports MacGregor's (1970) observations from her own clinical experience, that patients appeared to be more psychologically burdened by a relatively mild deformity than those with a more severe impairment.

Lansdown et al. (1991) compared parental reports of the frequency with which the public stared at the child, and impairment ratings of parents and unrelated children, pertaining to 27 children with facial deformities, including cleft lip (unilateral and bilateral), 26 unaffected siblings of the experimental sample, and 12 control control siblings (aged 6 to 15). A statistically significant relationship was found between the evaluators' perceptions of attractiveness, and the degree of public staring at the children. Following a battery of psychological tests, including the Piers-Harris Children's Self-Concept Scale (Piers and Harris, 1969), to parents and teachers, Lansdown et al. 1991, p.168) report:

The raters generally perceived photographs of children in a predictable way; that is, the more attractive children were seen to be, the more likely they were rated as happy, clever, friendly and easy to get along with. All predictions reached the < 0.001 level of significance.

Whilst Lansdown et al. did not detect an association between the severity of the impairment and the overall self-concept scores in the experimental group, it appears (although not statistically significant) that the mildly deformed possessed the poorest self-concept.

Therefore, there does not appear to be a predictable relationship between the severity of physical disfigurement and the social reaction the disfigured person receives to the impairment (Katz, 1981). As MacGregor et al. (1953) and Lansdown et al. (1991) document, it is those with relatively minor facial defects, who often experience the most problematic social relationships. Furthermore, the reviewed literature suggests that it is the child's social development and integration which are at greater risk than deviant personality development.

The quality of parenting and family interaction

The parenting and family interaction unique to each child, continues to influence his/her psychosocial development alongside the increasingly significant role of peers in socialization. Evidence suggests that a close association exists between families who are supportive, and the child's psychological adjustment to the disfigurement (Blakeney et al., 1990).

Cognitive development and educational achievement

In this section, particular attention is paid to the child's cognitive functioning, school performance and the school teacher's perception of the child's ability, since the literature reveals a significant association between these areas.

The cognitive functioning of the child with a cleft   Some literature alludes to the apparent intellectual deficit of the cleft population, as evidenced by lower intelligence quotient (hereafter referred to as IQ) scores compared to non-cleft subjects (for example, Lamb et al., 1973). However, the methodology of some of these earlier investigations is dubious. In other studies, although the IQ scores of cleft groups were statistically inferior to their noncleft peers, their mean scores fell within the average range of 90-100 (for example, Smith and McWilliams, 1968).

Richman (1980) investigated the incidence of language disability in 57 cleft subjects, whose IQ scores fell within the mean range, but who evidenced significantly poorer results on the WISC Verbal than Performance tests. Following assessment, two subgroups were discerned, namely those displaying a general language deficit, and those with impaired verbal expression only. Richman contends that the former subgroup presented with a specific language-based learning disability, showing more arithmetic and reading problems, and including more cleft palate only males. The latter subgroup, is thought to demonstrate underachievement associated with early speech difficulties and poor language stimulation.

Richman et al. (1988) investigated the prevalence of reading disability in cleft-impaired children aged (6-13 years). They found that those with cleft palate only may be more susceptible than their cleft lip and palate contemporaries, to general language disorders, resulting in long term reading difficulties. The latter tend to experience reading problems which resolve with maturation and reinforce the findings of Richman and Eliason (1984).

Following a literature review, Heineman-de Boer (1985) concludes that the cleft palate population exhibits average to upper average cognitive potential. Stengelhofen (1989) suggests that earlier findings of lower IQ levels in cleft palate groups, may not have controlled for variables such as socio-economic status, or parental intellectual abilities. The utilization of verbal assessments and sampling problems could be other compounding factors.

The school performance of the child with a cleft, and the school teacher's perception of the child's cognitive ability   On interviewing the parents of 175 cleft and 175 control subjects, Spriestersbach (1973) identifies trends relating to school performance, and suggests that both parents and teachers may harbour lower expectations for the cleft population. In summarizing the results of Spriestersbach, Richman and Eliason (1982, p.253) state that in comparison to the controls:

> ... twice as many cleft children were delayed in starting school, twice as many cleft children were considered (by their parents) to be nine or more months delayed in school achievement, twice as many cleft children repeated one or more grades in school, and mothers of cleft children were less likely to expect their children to attend college.

Kapp (1979) has emphasized the influence of self-perception on the school achievement of the cleft population. In assessing the self-concept of 34 cleft and 34 control subjects, the cleft female subjects perceived themselves as less successful than their cleft male and unaffected peers. The findings highlight the comparatively low self-esteem of the cleft female group.

Evidence suggests that the teacher's perception of the child with a cleft can exert considerable influence upon the pupil's school performance (or cognitive functioning). Clifford and Walster's (1973) study, emerging from the literature on physical attractiveness, investigates the impact of teacher expectations upon pupils. Reports on a fictitious child accompanied by photographs, depicting varying levels of facial attractiveness, were handed to 404 teachers, who were requested to estimate the child's future social and academic performance.

The relative attractiveness of the child was found to be positively and significantly related to the teacher's perceptions of the child's intelligence, the length of the child's anticipated school career, the child's popularity stakes with peers, and the extent to which the child's parents supported his/her education. These dramatic results were subsequently reinforced by

Salvia et al. (1977), who studied the end-of-year reports of school teachers. No differences were found in the objective evaluation of the individual's performance, which supports Clifford's (1975) hypothesis that, whilst physical attractiveness may fundamentally influence teachers' expectations, it lacks predictive value for pupils' long term academic achievement. The teacher's differential treatment of attractive and unattractive pupils, may actually provoke the latter into a role of deviant behaviour, which may effect poor interaction with peers (Clifford and Walster, 1973). In similar vein, (Stricker et al., 1979) document the influence of negative peer perceptions upon encouraging misbehaviour.

Shaw and Humphreys (1982) distinguish between 'unattractiveness' and 'disfigurement', since the latter may adversely affect academic success. Various investigations focus on the association between the visible disfigurement of cleft lip and the child's schooling (for example, Richman and Harper, 1978). Summarizing their outcome, Shaw and Humphreys indicate that although the cleft lip subjects exhibited normal IQ levels, their inferior attainment on objective assessment, suggests that teacher expectations engender a self-fulfilling prophecy. The teachers made less accurate ratings of the intellectual abilities of severely deformed cleft subjects, recording their behaviour as inhibited in the competitive classroom atmosphere, compared with their more normal-looking peers. Since classroom success may depend upon competition and independence, underachievement may be a consequence of inhibition (Richman and Eliason, 1982).

Shaw and Humphreys (1982) document the negligible influence of facial disfigurement upon teacher expectations, in examining the perceptions of 320 teachers of different dentofacial anomalies. They advocate that teacher expectations are generally determined by age and gender. Later investigations on teacher expectations undertaken in America, suggest that supplementary information on the child (such as his/her conduct), diminishes the discriminatory effect of attractiveness (Adams, 1977). In that the studies mentioned in this section focus on evaluations based upon teachers' first impressions, rather than personal experience of the children, their validity is limited.

In summary, whilst the cleft population tends to evidence a normal range of intelligence, their intellectual ability may be affected by speech, language and hearing difficulties, cleft type, sex and additional congenital impairments (Richman and Eliason, 1982). A trend towards middle to low achievement is evidenced (for example, Peter and Chinsky, 1974), but not endorsed by Lansdown and Polak's (1975) failure to find significant differences between the achievements of cleft and control subjects. Moreover, significant improvements can occur with time (Stengelhofen, 1989), which highlight the need to resist labelling children too young, especially since initially delayed development may be attributable to disruptions in their early childhood (Starr et al., 1977).

The adolescent stage: 13 - 17 years old

According to Erikson (1959) adolescence is characterized by the individual's search for identity during the teenage years. Whilst preoccupation with assimilation and self-examination helps to determine self-perception, peer perceptions exert a profound influence throughout this stage. Regarding disfigured adolescents, Strauss et al. (1988, p.355) suggest:

> Goffman's (1963) theory of stigmatization holds that persons with physical disabilities are socially discredited and have reduced self-esteem. They respond to the values and judgements of 'normals' by internalizing how they are socially 'seen' and thus develop negative self-perceptions.

The self-perception of the adolescent with a cleft

Richman and Eliason (1982) note the inconclusive evidence concerning the differences between the self-concept and self-satisfaction evaluations of cleft and non-cleft adolescent populations. Kapp (1979) found that cleft-impaired adolescents reported less satisfaction with their physical appearance compared with their unaffected contemporaries. The female cleft subjects alluded to a deeper sense of dissatisfaction and unhappiness than the male cleft subjects, which supports Harper and Richman (1978), and they also experienced greater anxiety and poorer school performance than the latter group.

In similar vein, Leonard et al. (1991, p.350) found distinct sex and age differences between the self-concepts of their subjects with cleft lip and/or palate (aged 8-11 and 12-18 years).

> Adolescent girls experienced lower self-concept in comparison to younger girls and adolescent boys experienced higher self-concept in comparison to younger boys on global scores and cluster scores denoting behavior, intellect and school status, appearance and attributes, and happiness and satisfaction. Anxiety and happiness and satisfaction were more problematic for females, regardless of age, than for males. Popularity was the only cluster score that fell below the mean norms for all subjects.

Offer et al. (1984) administered the Offer Self-Image Questionnaire to 1385 males and females, aged between 13 to 19 years. They found that girls expressed significantly more negative emotions than the boys. For example, the females were lonelier, sadder and more emotionally sensitive than their male contemporaries. Leonard et al. (1991) similarly document the finding and suggest that girls with a visible disfigurement, may be particularly at risk for depression. Allgood-Merten and Lewinson (1990) advocate that society's preoccupation with physical appearance contributes to adolescent female depression.

Although Strauss et al. (1988), failed to evidence significant gender differences in the appearance, speech and satisfaction ratings of their 102 cleft lip and/or palate (aged 13 to 19) and parent subjects, they did identify specific areas of anxiety. Concerns relating to facial appearance, rather than to speech were detected in a high proportion of the subjects, and reinforce the findings of Richman (1983) which suggest that social introversion is associated more with facial than with speech anomalies.

In surveying the anxieties and attitudes of 28 individuals with unilateral cleft lip and palate (aged 16 to 25), and their parents by postal questionnaire, Noar (1991) comments on the patients' overall satisfaction regarding their appearance and speech. However, they expressed less satisfaction with cleft-related features, namely profile, lips, teeth, nose and smile.

The literature suggests, that a minority of adolescents with clefts does experience adjustment problems. Clifford and Clifford (1986) describe this group as displaying characteristically low self-esteem, high social inhibition, and anxieties regarding personal relationships which may stem from early childhood (they cite Richman, 1983 amongst others). In this domain, Stengelhofen (1989, p.28) gleans from her clinical experience.

> The author has frequently met adolescent cleft cases who are extremely reluctant to communicate in most situations. They exhibit such behaviour as unwillingness to talk, situation avoidance, hiding behind their hair, head lowering and lack of use of eye contact. In their speech they may use low intensity and talk very quickly, hoping that if they do this they will not be noticed; in fact their whole demeanour and unintelligible speech draws attention to themselves ... Where the speaker is concerned about his facial appearance communication may be disturbed. The problem will be exacerbated by the presence of speech difficulties, especially if they lead to lack of intelligibility. Features such as nasal grimace will also be distracting for the listener.

Concerning the relevance of the social psychological literature on physical attractiveness in determining adolescent self-concept and self-esteem, the reader is referred to the group of studies reviewed in the previous section on childhood development. Another notable study in this area was conducted by Orr et al. (1989), who looked at the effect of social support upon the self-esteem, body image and depression of adolescent and young adult burn patients. Perceived social support from friends was the most crucial factor in adjustment to the disfigurement.

Peer perceptions of the adolescent with a cleft

The face is what one goes by, generally, remarked Alice. (Carroll)

Lerner and Lerner (1977) suggest that adolescents demonstrate a significant preference for befriending peers whom they perceive as attractive. 'Unattractive' peers are perceived as more antisocial. Adolescents and young adults are also found to be prejudiced towards competence and against physical disability (Sigelman and Singleton, 1986). The literature discussed in the preceding section focusing on the concept of attractiveness and peer assessments of physical appearance, is also pertinent here, since the majority of studies mentioned involve subjects who cross the age boundary of childhood-adolescence.

According to the literature, many cleft-impaired teenagers have particular anxieties about their social interactions, which may be hampered by concerns relating to self-perception, such as unsatisfactory appearance and speech (Kapp, 1979).

> This may explain why 75 per cent of these patients reported that they were teased because of their cleft and why over half of these patients felt that their cleft had affected them in getting a girlfriend or boyfriend and that they felt less confident than their friends because of their cleft. (Noar, 1991, p.282)

Similarly, Clifford and Clifford (1986) point out that some cleft-impaired adolescents may be especially prone to peer pressure and peer perceptions, if they feel unacceptable and stigmatized. They describe the accumulative effect of negative experiences for this minority group.

> Some patients with a childhood history of over-concern about the consequences of their clefts, accompanied by poor adaptation, can have their already low self-esteem depreciated even more in adolescence. Besides feeling personally inadequate, imagined and real rejections by the peer group can be devastating. These adolescents are particularly vulnerable to stigmatization by others and by themselves and are discounted or devalued by themselves or by others (Goffman, 1963). (p.117)

In view of the problems evidenced by some cleft-impaired adolescents, reference is made to pioneering work being currently undertaken in the wider field of facial disfigurement (Rumsey et al., 1986). The initiative is a positive response to the difficulties experienced by the disfigured regarding social interaction, particularly in initial encounters (Bull and Rumsey, 1988). With respect to the facially disfigured population, research has highlighted the significance of facial appearance to effective social functioning (Baron and Byrne, 1991). For example, members of the public tend to avoid those with a facial disfigurement Bull and Rumsey, 1988). Without appropriate intervention, a vicious circle can evolve which may result in social withdrawal and psychological dysfunction in adulthood.

The pilot study conducted by Rumsey et al. (1986) has shown that by enhancing the social skills of the facially disfigured, this population may be helped to take control of social situations, and function more effectively. Social skills training is proving to be an invaluable means of addressing the sensitive and challenging problems encountered by the facially disfigured (Partridge, 1992). The extent to which the training programme is applicable to the cleft population will be discussed in chapter eight.

The adulthood stage: 18 years and over

Whilst eighteen years of age marks the legal entry into adulthood, in psychosocial terms the demarcation is not as sharp nor as evident. Since adulthood is partially determined by the consequences of earlier development, it is conceivable that negative influences and experiences may stunt subsequent maturation in some way. For this reason, the subsequent literature is examined under the two predominant areas of psychosocial and cognitive functioning. In reviewing the literature, reference is made to Noar's (1991) caution against drawing parallels between the predominantly American-based studies and those emerging from the United Kingdom, since the attitudes of the populations may differ significantly. For example, more American patients may express satisfaction with their medical treatment in justifying their financial investment in the treatment (Clifford, 1991), which contrasts with the state provided National Health Service in Britain.

Psychosocial functioning - personality and social interaction

Heller et al. (1981) studied the psychosocial functioning of adult cleft subjects, and relate that 67% of subjects reported adequate functioning, 23% marginal, and the functioning of 10% was considered to be clearly inadequate. These findings are supported by Bjornsson and Agustsdottir (1987). Whilst the assessments did not significantly relate to the severity of the defect, nor to the extent of hospitalization or treatment, the strong correlation between functioning and expressed dissatisfaction with hearing and appearance, was particularly evident in the male subjects. Language and functioning were also significantly associated, compared with the weak relationships between inadequate functioning and lower socio-economic status, poor educational attainment, single marital status and larger sibships.

Furthermore, concerning the past social life of the adults, Heller et al. indicate that over half the subjects felt that their social lives had been adversely affected by the cleft, and almost one-quarter stipulated being teased regarding their speech or appearance. A minority related their earlier speech or appearance-related inhibitions. These findings are not supported, however, by Bjornsson and Agustsdottir's (1987) Icelandic study of 63 adults with cleft lip (some with additional cleft palate), in which the cleft was generally perceived to have had little significant impact upon the subject's lives. Although the female subjects were more self-consciousness about their appearance than the males, overall satisfaction with treatment was expressed, even if their expectations of surgery exceeded the outcome, which is reinforced by Noar's (1991) British study. Concerning their own research in this area, Bjornsson and Agustsdottir (1987, p.156) note:

> The relatively high expression of satisfaction is perhaps attributable to factors likely to be operating in a retrospective study like this one. Time 'heals wounds', and we tend to push painful experiences of

our childhood into the deeper recesses of the mind (Clifford et al., 1972; Edwards and Watson, 1980; Heller et al., 1981).

Similarly, Crocker et al. (1973) report the overall high body satisfaction reported by cleft-impaired subjects. The individuals expressed least satisfaction with cleft-related features, namely, lips, mouth, teeth, speech, voice and talking.

These results contradict those of Heller et al. (1981), who note the dissatisfaction with appearance of over half of the psychologically 'adequate' and 'marginal' subjects, and all of the 'inadequate' group. In interpreting these findings, McWilliams (1982) stresses that she encountered many young adults who hesitated to relate their dissatisfaction, for fear of offending their clinicians. Other research suggests that high expectations regarding the outcome of surgery can produce negative reactions (Pruzinsky and Edgerton, 1990). There does not appear to be a positive relationship between satisfaction with surgery and enhanced psychological adjustment. Lovius et al. (1990) found that orthognathic patients were as fearful post-operatively of other people's negative evaluations of them, as they were prior to surgery, despite believing surgery had diminished their disfigurement.

Dissatisfaction with present social life was expressed by 56% of Heller et al.'s (1981) sample, whilst approximately 33% were 'very satisfied'. Regarding friendships, 24% reported that they possessed few friends, half of whom socialized infrequently, compared with nearly 50% who claimed to pursue few leisure interests. Evidence of fewer friendships, less and disadvantaged social integration is also reported in other studies (such as Peter et al., 1975).

Van Demark and Van Demark (1970) found that their cleft subjects tended to feel socially inept, preferred one-to-one rather than group social interactions, and were inclined to observe rather than actively participate in life. The findings endorse those of Heller et al. (1981), and Peter et al. (1975), who note that cleft subjects selected more passive activities compared to controls.

Difficulties with socializing are evident in studies of other forms of facial disfigurement. For example, Porter et al. (1990) focused on patients with vitiligo and document their particular problems in meeting people for the first time, and establishing new friendships especially those with the opposite sex. Similar findings are reported by Rubinow et al. (1987) in their study of patients with cystic acne, and by Lanigan and Cotterill (1989) who looked at the psychosocial implications of port wine stains According to Porter et al. (1986), the facially disfigured feel discriminated against at work and in their private lives, and experience insulting and intrusive comments about their appearance.

MacGregor (1990, p.250) describes the catalogue of stigmatizing responses which may be experienced by those with facial disfigurement when encountering other people.

> ... in their efforts to go about their daily affairs they are subjected to visual and verbal assaults, and a level of familiarity from strangers ... naked stares, startle reactions, 'double-takes', whispering.

remarks, furtive looks, curiosity, personal questions, advice, manifestations of pity or aversion, laughter, ridicule and outright avoidance.

The fear of rejection by others is so strong for some people with facial disfigurement, that their only coping strategy is to withdraw from social situations altogether (Harris, 1992).

The previously cited literature on the implications of physical attractiveness for social functioning, is relevant to the adult cleft population. Berscheid et al.'s (1973) large-scale survey on adults, suggests that early adverse experiences (such as teasing), can have negative and long term consequences for body image.

Regarding the family life of the adult cleft population, Peter and Chinsky (1974) found prolonged dependence upon family members, which concedes with the findings of Heller et al. (1981) amongst others.

> ... 56 are still living with family members and only 17 (18%) are married, although 22 others were 'seriously involved.' (The corresponding census figure is 39% married among those aged 20 to 24 in metropolitan Montreal in 1976). (p.463)

Other studies examining the implications of facial disfigurement, have shown the tendency for the disfigured to spend a larger proportion of time with their families, and less time with non-family members (for example, Everett et al., 1993 and Gamba et al., 1992).

The literature also documents evidence of less frequent dating (Van Demark and Van Demark, 1970), and lower and later marriage trends in this population (Bjornsson and Agustsdottir, 1987). According to Peter and Chinsky 1974), individuals with cleft palate only tended to marry earlier than those with cleft lip and palate, which is endorsed by Heller et al. (1981). Moreover, the cleft population appears to experience more childless marriages, significantly fewer children, and produce less children per year than the control group (Peter and Chinsky, 1974). McWilliams (1982) refers to the anxieties attached to the possible recurrence of the deformity as a feasible explanation for the findings, which may be associated with the cleft population's inclination towards social inhibition, and constrained social relationships.

Cognitive functioning - education and employment

The notably sparse research devoted to the adult cleft population tends to be retrospective in nature. It includes Peter and Chinsky's (1974), finding that no significant differences emerged between the academic aspirations expressed by the cleft, sibling and control groups studied (aged 24 to 54), which supports Bjornsson and Agustsdottir (1987). However, the cleft subjects held lower aspirations, and fewer cleft subjects attended college than the control subjects. Familial factors offer one explanation for these results. Other investigations evidence underachievement (Richman, 1976). On telephone interviewing 96 young adults with cleft lip and/or palate

50

(mean age 22.5 years), Heller et al. (1981, p.462) report:

> About 25% stated that they had school problems during their youth, and nearly 40% had actually repeated one or more grades. About one in ten required special help, and at least the same proportion thought that, in general, their condition had an adverse effect on their schooling ... only 8% were completely without jobs. Of the 80 with jobs that could be classified, a high proportion (54%) were in professional or white-collar occupations. This figure is similar to that of the general population of the city ... nearly 30% reported having had some difficulty finding employment, and less than one-half (45%) were enthusiastic about their present jobs.

These data contrast with Peter and Chinsky's (1974) claim that adult cleft subjects (in America) actually earned less than the control subjects. Peter et al. (1975) also found that unlike their sibling controls, males with clefts were not upwardly socially mobile although both groups were dissatisfied with the suitability of their employment. In addition, the latter expressed higher career aspirations than either the siblings or unaffected controls, a finding reinforced by Van Demark and Van Demark (1970). McWilliams and Paradise (1973) document that although cleft and sibling control subjects attained higher academic achievement than their fathers, neither group exceeded their father's occupational status. These results suggest a disharmony between achievement and capability, which may exist in the cleft population (McWilliams, 1982).

The persistence of language impairment within the adult cleft palate population is documented by Pannbacker (1975). In comparing cleft and unaffected adult subjects, the former generally used shorter responses, and significant correlations were found between mean length of utterance and intelligibility. However, differences concerning syntax and vocabulary were not apparent. Stengelhofen (1989) attributes the lack of evidence of language delay in recent studies to changed methodology, or a positive indication of the efficacy of early diagnosis and language intervention. Leder and Lerman (1985) document the long term, adverse effect of compensatory articulation in inappropriate vocal fold adduction, evidenced by the increased incidence of vocal abuse and vocal nodules in the adult cleft palate population (for example, Bronsted et al., 1984).

In summary, the adoption of a developmental approach in reviewing the literature, has enabled the particular challenges faced by the cleft population at different stages, to be put into perspective. Whilst it is hazardous to attempt to draw any cause-effect conclusions, the literature does suggest that difficulties (and their consequences) which have not been resolved in childhood may well persist into adulthood. In doing so, it appears that they become increasingly resistant to effective intervention.

About 25% stated that they had school problems during their youth, and nearly 40% had a twelve-repeated their schooling grades. About one in four reported special help, and at least the same proportion (note that by certain specifications had an adverse effect or correcting ... could have are completely without help. Of the 85 ... who that could be classified a high proportion ... were in some work or without discontinued ... This higher number of that the general population. In addition, nearly 40% reported having had some difficulty in their employment and less than one half (45%) were extinguished about their present jobs.

Here is in contrast with Peter and Ohlms ... claim that adult clients in certain ... actually control less than ... control settings, they are as have also noted that unless ... has no control, made, only little more ... probability sociably mobile although both groups were dissatisfied with the variability of their employment. In addition, if clients expressed more ... to speak less than either the things or uncontrolled control. A finding confirmed by ... Durham and Van Lumme... (1970), ... Williams and Radleen (1973) document that adult of cleft and stamp could subjects maintained higher academic achievement than their highest status ... extent than either occupational status. These results suggest a similarity between employment and variability ... that is of in the 1970s population (Van Lumme...).

The past several latest is uncommon in within the adult cleft palate population, documented by ... Tambacke (1970). In comparing cleft and non-cleft adult subjects, the author generally used shorter sentences, and shorter utterances. Van Lumme... found ... mean length of utterance and intelligibility. However, differences concerning syntax and vocabulary were not were as significant. These subjects had elevation ... language, in terms quality is in their verbal pathology, or indicators of the differences may present in and language the studies. Taylor and Tambacke (1970) noted that long sentence structure compensation articulation. In the normative vocal child, articulation evidenced by the increased intelligence and communication vocabulary in the adult cleft palate population (for example Brennich et al., 1970).

In summary, the author provides development in speech child receiving of therefore has been the particular challenge faced by the cleft population at different stages to be put into perspective. While it has been debated to attempt to draw any causative conclusions, the literature does suggest that difficulties faced their consequences, which have a bearing resolved in childhood and may well persist into adulthood. The longer so it appears that they become increasingly resistant to effective intervention.

3 Design of the study

Research design is the point at which questions raised in theoretical or policy debates are converted into operational research projects and research programmes which will provide answers to these questions. (Hakim, 1987, p.xi)

Stage one: the formulation of the research proposal

Introduction - methodological and ethical considerations

The design stage of a research project not only directly determines the ultimate success of the study, but as Hakim (1987) suggests has a pivotal role to play in putting theory into practice. Thus, if the researcher is prepared to invest time and thought into mapping out the most expedient course for the investigation, his/her efforts are more likely to be rewarded in reaching the desired destination.

In order to reach that destination, however, the following criteria must be satisfied if the potential obstacles are to be overcome.

- The chosen strategy must be valid, that is it must be conducive to the objectives of the research.

- The strategy must also be reliable in that it enables the elicitation of consistently pertinent data.

- The limitations of the strategy should be identified, as far as possible, before its adoption, with some foresight as to how the limitations might be overcome during the course of the research.

- The selected strategy must be the most feasible given the practical constraints surrounding the ideas, and researcher(s) involved.

In addition, the proposed research must withstand the scrutiny of ethical justification. Indeed, this is so integral to research involving humankind, that an alertness to the possible ethical implications of undertaking the research, should become a 'nagging conscience' in the mind of the researcher. To consider the ethical issues of research, is to consider the researcher's responsibility, obligation towards and respect for those who are to be involved in the research project.

In the case of research undertaken in conjunction with medical treatment, there is a sharp distinction to be made between involving so-called 'healthy' volunteers and patients. Wall (1989, p.11) proposes a useful definition of patients as: '...people whose health requires the help of others with special skills. The patient may ask for this help or be perceived by others as needing it.' Thus, the patient is dependent upon others for his/her healthy well-being, whereas the healthy volunteer is comparatively independent for his/her well-being. Whilst obvious, this difference has far-reaching implications in undertaking research, not least because the patient has the added complication of being reliant upon medical attention at the same time.

Aware of the potential difficulties of conducting research with patients, the Royal College of Physicians in 1967 recommended that such research should be subject to ethical review. This recommendation has instigated the introduction of local Research Ethics Committees in National Health Service hospitals throughout the country, which are sometimes jointly attached to universities. The Royal College of Physicians published a document entitled *Guidelines On the Practice of Ethics Committees In Medical Research* in 1984, which was revised in 1990. Any research proposal which envisages the involvement of patient subjects is now strictly scrutinized by the appropriate Research Ethics Committee before it can proceed further.

In view of these guidelines, the study being presented on this occasion constitutes (para)medical research, since it aims to have direct implications for the clinical treatment of the patient population represented in the research. For this reason, the researcher is familiar with the code of conduct outlined by the Royal College of Physicians concerning both medical practice and medical research and their different nuances. Since the therapeutic intervention provided by speech therapy tends to adhere to the ideology of the medical model of patient care, reference to the medical code of conduct is apposite on this occasion.

Although the investigation does not involve methods of treatment experimentation (such as drugs trials), the predominant ethical concern of possible psychological intrusion of the participants has had to be addressed. In doing so, the potential damage to the participants was assessed as being of minimal risk, and was stated as such in submitting the research proposal to the Research Ethics Committee.

The research proposal was unanimously approved by the local Research Ethics Committee with no suggested amendments, on the understanding that a progress report would be submitted to the Committee six months after the commence of the study. This was undertaken, and no recommendations or comments have been received by the researcher following the Committee's inspection of the report.

A further consideration concerns the protection of data under the Protection of Data Act 1984, which seeks to give individuals the legal right to have access to the data recorded on computer which concerns them. Data held for the sole purpose of undertaking research are exempt from the Act, and it is understood that the participants will not be identified in the reporting of the research findings. The data of the current study thus fall into this category.

The research proposal

With respect to the present study, the availability of an extensive, largely raw data base (as delineated in chapter one) relating to the cleft population, offered the writer the opportunity to undertake a retrospective follow-up study. The number of participants followed-up has been determined by the successful location of their current whereabouts. All of the individuals involved in the research (aged between 20 and 42 years), received cleft-related treatment at the Wessex Centre for Plastic and Maxillo-Facial Surgery, Odstock Hospital, Salisbury. In each instance, soft palate repair surgery was undertaken prior to 30 months of age.

It should be noted that BNH extended her own survey to include 60 children whose palates were either repaired at Odstock Hospital at a later age, or at a plastic surgery unit elsewhere. Since the variables inherent in this group of children are very diverse, and in view of the constraints of time and financial resources, they have not been incorporated into the writer's study.

Regarding the proposed objectives of the follow-up investigation, the reader is referred to the hypotheses as stipulated at the end of chapter one.

Given that the majority of adults tend not to live at their parents' home, the process of tracking down the (ex-)patients has been hampered. Moreover, as cleft-related treatment generally ceases for the patient during adolescence, the parental address as recorded in the hospital records was the last known place of contact for the 501 potential participants. Thus, in tracing those involved in BNH's study, reliance upon parental co-operation has been paramount. The necessary involvement of a 'third party' in this way is clearly a disadvantage, particularly in an investigation focusing upon parental attitudes towards their cleft-impaired offspring, amongst other aspects.

Ignorance of the present marital status of the females concerned has proved a further hindrance. Consequently, correspondence with these individuals has deployed their maiden names, which is unsatisfactory given that some of the females have been married for over twenty years.

The research strategy adopted for the follow-up study comprises four different approaches to data collection, which are detailed below. Before examining the research design, mention must be made of the alternatives which have been considered, but duly dismissed as inappropriate in failing to fulfil the research objectives.

Aternative methodologies for conducting the proposed study

Whilst the use of a control group can enhance the impact of the research findings in gauging the effects or non-effects of particular variables, it does not have universal application to all research objectives. As the term suggests the 'control' group is characterized by vigilance to tightly controlled variables.

Thus, in a study which seeks to gain insight into individual differences and experiences, the imposed structure would limit the scope of the variables investigated. Indeed, in the current study the inclusion of a control group would hinder rather than facilitate, the aim of obtaining the maximum number of participants in the study as possible.

A further alternative to be considered was the value of a case study approach. However, this methodological framework was also discarded in view of the number of participants involved. Having perused the possible methodologies, in view of the research objectives the most expedient strategy was to undertake a retrospective follow-up study.

Stage two: the nature and process of data collection

The design of the retrospective follow-up study

The follow-up study which is necessarily retrospective in nature, comprises the following four parts, which combine both quantitative and qualitative methodologies. It should be noted that they are arranged in a broadly chronological order to reflect the developmental paradigm of the research. Thus, whilst BNH's data (Part A) details the participants' development during their formative years, the interviews (Part D) with a selection of the adult participants comprise the most recent data.

> *Part A*   The legacy of data collected by BNH
> *Part B*   Examination of speech therapy and plastic surgery records
> *Part C*   Administration of a postal questionnaire
> *Part D*   Conducting of personal interviews

Part A - the legacy of data collected by BNH

The nature of the legacy of data left by BNH was elucidated in chapter one. For this reason, it will not be detailed further in this chapter, other than to state that for the purposes of the current study, the writer has converted the available data into discrete variables. This practice has enabled BNH's data (Part A), to be incorporated into the same computer software as the later data sets (Parts B and C), collected by the writer, thus permitting cross-tabulation of data. Part D does not necessitate computer analysis. The composition of the variables relating to BNH's data, will be defined in reporting the findings in the subsequent chapter (the developmental years).

Part B - The examination of speech therapy and plastic surgery records

An in-depth examination of hospital records was undertaken, to obtain as full a profile as possible of each participant in the study, and to supplement other data. The utilization of hospital records requires attention to a further ethical implication. The issue emerges where the researcher takes off her professional 'hat' to don the researcher's 'hat'. Happily, the dispute is resolved by the fact that the researcher was employed at the same hospital, at the time of the study with the interests of both the hospital and patients at heart. Therefore, the potential problems faced by the outside researcher seeking access to hospital records is not an issue on this occasion. Moreover, as the researcher worked at Odstock Hospital, the individuals approached for completion of the questionnaire (Part C to be detailed in due course) would expect the researcher/therapist to have access to their hospital records. Providing the information gleaned from hospital documents is treated with respect and in confidence, it can be used for the purposes of medical research without the explicit consent of the patients (*A Report of the Royal College of Physicians, Research Involving Patients*, 1990).

The rationale for data collected by the examination of hospital records By way of supplementing the information gathered by BNH, the examination of hospital records focused upon references made to the individuals' psychosocial development and functioning. For this purpose, a data collection form was compiled (please see Appendix 3a), which was pre-coded as far as possible for ease in later data analysis. The rationale for items included on the form is outlined below.

Section A - Background details

Item 1 - Source of information
To ascertain whether the information is gleaned from the speech therapy records or the Plastic Surgery Unit medical records only, or from a combination of the two sources, depending upon the availability of the information.

Items 2 and 3 - The patient's sex and date of birth (respectively)
For identification purposes.

Item 4 - Home area
Town or City in which the Cleft Plate Team's peripheral clinics are held within the Wessex Region.

Item 5 - Extent of cleft
To enable the classification and analysis of data according to the variable of cleft type.

Item 6 - Maternal complications
Information pertaining to difficulties experienced by the patient's mother during the ante-, peri- and/or postnatal stages of the patient's birth are noted here. A problematic pregnancy or labour could have connotations for the way in which the mother perceives motherhood, and her subsequent parenting skills. This information is also valuable in indicating the general health of the patient's mother.

Item 7 - Medical complications
Any additional medical problems of the cleft-impaired individuals are included in this item. For example, these may be directly related or unrelated

to the cleft condition. Such complications have implications for possible further hospitalization, school absence, and overprotective parenting, amongst other aspects. Moreover, cleft-related treatment may be regarded as low priority by the parents, if the patient has a life-threatening condition.

Item 8 - Composition of the patient's family
The position within the family of the cleft-impaired child is of significance regarding his/her psychosocial development. For example, in the amount of attention he/she receives from other family members. If the child is the youngest in a large family, there is a greater chance that child may be spoilt and 'babied' by older siblings as well as the parents. On the other hand, if the first child has a cleft, the parents are more likely to place higher demands and expectations upon the child. The sex of any siblings provides further information.

Section B - NHS (National Health Service) hospital treatment

Item 9 - Number of hospital admissions
An indication of the extent of hospitalization experienced by the child and his/her family in the treatment of the cleft. The associated aspects of trauma, maternal separation, missed schooling and of feeling 'different' to peers all need to be taken into account in considering the psychosocial implications of having a cleft.

Item 10 - Correspondence relating to non-attendance at hospital follow-up clinics or speech therapy appointments
The extent to which non-attendance is or is not explained, may reflect the parents' interest in the child and his/her treatment programme. For example, a series of unexplained non-attendances may suggest indifference if the parents consider treatment to be of low priority.

Item 11 - Other agencies involved
The involvement of other agencies or services in treating the patient with a cleft is recorded here. That is, services other than surgery, speech therapy and orthodontics which form the core provision by the Cleft Palate Team. The nature of the additional services involved suggests the extent of the patient's needs, which tend to vary from individual to individual.

Section C - Psychosocial development

Item 12 - Reference to the family environment
The focus here is upon the patient's home life, and includes attention to the home environment, parenting style, parental attitude towards the child and the interest shown by the parents regarding the child's hospital treatment.

Item 13 - Reference to pre-school years (0-approximately 5 years old)
Attention is given to the patient's early socialization and personality development, which largely takes place in the home context before commencing pre-school education (such as playgroup or nursery school).

Item 14 - Reference to pre-teenage years (5-12 years old)
References made to socialization and to personality development during the pre-teenage years are noted here, such as subjection to teasing.

Item 15 - Reference to teenage years (approximately 13-17 years old)
As for item 14 above where applicable to adolescence.

Item 16 - Reference to adulthood (18 years and above)
As for item 14. above where applicable to adulthood.

Section D - Details of hospital discharge

Item 17 - Age at discharge from speech therapy and plastic surgery
This information indicates the extent of the treatment required, which reflects the hospital resources consumed in providing that treatment.

Item 18 - Situation regarding treatment according to last entries on records
The degree to which the treatment programme has been completed, and on what terms the discharge took place are noted. For example, whilst some discharges follow completion of all treatment, others are made following a series of unexplained non-attendances.

It should be noted that the aforementioned data sets (Parts A and B), entail information which has been gleaned by BNH (and her colleagues) and the writer. Therefore, data collection has not necessitated the writer's direct involvement with the individuals concerned. However, the following two data sets (Parts C and D) are fundamentally different in nature, in that they both require personal contact with the participants. That is, whilst the postal questionnaire entails corresponding with potential respondents, the conducting of personal interviews compels face to face interaction with a selection of them. It is to the former of these that attention is turned now.

Part C - the administration of a postal questionnaire

The rationale for the proposed use of a postal questionnaire In view of the potential size of the proposed study, the advantages of using a postal questionnaire were considered to far outweigh the inevitable disadvantages of its use.

The advantages of implementing a postal questionnaire:

- This method is expedient for widespread distribution.

- It is economical on time and cost, e.g. travel is not necessary.

- The study is centrally controlled.

- Interviewer/researcher biasing effects are eliminated.

- Respondents have time to respond without feeling pressurized and under observation whilst doing so.

The disadvantages of implementing a postal questionnaire:

- The literacy and intelligence of the respondent are assumed.

- As there is no opportunity for explanation, the postal questionnaire must be necessarily simpler and less flexible in form and content, than if engaged in face to face contact with the target population.

- The researcher has no control as to how the questionnaire is completed. For example, the actual respondent may not be the intended respondent, and/or the order in which the questions are answered may be inconsistent across respondents, having a possible biasing effect.

The rationale for questions comprising the postal questionnaire In accordance with the considerations cited above, this section expounds the rationale behind each of the questions comprising the postal questionnaire, a copy of which is available in Appendix 3b. The subsequent explanations relate to the various sections of the questionnaire, and the questions asked under each section heading.

Section A - Personal details

Questions 1.-4.
Elicit background information (such as sex and date of birth).

Question 5.
Indication of family history or isolated incidence of cleft. This is significant regarding parents' prior knowledge of the cleft condition before the birth of the cleft-impaired child. Familiarity with the condition may have implications for parental attitude towards the baby and the defect.

Section B - Education

Question 1.
The number of years spent in full-time education is a broad indication of intellectual ability. As this question is taken from a study by Clifford et al. (1972), the data can be directly compared with the published findings.

Question 2.
Further information relating to intellectual achievement and aspirations. Various authorities (e.g., Lansdown, 1981), report lowered school attainment and aspirations in individuals having a cleft, suggesting impoverished self-esteem.

Question 3.
Perceptions concerning how the respondent felt about having a cleft at

school are sought here. Concern or lack of concern can provide insight as to the extent to which the cleft influenced the individual's school life and socialization with peers.

Question 4.
With respect to question 3. above, the respondent is asked if his/her perceptions have now changed with time and experience. This suggests the stability of the respondent's perceptions about him or herself with maturity, and the development (or absence) of coping mechanisms.

Section C - Employment

Question 1.
Details of the respondent's current employment situation purport to his/her career choices, level of intellectual attainment and broadly indicate socio-economic status, all of which are discussed in the literature. The extent to which a cleft condition affects chances and choices of employment can begin to be evaluated from responses made to this, and the subsequent two questions.

Questions 2. and 3.
Information elicited by these two questions relates to the respondent's satisfaction with present employment (if applicable), and aspirations for the future. Clifford et al. (1972), published their findings in this area using the same rating scale as in question 2. Direct comparisons can thus be made. Aspirations may be seen to reflect self-concept and self-esteem.

Section D - Speech and appearance

Question 1.
Although reference can be made to the respondent's medical notes for information regarding speech therapy, some respondents may be unaware that they received this form of intervention. This question seeks insight into their perception on this matter.

Question 2.
The 'looks versus speech' issue is touched upon in this item. Appearance is often a sensitive subject to adolescents. Those with a cleft lip and/or palate may have additional concerns as to how they look and/or speak. Undue self-consciousness can exacerbate low self-esteem, and its negative connotations regarding psychosocial functioning.

Questions 3. and 4.
The rating scales used in these questions derive from the published findings of Clifford et al. (1972). Comparisons can be therefore made. Satisfaction with both current speech and appearance may indicate the development of personal coping mechanisms, which are fundamental to functioning effectively.

Section E - N.H.S. treatment for your cleft lip and/or palate

Question 1.
This open-ended question seeks the respondent's opinion concerning the follow-up clinics for cleft-related treatment. The responses elicited offer insight into attitudes towards the treatment received.

Questions 2. and 3.
The rating scales are taken from Clifford et al. (1972), to ascertain the respondent's present satisfaction with the surgery and orthodontic treatment received at Odstock Hospital. Comparisons can be made with the published findings.

Section F - How you see yourself now

Question 1.
This personality profile derives from the work of McCrae and Costa (for example. 1987). A measure of personality needs to be incorporated if a comprehensive picture of the individuals' personal and social functioning is to be obtained. By including a personality profile in the questionnaire, the controversial existence of a 'cleft personality' can be addressed.

Question 2.
The self-esteem scale included in the questionnaire was compiled by Rosenberg (1965), and continues to be used extensively in a variety of contexts. The literature suggests that the cleft population evidence lower levels of self-esteem than non-affected individuals. By including the scale this matter can be addressed.

Section G - Your experience of having a cleft lip and/or palate

Question 1.
This question seeks to discover how actively involved the respondent and his/her family are or have been in the self-support Cleft Lip and Palate Association (CLAPA). It could be postulated that those who have/had close links with this group, are those who are/were in most need of support offered by the association.

Question 2.
This question offers the respondent an open forum in which to express his/her perception of earlier cleft-related treatment at Odstock Hospital. The responses reflect the respondent's recollection of both the intervention and nature of his or her cleft condition.

Question 3.
Teasing appears to be one of the most stigmatizing aspects for the

individual with a cleft. Frequent teasing can, therefore, have a potentially damaging effect upon the personal and social development of those subjected to it. The data elicited here will indicate the extent of this problem amongst the respondents.

Question 4.
The perceived influence of the cleft upon the individual's life is addressed in this question, using the rating scale of Clifford et al. (1972). Direct comparisons can be made. The profile obtained is invaluable as an indication of how far the individual feels hampered, and even handicapped by his or her cleft.

Questions 5. and 6.
As for question 2. (Section G) above.

Part D - The conducting of personal interviews

The inclusion of interviews in the overall research design of the current study, reflects the researcher's realization that interviews can offer a unique means of data collection. Moreover, when used in addition to other methods interviews not only prove an invaluable way of supplementing the existing data base, but a rich source of data in itself. In conjunction with the methodologies adopted for the postal questionnaire and the examination of hospital records, the researcher undertook a series of personal interviews with a selection of the questionnaire respondents. This decision was based on the belief that interviews were the most pertinent means of gaining the required anecdotal information.

The rationale for undertaking personal interviews In drawing up the objectives, the interviews have been perceived in terms of a 'sounding board' for the discussion of issues arising from the postal questionnaire, as well as a means of gathering further data.

The value of personal interviews in action research In view of the objectives of the present study, emphasis is placed upon providing convincing evidence which has the potential for improving current management of the cleft population (where applicable). The presentation of recommendations (chapter nine) based upon the findings, reflect the intention, as well as the challenge for the researcher to combine theory and practice with a new perspective for the future. This paradigm has been identified by social scientists as 'Action Research', which Breakwell (1990, p.70) amongst others, defines as:

> ... a piece of research designed to initiate some change in the people, the organisations, or the procedures, studied. In other words it has an objective, normally to produce development or improvement. It is not simply aimed at producing a description of what already exists; it is aimed at changing it.

The presentation and format of the interview schedule The interview schedule was displayed using a single pocket photograph album, with one index card inserted into each pocket, with a maximum of two cards being visible at any given time. Since the objective was to lay the interview schedule in a position accessible to both the interviewer and the interviewee, this form of presentation actively encouraged the adoption of a partnership role with the interviewee. That is, discussion of the questions was sought rather than conducting the interview on a purely question-answer level of interaction.

Concerning the contents of the interview schedule, data elicited by the postal questionnaire was written on an index card and placed in the left hand side pocket of each 'page'. The data were related to the question(s) presented in the opposite right hand pocket. This method encouraged a semi-structured form of interviewing, and proved an effective way of engaging the interviewee in conversation. The questions directly correspond to the areas of interest encompassed in the postal questionnaire with the exception of gathering personal details.

In view of the one hour allocated for each interview, in devising the schedule the interviewer did not intend to cover all of the questions in the schedule. One of the main features of the shared access to the schedule is that the book form allows both the interviewer and the interviewee to scan the questions on each page, and to select those which are considered most pertinent to the experiences of the interviewee. As the number of interviews undertaken increased, the interviewer was able to focus upon particular question areas in order to acquire a comprehensive and balanced set of data.

The contents of the interview schedule The contents of the interview schedule are presented below in chronological order. Details of the questions asked have been placed in Appendix 3c. In order to gain maximum rapport and outcome, the questions were posed in such a way that each interview commenced with eliciting general information (public), before verging into the more personal, and possibly more threatening areas of experience (private).

- Introduction: views on receiving the postal questionnaire
- NHS treatment for your cleft
- Parents, home environment and siblings
- Imagining situations (e.g. parenting a child with a cleft)
- Perceived influence of the cleft upon life
- Personal experiences: having a cleft at school
- Perceived change since leaving school
- Experiences of being teased
- Perceived change since teenage years
- Perceived developmental changes: personality and self-esteem
- Employment
- Advice based upon personal experience of cleft
- Maturation and the development of coping skills
- What of the future ?
- Recommendations emerging from the questionnaire data

Definition of the research population

As the research population of the current study is ultimately determined by the response rate regarding postal questionnaire returns, attention has been given to features universally identified for maximising this percentage (for example, Baumgartner and Heberlein, 1984).

- population
- confidentiality (and anonymity)
- introductory or covering letter

Population The population for whom the postal questionnaire has been devised, comprises those who have been born with either a cleft lip and palate or cleft palate only. Therefore, the questionnaire has not been randomly distributed to the cleft population. More specifically, it has been sent exclusively to those who fulfil the specific criteria of being involved in BNH's survey at Odstock Hospital, and whose present location could be traced.

Confidentiality (and anonymity) The guarantee of confidentiality must be assured when enlisting the participation and co-operation of respondents in a survey or interview. As all of the participants received cleft-related treatment at Odstock Hospital, there is no breach of confidence in acknowledging their status as patients or ex-patients. Indeed, since the researcher was employed at the same hospital, and therefore, had access to their hospital records, the participants have no grounds for suspecting anything other than guaranteed confidentiality.

With respect to the questionnaire, no findings nor responses should be published if there is any possibility of tracing them back to the individuals concerned. Indeed, the promise of confidentiality may be instrumental in eliciting sincere responses, and may discourage the respondent who may be inclined to give socially desirable responses.

Whilst confidentiality was assured to the respondents in administering the postal questionnaire, anonymity has not been mentioned. Regarding terminology, 'confidentiality' infers the keeping of one's confidence. 'Anonymity', however, implies that the respondent's identity is not known to the researcher. If the aims of the retrospective follow-up study are to be fulfilled, anonymity of the respondents would be abortive. Furthermore, whilst the code of ethical conduct for research involving patients (*A Report of the Royal College of Physicians*, January 1990), stipulates the need for confidentiality in gathering data, it does not appear to refer to the need for anonymity.

A potential obstruction to total confidentiality has been the necessity to send the postal questionnaires to the individuals via their parents' home address, since in most instances this was the last known address of the individuals concerned. It must be stressed that the envelope in each case was addressed to the potential participant, and it would, therefore, be the parents' breach of confidence to open the correspondence. Moreover, as the cleft deformity is congenital, and as the parents would have been involved in the hospital treatment for their son's or daughter's cleft, the parents would be fully aware of the cleft's existence. Thus, again this does not constitute a breach of confidence by the researcher.

On completing the questionnaire, respondents were not requested to sign their forms or to supply their names, but they were encouraged to give their date of birth and sex. This was one method of identification used in the study. A further means of identification entailed coding the date of administration of the questionnaire in various ways. With hindsight, it is notable that many of the respondents either signed their forms, or voluntarily gave their names and addresses.

Introductory or covering letter In considering the methodology to be adopted, the frequent need for compromise has been a pressing concern on three different counts. The first of these issues relates to the principle of informed consent. Whilst every code of conduct would stipulate that the participants in a research project should consent to their subsequent involvement in the project, there do appear to be some exceptions. In the present study, the notion of obtaining the written consent of so large a group of individuals whose current whereabouts was itself uncertain, in order to then send each individual a postal questionnaire, appeared to be of questionable value. Hence, the importance and relevance of this principle to the potential participants, had to be weighed against the most efficient use of time and resources. Needless to say, there is no indication that such methodology is superior to the use of an introductory covering letter.

Given that in the first instance, the participants were to be involved by means of a postal questionnaire (and an explanatory covering letter), which they could refuse to complete and return, the choice to participate or not to do so lay directly in their hands. Thus, the sending of a postal questionnaire to each of the individuals whose whereabouts had been traced, served to invite the recipient to participate in the study. Indeed, the *Guidelines On the Practice of Ethics Committees In Medical Research* involving human subjects state: 'The fact that the subject completes the questionnaire can be taken as consent' (*A Report of the Royal College of Physicians*, January 1990, p.22). Therefore, those who wished to become involved returned their forms, whilst those who wished to remain uncommitted to the research have not done so.

Since the questionnaire was the first means of contact between the researcher and the recipient, careful attention has been paid to the nature of the accompanying introductory or covering letter. This letter serves to introduce the study and to explain its objectives, and may determine whether or not the individual chooses to participate in the study. It is crucial to provide sufficient explanation, encouragement and gratitude at this stage to gain the recipient's interest.

For the purposes of the current investigation two different covering letters were composed. The first of these was sent with the initial questionnaire. The second letter accompanied the same questionnaire when it was necessary to issue reminders to certain respondents.

It should be pointed out that as the researcher had no insight as to the present marital status of the females to be appoached, the covering letters were hand-addressed using the 'Ms.' title followed by their maiden names

66

(as recorded in the hospital notes). In addressing each individual in the covering letter, alongside 'Dear Ms. X' was placed the request 'please let us know if your name has changed' in parentheses. This proved an effective approach as several respondents volunteered their married surname and their current address. These details were useful in selecting potential interviewees.

Tracing the (ex-)patients

Whilst efforts were made to maximize the response rate regarding the postal questionnaire, in the first instance, the administration of the questionnaire depended upon the 'success' with which the potential participants could be traced.

The first phase of the tracing process Before commencing the follow-up study, it was necessary to ascertain the current whereabouts of the original 501 individuals. The procedure adopted is summarized below.

- It was possible to deduct 39 (7.8%) names from the total of 501 at the start since they were still on the 'current' hospital patient records. The addresses were, therefore, assumed to be correct.

- The last known address of each person was noted from hospital records. The vast majority of cases had been discharged from further treatment. Although most of these addresses were encompassed within the region of Wessex, 53 (10.6%) fell outside the boundaries. For ease of access and practicality, only Wessex addresses were subsequently followed up. This criterion decreased the total from 462 to 409 names and addresses.

- The first source to be tapped was the relevant telephone directory for each address. The matching of the last known address with the patient's surname proved fruitful in 90 (22.0% of 409) cases. The assumption was made that if the address and surname found in the telephone directory were consistent with those in the hospital records, it seemed likely that this was also the present parental address of the person concerned.

The researcher was aware at this stage that tracing individuals via the telephone directory elicited an undesirable bias, since it incorporated only those who were registered users of the telephone. Moreover, even the criterion of telephone user is misleading, as there may have been a proportion of users who chose to be ex-directory. A further assumption underlying the whole procedure was that the address, and even the surname of each patient had been accurately recorded on the hospital notes.

- Those whose last known address and surname could not be found in the current issue telephone directories (n=319) were sought via the Electoral Register. A further 80 (19.6%) cases were traced through this source, leaving a residual 239 of the 409 individuals not as yet located.

Whilst perusing the two sources of reference for current addresses, the value of some of the addresses found was questionable. That is, in 32 (7.8%) cases, the last known address recorded in the hospital notes differed slightly from that displayed in the telephone directory, or the Electoral Register. For example, although the street name matched, the number of the house in that street differed to that of the last known address. Where such incongruity occurred a note was made by the researcher, and these addresses were subsequently kept separately from those which appeared to tally exactly with the hospital records. This was deemed necessary since the questionable addresses warranted further confirmation before sending the questionnaires.

The second phase of the tracing process Having pursued the most economical and expedient methods of tracing the individuals, in terms of time and limited financial resources, there remained a total of 292 (58.3%) of BNH's 501 patient-subjects whose current whereabouts was still uncertain. Whilst the postal questionnaire was sent to the traced names and addresses, attention was turned to alternative sources in locating the remaining individuals. namely the Family Health Service Authorities (hereafter referred to as FHSAs), general practitioners, and the Central Register (at the Office of Population Censuses and Surveys, London).
Since travel was not necessary in tapping these sources, the geographical restraints placed upon the first phase of the tracing process

in keeping to the boundaries of the Wessex region, were lifted. Thus, FHSAs throughout the country were involved in the identification of (ex)patients. The only criterion for elimination during the second phase of tracing was where individuals were known to be living outside the United Kingdom (n=5, 1.0% according to the hospital records). At this stage, the location of 287 (57.3% of 501) individuals was still uncertain.

Once additional financial support had been secured, the second phase of the tracing procedure began in earnest, as outlined below.

- FHSAs were approached for their assistance in locating named individuals, on the basis of date of birth and last known name and address (as noted on the hospital records). It should be noted that the FHSAs are in a position to provide details pertaining to the individuals' general practitioners only, and not the present home address of the individuals. However, the FHSAs were permitted to give the marital surname of females if applicable.

- The subsequent correspondence received by the researcher from the FHSAs, was placed in one of three categories depending upon the nature of the reply. The categories are outlined below.

68

Group A   Ex-patient identified and the name, address and telephone number of his/her current general practitioner supplied.

Group B   Ex-patient no longer resident within the boundaries of the particular FHSA approached. Details of the 'new' and present FHSA were provided on these occasions, which meant that the specified FHSA could then be contacted.

Group C   Ex-patient not traced, and an alternative FHSA not recommended by the first FHSA to be considered.

• For the individuals whose current general practitioner's name and address had been supplied by the relevant FHSA, the researcher was in a position to correspond directly with that professional. A covering letter was sent introducing the general practitioners to the study, and to request their co-operation in forwarding the postal questionnaire to the named person (with date of birth provided).

A stamped envelope addressed to the general practitioner.
A covering letter addressed to the general practitioner.
A stamped addressed envelope for forwarding the questionnaire.
A copy of the postal questionnaire.
A covering letter to the individual to be included in the study.
A stamped addressed envelope for return of the postal questionnaire.

Since the administration of each questionnaire had to be facilitated by the general practitioner, a prompt return of the questionnaire was precipitated by using first class stamps on all three envelopes used. With the assistance of FHSAs and general practitioners, a further 170 (33.9% of 501) individuals were traced. This figure excludes 4 (0.8%) individuals whose death was reported by the FHSAs, leaving 113 (22.6%) potential participants to track down by other means.

• Where the pertinent FHSAs had not been able to identify the specified names and addresses (n=113), a further source of tracing was necessary. This entailed applying to consult the Central Register held at the Office of Population Censuses and Surveys, London. As the Central Register can only provide details of the name and address of individuals' present general practitioners, the timely process of approaching the relevant FHSAs outlined above had to be reinstated.

It is regrettable that although the writer's application to consult the Central Register was accepted, due to the length of time taken to secure the information from the FHSAs, this procedure had to be abandoned. Thus, 113 (22.6%) of BNH's 501 patient-subjects have not been located.

The outcome of the tracing procedure   Having completed the search for individuals involved in BNH's research (n=501), the outcome of the tracing procedure is summarized as follows.

Table 3.1
The outcome of the tracing procedure

Outcome	n	%
Current patient (tracing unnecessary)	39	7.8
Traced via local telephone directory	90	18.0
Traced via Electoral Register	80	16.0
Traced via FHSA	170	33.9
Eliminated as living abroad	5	1.0
FHSA reported death of individual	4	0.8
Location remains unidentified	113	22.6
Total	501	100.1

The association between the percentage of individuals traced and those incorporated into the present follow-up study, will be detailed in discussing the response rate obtained for the questionnaire (Table 3.2).

The criteria for the selection of interviewees

It is with the implications of Action Research in mind (delineated earlier), that the personal interviews were planned. The criteria for the selection of those to be interviewed are outlined below.

Having coded the completed postal questionnaires for data analaysis, the forms were divided into three groups as specified below, according to the type of information (if any) volunteered by the respondents.

Group 1 Those who offered further involvement in the study or who requested further information, and gave their name and address (or telephone number).

Group 2 Those who gave their current address, with no additional information.

Group 3 Those who did not fall into either group above. That is, those who volunteered no further information of any description.

Respondents incorporated into the first two groups were then examined in more detail. The apparent wish of the third group for privacy with no additional involvement in the study was respected. Therefore, regarding the selection of interviewees this group was not considered further. In order to filter out a representative sample for interviewing from groups 1 and 2, the data pertaining to each individual were looked at according to specific variables. The variables were considered by the researcher to be of direct relevance to the emerging implications of the study for improved clinical practice, and are listed as follows.

- Sex
- Year of birth
- Marital status
- Current employment situation
- Experience of being teased
- Whether or not a contact telephone number was given
- Resident inside or outside the boundaries of Wessex

The respondents were categorized according to how far they fulfilled three particular criteria. These criteria were namely, whether or not they had reported incidences of being teased, supplied their current address and were resident in Wessex. The new groupings consisted of those who fulfilled all of these criteria (n=23), those fulfilling only two criteria (n=12), and those fulfilling one criterion only (n=14). In this way, the possible candidates for interview were prioritized.

If the selected group of respondents for interview are to be representative of the respondents involved in the study, its composition should reflect the same ratio of males to females as the larger group of respondents (53.5% and 46.5% respectively). In order to obtain a similar ratio amongst the interviewees, 13 individuals (7 males and 6 females) from the three criteria group were initially invited for interview. The researcher sought approximately twelve acceptances for interview.

Having established to whom interviews should be offered, a letter of invitation was despatched. The letter thanked the respondent for his/her contribution in returning the completed questionnaire. It also explained the purpose of the interview in view of the research project. A form was attached to the letter requesting the recipient's response to the invitation, and to indicate the most convenient dates and times if the respondent wished to participate in the interview. A stamped, addressed envelope was provided for the swift return of the completed form. To enhance efficiency, the outgoing and return envelopes were mailed first class.

Regarding the 13 respondents invited for interview, the subsequent response demonstrated that twelve respondents (6 males and 6 females) were willing to be interviewed. The thirteenth individual replied that he did not wish to be involved. Thus, a 92.3% compliance rate was obtained. The interviewees approximated the sex ratio of the main study (n=217).

Data collection - the pilot study

Piloting the postal questionnaire With regard to the current study the main objective of the pilot study was to test the method of data collection, in order to ascertain if it elicited the appropriate data. The analysis and presentation of the data were not pursued on this occasion. Taking the practical constraints of time and resources into account, the postal questionnaire was piloted by selecting 5 of the 217 individuals who returned a completed questionnaire. The five chosen were all living in the vicinity of Salisbury, to enable the ease of personal follow-up if necessary. Those selected for the pilot study can be described as follows.

Sex	2 Females (1 single and 1 married with children)
	3 Males (all single)
Age	Year of birth ranged between 1952-1970

The pilot questionnaire comprised 41 questions and 8 sections of interest.

- Section A - Personal details
- Section B - Education
- Section C - Employment
- Section D - Speech
- Section E - Appearance
- Section F - How you see yourself now
- Section G - NHS treatment for your cleft lip and/or palate
- Section H - Your experience of having a cleft lip and/or palate

In administering the pilot questionnaire, attempts were made to maximize the response rate by adopting the following practices.

- Personalizing the material where possible. For example, both the addressed and self-addressed envelopes were handwritten. The covering letters were also personalized. Both sets of envelopes were stamped in accordance with Scott's (1961) finding that stamped self-addressed envelopes for the return of the requested information elicit a higher response rate, compared with business reply envelopes. In addition, two signatures concluded the covering letters, namely that of the researcher and of her supervising medical Consultant.

- The questionnaires were sent by first class post, and the stamped addressed envelopes enclosed were returned via second class post.

- As the ultimate response rate relied almost entirely upon the co-operation of respondents' parents to re-direct the questionnaire to their son/daughter (with the exception of the few respondents still living at their parents' address), a handwritten request was made on the envelope to 'Please forward if necessary'.

- In the pilot questionnaire, a reference code number was placed discreetly on the final page, since the study necessitates the identification of the respondents.

The outcome and the revision of the pilot postal questionnaire Having sent out a total of five questionnaires with only one return after a period of three weeks, four reminders were despatched to the relevant respondents. Six weeks from the launch of the pilot study, a response rate of 80% (n=4) had been secured.

Analysis of the returned questionnaires indicated that the series of questions needed to be reduced, and that several questions could be abandoned altogether, in view of the data they elicited. The revised questionnaire used for the main study comprises twenty-seven questions, which fall into six areas of interest. These areas are the same as for the pilot instrument, apart from the combination of Speech and Appearance (section D). Only one question appears in the revised format but not in the pilot questionnaire. That is, as a result of the pilot study, a question concerning teasing was considered essential and, therefore, has been included in the main study questionnaire (question 3, Section G).

Since the main study contains twenty-six of the questions (in identical format) used in the pilot questionnaire, the four completed pilot questionnaires have been incorporated into the data base of the main study. The two sources of data can be distinguished where necessary.

Following the pilot study, the covering letter accompanying the second, reminder questionnaire was re-drafted. It was then typed, as the handwritten form of the letter used in the pilot study was deemed impractical for the mass distribution necessary for the main study.

Follow-up contact Subsequent to the piloting of the questionnaire, it was intended that the main study follow-up questionnaires would also be sent after a period of three weeks. However, this required revision since a proportion of the first batch of initial questionnaires of the main study were still being returned some four to five weeks later. Thus, the period between administrating the first and the follow-up questionnaires was extended to about six weeks. Reminders were sent, therefore, to all respondents for whom a returned questionnaire or envelope (where the address was not known), had not been received after about six weeks.

The follow-up procedure adopted by the researcher was identical for all respondents whose current whereabouts had been traced by the telephone directory or the Electoral Register. That is, the same questionnaire was sent again, in addition to a stamped addressed envelope, and a covering letter which differed slightly from that sent with the initial questionnaire. First class postage was again used on the outgoing mailing, and second class postage for the return of the questionnaire. The exception to this procedure affected the final forty-two questionnaires, which were given first class stamps for a speedy return before embarking upon the second phase of the tracing process.

Regarding the group of ex-patients who were not successfully traced in the first phase of the tracing procedure (via the telephone directory or the Electoral Register), the subsequent involvement of general practitioners in redirecting the postal questionnaires obviated follow-up contact for several reasons. These are outlined below.

Given that the ex-patient could not be approached directly by the researcher, any follow-up contact with him or her would have to be undertaken through the mediation and co-operation of the general practitioner. Thus, it was not possible to distinguish between the non-responsive general practitioner in forwarding the postal questionnaire, and the non-respondent receiving the questionnaire. Moreover, it is conceivable that the 'non-respondent' did not actually ever receive the questionnaire from the general practitioner. It is acknowledged that the medical professional's pressurized caseload may determine whether or not the questionnaire is forwarded, rather than his or her deliberate obstruction in the procedure.

Even if the necessary financial resources had been available to send a return slip to each general practitioner with the postal questionnaire, there was no guarantee that the slip itself would be returned to the researcher. This might confuse the situation further since a non-returned slip would not indicate whether the postal questionnaire had or had not been forwarded to the named individual by the doctor as requested.

An alternative means of ensuring the co-operation of the general practitioner in re-directing the postal questionnaire, would be to telephone the doctor's surgery in order to establish his or her intentions regarding the questionnaire. In view of the fact that doctors' surgeries are excessively busy places, and that the doctors themselves are in constant demand, it is likely that a telephone call regarding this administrative matter may not be given first priority.

The process of data collection

Data collected by BNH Having established the potential research population on the basis of the tracing process outlined above, the details collected by BNH pertaining to each of the individuals traced were singled out for the writer's further examination. By implication, therefore, the participants in BNH's survey whose current whereabouts could not be identified were excluded from the follow-up study. It should be noted, however, that the tracing process defined only the potential research participants, since the actual participants comprised those who completed and returned the postal questionnaire.

Regarding the process of data collection, since the information has been gathered already by BNH, further discussion of this particular data set will be preserved for the subsequent chapter (the developmental years).

Data collected on examining the hospital records Only the hospital records of those individuals who had completed and returned the questionnaire, were included in the study. That is, the speech therapy and plastic surgery records held at Odstock Hospital of the individuals traced, were consulted to the exclusion of non-traced potential participants. Needless to say, it is regrettable that following the process of tracking down BNH's survey subjects, those who were potential participants in the present study, had to be excluded from further investigation. Having distinguished the participants for the follow-up study, the process by which the second set of data were elicited is outlined as follows.

In the first instance, permission was secured to consult the speech therapy records, held in the Speech and Language Therapy department archive of Odstock Hospital. Since BNH was directly responsible for maintaining the speech therapy records relating to patients with a cleft, in conjunction with her role on the Cleft Palate Team (before the advent of other colleagues' involvement with the clinics), the speech therapy documents were consulted prior to the plastic surgery records.

It should be noted at this stage, that in line with management policy for patients with a cleft, the plastic surgeon's observations and recommendations at the time of the clinic are entered into the speech therapy records, albeit on a separate side or sheet of paper. Similarly, the speech therapist's comments and advice appear in the patient's plastic surgery records. The historical reason for this duplication of notes is that when either the speech therapist or the plastic surgeon is not available for consultation, the other professionals on the Cleft Palate Team have immediate access to the patient's treatment programme. Furthermore, this practice highlights the close relationship which exists between the patient's therapeutic and surgical treatment plans.

Having completed the examination of the appropriate speech therapy records, attention was turned to the plastic surgery records. This latter set of records is held in a separate hospital archive. Permission was again sought before embarking upon this exercise. Although, as stipulated earlier, the plastic surgeon's comments are added to the speech therapy notes, direct consultation of the plastic surgeon's own records was deemed of fundamental importance for two reasons. Firstly, the plastic surgery notes serve as an invaluable means of checking the accuracy of the details collected from the speech therapy records. Secondly, reference to an additional source of information, enables the opportunity for further data to be collected where available. The information gleaned from hospital records was then coded and analysed.

Administration of the postal questionnaire With the names and addresses of the potential research population identified during the course of the tracing process, the postal questionnaire was despatched to the individuals concerned. The response rate determined which of the individuals studied by BNH, were to be included in the current study.

Data elicited by conducting personal interviews Concerning this final stage of data collection, consideration was given to factors which would enhance the quality of the data gathered. To enable the atmosphere during each interview to be as relaxed and focused as possible under the circumstances, a tape recording of the entire interview was considered to be a more conducive method of data collection than continuous note-taking. With the exception of one occasion when the female interviewee particularly requested that the tape recorder should not be used, taped recordings were made in preference to written notes. Whilst transcription was more time-consuming for the researcher than taking rigorous notes, the means clearly justified the rich and spontaneous data which were thereby collected.

Following each interview, the researcher made a full transcription of the interview, whilst the interaction was still fresh in her mind. This was deemed to be particularly important since in some cases, the cleft-impaired speech of the interviewee made the accurate transcription from a taped recording a challenging exercise for the transcriber. It was for this reason, that the interviewer wished to transcribe the interviews personally, rather than engaging an audio typist.

Delineation of the data base upon which the current study is founded The data base emerging from the process of data collection previously outlined, comprises four independent data sets as follows.

Data set 1   data collected by BNH (1970s survey, Odstock Hospital).
Data set 2   data obtained from the Odstock Hospital records.
Data set 3   data elicited by postal questionnaire.
Data set 4   data gathered by conducting personal interviews.

Response rate for the return of completed postal questionnaires   The response rate obtained for the postal questionnaire determined the number of participants involved in the investigation.   Dillman et al. (1984, p.55) offer a concise definition of the term, which is universally accepted: 'The response rate (number of usable returned questionnaires divided by number mailed).'

Table 3.2
Designation of BNH's 501 subjects for the current study

Outcome	Sex of individual		
	Male	Female	Total
Questionnaire sent			
Returned and completed, included in study	116	101	217
	23.2%	20.2%	43.3
Returned too late to be included in study	5	3	8
	1.0%	0.6%	1.6%
Completed by mother of intended recipient	0	2	2
	0%	0.4%	0.4%
Learning difficulties, unable to complete	2	5	7
	0.4%	1.0%	1.4%
Informed of individual's death	1	1	2
	0.2%	0.2%	0.4%
Returned blank / not known at address	15	5	20
	3.0%	1.0%	4.0%
Not returned	83	40	123
	16.6%	8.0%	24.6%
Questionnaire not sent			
Living abroad	3	2	5
	0.6%	0.4%	1.0%
FHSA recorded death of individual	2	2	4
	0.4%	0.4%	0.8%
Untraced (candidates for Central Register	57	56	113
	11.4%	11.2%	22.6%
Total	284	217	501
	56.7%	43.3%	100.0%

Table 3.2 above shows that a total of 217 (43.3%) of the original 501 patient-subjects have been incorporated into the follow-up study.

However, since not all of BNH's subjects were sent questionnaires, the response rate is calculated from those that were distributed (n=379) and usable on their return. On this basis, it transpires that a 57.3% response rate has been obtained. If the forms (n=8) which were received too late to include in the study are incorporated, this figure rises to 59.4%.

One of the disadvantages of using postal questionnaires is that they produce lower response rates than other methods, such as personal interviews. Glastonbury and MacKean (1991, p.229) indicate:

> Self-completion questionnaires, especially postal ones, can be sent to much larger samples, even though the proportion who respond will be lower. While you might aim for a 75 per cent response rate from an interviewed sample, 50 per cent is more realistic through the post, though of course these will depend to an extent on the subject of the study and who makes up the sample.

Issues concerning non-response Discussion of the matter of non-response invites speculation, in that the researcher attempts to account for the lack of a 100% response rate. Realistically speaking, there may be diverse explanations for non-response which range from indifference towards the questionnaire sent, to more practical factors such as lack of time, illness or even forgetfulness. In many respects, therefore, it is hazardous and misleading to attribute possible causes for non-response. Indeed, in the case of the current study there may be seasonal reasons, since many of the questionnaires were sent out during the summer which is the peak holiday period.

Apart from the obvious sex difference between male and female non-respondents (Table 3.2: n=83 and n=40 respectively), there do not appear to be any significant factors, such as age or geographical location which distinguish the respondents and non-respondents. Whilst one could surmise that females may feel more obligated to respond or are more interested in divulging personal matters, this cannot be substantiated. In view of this, it could be advocated that greater importance is attached to the extent to which the 217 participants in the study, are seen to represent the wider cleft population. This consideration is addressed throughout the ensuing chapters, and in the use of published scales in the questionnaire itself.

Stage three: the analysis of data

Ethical considerations associated with data analysis

Data analysis entails interpretation. If the researcher's interpretation is regarded by others as accurate, reliable and valid, the research will have greater potential than if dismissed as faulty, deceptive and of little consequence.

One of the most significant determiners of the outcome of a study, is the extent to which it can or cannot be discredited on ethical grounds. For this reason, the writer has devised the following four-point code of ethical conduct as a means of avoiding the common pitfalls in the interpretation of data.

- Beware of bias
- Beware of error
- Beware of manipulation
- Beware of desired outcome versus real outcome

The four points are linked by the notion of responsibility towards the patient-subjects. Bias is exemplified by a tendency towards weighting the results in some way in order to produce more significant findings. An additional obligation towards the participants infers eliminating errors as far as humanly possible, since misrepresentations may be made if errors remain unchecked. Similarly, credence is lost by the fine manipulation of data in the hope that such tampering will not be detected. Other carriages of unethical practice involve the conflict between the ideal and the real implications of the research. A keen awareness of the potential consequences of such a conflict can help to stall its acceleration, and facilitate compromise.

The process of data analysis

In order to enable the comparison of data, information gleaned from the four data sets was converted into variables, to enable implementation of the Survey Analysis Package (SNAP2, 1988). This computer software was devised by Mercator Computer Systems Limited of Bristol, England, for the analysis of survey data. It should be noted, that given the predominantly quantitative nature of the first three data sets, and the qualitative nature of the fourth data set (personal interviews), the computer software was used for the former only.

Since the primary objective of undertaking the interviews was to gain insight into the interviewees' present day perceptions of their experiences, the data elicited were not intended to be subjected to detailed quantitative analysis. Thus, a descriptive method of analysis has been employed, which takes the form of a qualitative, thematic presentation of the data (as detailed in chapter seven).

In considering a developmental framework for processing the interview data, the research objectives again preclude such methodology. That is, the focus upon chronological ages and stages of development would deflect attention away from the 'themes' emerging during the interviews, to which importance was obviously attached.

Stage four: structure of the report of research results

Ethical considerations associated with reporting research results

The pertinent ethical issues in reporting the research findings, are largely the same as those already considered for data analysis. However, since reporting the results is, often the culmination of the research project, the researcher must be particularly sensitive to the information he/she is now making public. Again, a keyword is responsibility of the researcher to protect the interests and privacy of the participants, and the four-point code of conduct outlined above, is extended to include a further point.

- Beware of breaches of confidence

The presentation of data

The data collected by BNH, the examination of hospital records and postal questionnaire, are primarily quantitative in nature. The findings pertaining to analysis of these data are presented in chapters four and five. In each of these chapters, the presentation of data is followed by a section highlighting the most notable results of the relevant data set. In chapter six, the core variables of the three data sets are compared and cross-tabulated to enable further insight into the findings.

With respect to the qualitative analysis of the data elicited by personal interview (chapter seven), the information is presented in accordance with the section headings incorporated into the postal questionnaire, and is documented in chapter five (the adult years).

Having presented and analysed the data, the implications of the most notable findings are discussed in chapter eight in relation to the research objectives, and the published literature. The final chapter concludes the study by offering recommendations for improved clinical practice in the management of clefts.

Stage five: method of handling conclusions and recommendations for clinical practice

In the sphere of medical and paramedical research, the value of the research may be measured by the extent to which it offers relevant and applicable recommendations for improving clinical practice in a particular area. This is clearly the case in the current study, since it culminates by advocating recommendations for improved clinical practice (chapter nine).

With respect to the writer's study, many participants were willing to commit themselves to the research in various ways, in the hope that, by doing so, others in their position might be helped. As a group, the participants demonstrated an acute sense of wishing to 'pay back' the health service for their earlier cleft-related treatment. Therefore, in terms of a risk/benefit analysis of the research, the participants were apparently prepared to countenance any potential risk in maximising the benefit of the study to others. Nevertheless, some interviewees expressed their appreciation of the opportunity to discuss their feelings about having a cleft, and clearly felt that they had personally benefited from the experience.

If the researcher wishes to advance clinical practice in some way, his/her research will have to withstand the rigorous scrutiny of the relevant clinicians. That is, when the day of accountability dawns, the researcher will be held responsible for the way in which he or she chose to conduct the investigation.

4 The developmental years

It is a capital mistake to theorize before one has data. (Conan Doyle)

Introduction

The nature of the data bequeathed by Beryl Hammond (hereafter referred to as BNH), was outlined in chapter one. The way in which BNH's data have been analysed for the current study was detailed in chapter three (design of the study). This first set of data has been instrumental in determining the composition of the three later data sets, gathered by the writer. Only the data relating to those who completed and returned the postal questionnaire, is included in the first data set. This criterion reduces the number of participants from 501 (BNH's survey) to 217 in the present study.

Having analysed BNH's data, this chapter reports findings which relate to the participants' developmental years (0-18 years). In order to gain maximum insight, the data are discussed under separate sections. The subsequent section presents the classification of BNH's data. To enable comparison of these data with the three later data sets, the writer has converted the information into variables. Attention is then turned to the cross-tabulation of core variables endemic to the BNH data set. The following sections look at data elicited from the hospital records.

The classification of data collected by BNH - Results I

In their original form, the data gathered by BNH were arranged according to a list of assessments, and labelled 'items' (numbered 1-36). For ease of reference, the writer has grouped the 'items' according to the age and stage of the patients at assessment (Tables 4.1-4.6). In presenting the findings, the wording used by BNH in describing the assessments has been preserved as far as possible. In doing so, the reader will encounter instances when the terminology used by BNH seems out of vogue regarding present day usage. For example, Item 12 (Table 4.3) seeks to assess the patient's 'mental ability'. This term has now been superseded by other more acceptable descriptions, such as 'intellectual ability'. Moreover, amongst the response options for this assessment, BNH includes the category 'mentally handicapped', a label which is currently denounced by those acquainted with this population.

In similar vein, the writer takes this opportunity to highlight the implications of citing research undertaken over two decades ago. In the course of referring to BNH's work, it is apparent that the language used by BNH in describing her findings, may be considered authoritarian in current day parlance. For instance, in categorizing parental attitude towards the cleft-impaired child, she distinguishes between a 'detrimental' influence and that which suggests parental encouragement and 'co-operation'. Whilst such terms may have been acceptable at the time, their usage now conveys undesirably judgemental nuances. For this reason, the writer wishes to acknowledge that the style of language used by BNH does not necessarily reflect her own.

Regarding BNH's 'items', whilst the number allocated to each one remains unaltered, it has been necessary to rearrange their original sequence in order to present them according to a developmental paradigm. Thus, in view of the subject-matter, the final four items (numbered 33-36 by BNH), have been incorporated into the initial 'personal details' section below (Table 4.1).

Table 4.1
Personal details (applicable from infancy)

Item	Assessment made by BNH and colleagues
1.	Survey series I - primary palatal closure at Odstock prior to 30 months old
2.	Sex of patient
3.	Year of birth of patient
4.	Speech Therapy Department reference number
5.	Plastic Surgery Unit reference number
6.	Extent of cleft
33.	Personal aspects considered to be relevant
34.	Other factors of possible significance - further surgery offered but refused
35.	Other factors of possible significance - patient not seen at this Centre for a period in excess of two years, but received treatment elsewhere
36.	Other factors of possible significance - patient not seen at this centre for a period in excess of two years, and no treatment given elsewhere during this time

Table 4.2
Assessments pertaining to the soft palate

Item   Assessment made by BNH and colleagues

7. Age in months of primary closure of the soft palate
8. Operative procedure of primary closure of the soft palate
9. Early surgical complications relating to primary closure of the soft palate

Table 4.3
Assessments pertaining to the period between primary closure of the soft palate and School Age Assessment (SAA)

Item   Assessment made by BNH and colleagues

10. General physical condition
11. Environmental aspect
12. Mental (intellectual) ability
13. Further surgery between primary closure of the soft palate and SAA

Table 4.4
Assessments pertaining to School Age (SAA) (4.5-5.5 years old)

Item   Assessment made by BNH and colleagues

14. Speech at SAA as agreed by surgeon and speech therapist
15. Condition of soft palate noted by surgeon at SAA
16. Hard palate at SAA
17. Skeletal and dental aspect at SAA
18. Lip and/or nose at SAA
19. Hearing at SAA
20. Some indication of the extent of speech therapy given both pre- and post-SAA

Table 4.5
Assessments pertaining to the period between
School Age Assessment (SAA) and Latest Speech Assessment (LSA)

Item	Assessment made by BNH and colleagues
21.	Surgery to achieve adequate palato-pharyngeal closure given between SAA and LSA
22.	Surgery to correct hard palate fistula given between SAA and LSA
23.	Procedures to correct skeletal and dental abnormalities given between SAA and LSA
24.	Plastic surgery to lip and/or nose between SAA and LSA
	Treatment by otolarygologist between SAA and LSA
25.	Treatment by otolarygologist between SAA and LSA

Table 4.6
Assessments pertaining to Latest Speech Assessment (LSA)
(5-26 years old)

Item	Assessment made by BNH and colleagues
26.	Age and speech at LSA
27.	Assessment of soft palate at LSA
28.	Condition of hard palate at LSA
29.	Skeletal and dental aspect at LSA
30.	Cosmetic and/or functional aspect of lip and nose at LSA
31.	Hearing at LSA
32.	Dispersal following LSA

The analysis of data collected by BNH

The opportunity now arises to extract specific variables within BNH's data set, which warrant further attention. Certain variables (in the form of assessments) have been isolated by the researcher as having particular relevance to the psychosocial impact of being born with a cleft.

At this point, the variables which have been identified for extended study, will be cross-tabulated with only those data pertaining to the BNH data set. Where variables from this first data set have been cross-referenced with variables from the second (hospital records), and third (postal questionnaire) data sets, the results will be reported in chapter six. Since the individuals involved in BNH's research were still receiving hospital treatment, they are referred to as 'patients' rather than 'participants', which is the more apt description following their hospital discharge as used in later chapters.

The process of identifying the most pertinent variables to pursue, is an exacting task requiring not only self-discipline, but also a realistic perception of both the limits and the potential of the findings. This becomes especially apparent in the realization that an exhaustive presentation of cross-tabulations is not feasible, and that careful selection must therefore be made.

With respect to the first data set, the core variables are incorporated under two separate headings according to their subject-matter. The purpose of this categorization is to clarify and to highlight the main 'themes' or considerations, which emerge from the findings. As such, the themes form the germinal material upon which the discussion (chapter eight), and the recommendations (chapter nine) of the study are based. As will become evident in the course of the study, comparatively greater attention is given to data alluding to the participants' psychosocial functioning, than to aspects of their cleft-related treatment. The two considerations to be addressed in this section are outlined below, prior to addressing each one of them in conjunction with the relevant data.

- Factors influencing the patients' early psychosocial development.

- Manifestations of the cleft at different stages of the patients' psychosocial development (potentially audible and/or visible defects).

Factors influencing the patients' early psychosocial development

Predisposing factors In research methodology, the variables of sex and age are essential in explaining trends evidenced by human subjects. Their importance lies in their status as predisposing factors (apparent from birth), and therefore, not determined by confounding environmental influences. Congenital cleft lip and/or palate also fulfils this criterion, and is cross-tabulated with the variables of sex and age (Tables 4.7.-4.9).

Table 4.7
Sex and age (year of birth) of participants

Year of birth	Sex of participants		
	Male	Female	Total
Before/in 1950	1	2	3
1951-1955	17	18	35
1956-1960	24	20	44
1961-1965	31	29	60
1966-1970	43	32	75
Total	116	101	217

Table 4.8
Extent of cleft and sex of participants

Extent of Cleft	Sex of Respondents		
	Male	Female	Total
Soft palate only	15	21	36
Soft and hard palate only	21	29	50
Incomplete cleft lip and palate	11	7	18
Complete unilateral cleft lip and palate	53	35	88
Complete bilateral cleftlip and palate	16	9	25
Total	116	101	217

In undertaking the cross-tabulations, it is notable that no significant relationships emerge between the three factors. Therefore, it can be deduced that the extent of clefting presented by the individual, is not statistically related to gender nor to age, and that there is no significant correlation between sex and age on this occasion.

Table 4.9
Extent of cleft and age of participants (year of birth)

Extent of cleft	Year of birth					
	Before / 1950	1951-1955	1956-1960	1961-1965	1966-1970	Total
Soft palate only	1	3	4	13	15	36
Soft and hard palate only	0	5	9	16	20	50
Incomplete cleft lip and palate	0	2	5	6	5	18
Complete unilateral cleft lip and palate	0	20	18	21	29	88
Complete bilateral cleft lip and palate	2	5	8	4	6	25
Total	3	35	44	60	75	217

Although BNH and her colleagues assessed the 'extent' of each individual's cleft, further insight can be obtained by tabulating the data according to the visibility of the defect. For the purpose of this study, this dimension of the cleft will be referred to as the 'type' as distinct from the 'extent' of the defect. It transpires that those with soft palate or soft and hard palate only, have a comparatively 'non-visible' defect, compared with those who are born with an additional and visible cleft lip.

Table 4.10
Type of cleft according to visibility of defect

Type of cleft according to visibility of defect	n	%
'Non-visible' cleft palate		
(soft or soft and hard palate only without additional cleft lip)	86	39.6
'Visible' cleft lip and palate		
(all forms of cleft palate with additional cleft lip)	131	60.4
Total	217	100.0

It will become increasingly apparent in examining the findings, that the visibility of the deformity has significant implications, regarding how the cleft is perceived by both the patient and other people. As Table 4.10 above shows, these implications potentially apply to 60.4% (n=131) of the participants presenting with some degree of visible impairment.

Association between predisposing factors and influences upon the participants' psychosocial development In view of the need to focus upon core variables in this section, attention has been given to identifying data specifically pertaining to the patients' psychosocial development. In doing so, the adherence of BNH's data to the medical model becomes increasingly apparent. To appreciate this partiality, one needs only to study the range of assessments, which allude to the various medical and paramedical aspects of cleft-related treatment, with comparatively little reference made to psychosocial concerns. Consequently, only a small proportion of relevant data is available at this juncture.

The two core variables which especially reflect influences upon the individuals' psychosocial development, are the patients' environmental and personal aspects (Items 11 and 33 respectively). The former refers to the nature of his/her home background, as tempered by the parents, whilst the latter incorporates information relating to the way in which the individual was assessed as coping with the cleft. Each of the aspects will be now examined further, in the light of cross-tabulation with other data, with particular attention being paid to instances of potential disadvantage and detrimental influences.

Given the relevance of the item 'personal aspect' to the concerns of the present study, it is regrettable that data is absent for 23.5% (n=51) of the participants involved. Although BNH stipulates that on this occasion no data can be equated with no adjustment problems, such a presumption is viewed with some caution by the writer in implicating facts which cannot be substantiated. Thus, it should be noted that for the purposes of statistical analysis, the instances of no data have been omitted in all subsequent references to personal aspect in this section.

With respect to data relating to the patients' gender and personal adjustment to the cleft, it appears that difficulties were encountered by more males (n=34, 29.3% of males) than females (n=24, 23.8% of females). Closer scrutiny, however, suggests that major problems were apparent in the same number of males as females (n=6, 5.2% and 5.9% respectively).

The seemingly more problematic life experiences of males compared with females, is reinforced by the relationship between home environment and gender. In this instance, 17.2% (n=20) of the male population and 13.9% (n=14) of the female population, were identified as living in 'detrimental' circumstances. Although these relationships are not statistically significant, the extent to which the apparent gender difference persists into adulthood, will become evident in subsequent analysis of the data.

Insight into the characteristics of those experiencing personal cleft-related problems, is enhanced by considering the association between personal aspect and the type of cleft with which the individuals were born, according to the visibility of the impairment (Table 4.11). In doing so, there is a statistically significant relationship ($p < 0.05$) between the visibility of the cleft, and the patients' adjustment to the defect. That is, whilst a total of 50% (n=24) of those with non-visible disfigurement were assessed as displaying some or major adjustment problems, only 28.8% (n=34) with visible defects fell into this category. By implication and contrary to expectation, it would seem at this stage, that visible clefting does not necessarily infer greater personal difficulties than non-visible clefting.

Table 4.11
Personal aspect and type of cleft according to visibility of the defect

Personal aspect	Type of cleft		
	Non-visible (cleft palate)	Visible (cleft lip & palate)	Total
Good, co-operative patient	24	84	108
Some difficulties in adjusting to defect	19	27	46
Major problems manifested by patient / major detrimental environmental situations	5	7	12
Total	48	118	166

NB: $p < 0.05$

A different picture emerges, however, when the individuals' home environment is contemplated alongside type of cleft, as evidenced by Table 4.12 below.

88

Table 4.12
Environmental aspect and type of cleft according to
visibility of the defect

Environmental aspect	Type of cleft		
	Non-visible (cleft palate)	Visible (cleft lip & palate)	Total
Satisfactory	78	105	183
Detrimental	8	26	34
Total	86	131	217

With respect to those incorporated into the 'detrimental' category, it appears that most of the patients concerned (n=26, 76.5%) presented with visible clefting, implicating cleft lip and palate. However, it transpires that the majority of those with 'satisfactory' parents (n=105, 57.4%) also have a visible cleft. The implications of this statistically non-significant finding will be more fully addressed in relation to other data in due course. Suffice it to say at this point, that the extent to which the visibility of the deformity actually affects the environment in which the patient is raised, is a matter of speculation. For example, it could be argued that a visible anomaly may exert an adverse effect upon the individuals' parents (or caregivers), if the latter perceive it to be a constant reminder of their failure to produce the proverbial 'perfect' child. The type of cleft may be seen to influence parent-child interaction.

A clearer understanding of the disadvantaged circumstances affecting some patients' psychosocial development, is gained when information relating to personal and environmental aspects is considered (Table 4.13).

Table 4.13
Personal aspect and environmental aspect

Personal aspect	Environmental Aspect		
	Satisfactory	Detrimental	Total
Good, co-operative patient	98	10	108
Some difficulties in adjusting to defect	31	15	46
Major problems manifested by patient / major detrimental environmental situations	6	6	12
Total	135	31	166

NB: p < 0.01

In studying the correlation between personal and environmental aspects, the findings tend to support predictions. That is, the majority of 'co-operative', well-adjusted patients were raised in a 'satisfactory' home environment (n=98, 72.6% of the 'satisfactory' group). At the same time, however, the preponderance of individuals raised in what is described by BNH as a 'detrimental' home environment, presented with some form of maladjustment to the cleft deformity (n=21, 67.7% of the 'detrimental' group). These associations are statistically significant at the 1% level.

In profiling the characteristics associated with the two core factors relating to personal and environmental aspects, mention must be made of a cluster of variables which impinge upon the psychosocial development of the patients. The first of these, which concerns intellectual ability serves to reinforce the as yet predictable pattern of results (Table 4.14).

As Table 4.14 below suggests, patients who were deemed to be of average or above intelligence were generally 'co-operative' and well-adjusted (n=101, 75.4% of the 'above average or average' intelligence group). In contrast, the majority of those exhibiting below average intelligence or with special educational needs, experienced some form of personal difficulty (n=25, 78.1% of the 'below average or special needs' group). A significance level of 1% is reached in cross-tabulating these data. Thus, it would seem that an association exists between intellectual ability and personal adjustment to the cleft.

Table 4.14
Personal aspect and mental (intellectual) ability

Personal aspect	Mental (intellectual) ability		
	Above average / average	Below average / special needs	Total
Good, co-operative patient	101	7	108
Some difficulties in adjusting to defect	26	20	46
Major problems manifested by patient / major detrimental environmental situations	7	5	12
Total	134	32	166

NB: p < 0.01

Table 4.15
Environmental aspect and mental (intellectual) ability

Environmental aspect	Mental (intellectual) ability		
	Above average / average	Below average / special needs	Total
Satisfactory	163	20	183
Detrimental	15	19	34
Total	178	39	217

NB: p < 0.01

In similar vein and as anticipated, a statistically significant relationship at the 1% level exists between environmental aspect and intellectual ability (Table 4.15). For example, the vast majority of children who were raised in a 'satisfactory' home environment, were of average or above average intelligence (n=163, 89.1% of the 'satisfactory' environment group), whilst over one half of those having a disadvantageous home background, exhibited below average intelligence or special educational needs (n=19, 55.9% of the 'detrimental' environment group). Table 4.15 above indicates the cross-tabulation of these data. These findings suggest a close correspondence between the climate of the home and the youngster's intellectual functioning.

With reference to other pertinent variables in the BNH data set, those relating to the patients' general physical condition, age at primary palatal surgery and dispersal following Latest Speech Assessment (LSA) were identified by the writer as being of potential interest to this section. However, on closer analysis they yielded no notable relationships in conjunction with the predisposing factors of age, sex and type of cleft, and the two core variables of personal and environmental aspects.

Thus, in view of the findings concerning the factors influencing the patients' early psychosocial development, a predictable and unremarkable picture emerges. One could speculate at this preliminary stage, that it is precisely the realization of predictions which will enable identification of an 'at risk' group amongst the cleft-impaired. This fundamental issue will be addressed in due course.

Manifestations of the cleft defect at different stages of the patients' psychosocial development (potentially audible and/or visible impairments)

Having identified potent predisposing and personal influences upon the individuals' psychosocial development, consideration can be given now to the way in which the type of cleft is presented to the 'outside' world. That is, in the case of the non-visible cleft palate, the primary evidence of its existence is impaired speech. Therefore, the outward manifestation of cleft palate only is potentially an audible defect. It should be noted, however, that the palatal defect can, in some instances, effect visible nasal grimacing. This cleft-related feature occurs where the person uses facial tension to restrict the anomalous nasal airflow. It is unfortunate that BNH does not refer to such occurrences in her data.

With respect to cleft lip, the deformity is evidenced by a visible defect. In the present study, all of the patients with cleft lip have additional cleft palate, implicating that conceivably, this group of individuals have both audible and visible symptoms of clefting.

Whilst it is the anatomical malformation of the physical features caused by the cleft, which determines the defects (and hence the diagnosis of type of cleft), the extent to which speech and/or appearance are impaired, is largely a matter of subjective, perceptual judgement. Thus, in isolating the core variables which reflect the presence of audible and/or visible defects, attention is turned to the perceptual assessments made by BNH and her colleagues of the patients' speech and appearance.

Manifestations of cleft palate affecting the patients' speech It was established earlier in this chapter, that assessment of speech specifically that of nasality and articulation, was undertaken at two different stages, namely School Age Assessment (hereafter referred to as SAA), and Latest Speech Assessment (hereafter referred to as LSA). In elucidating further upon those whose speech was impaired, and the implications of the impairment upon the psychosocial development of the individuals concerned, almost exclusive attention is given in this section to instances where the nasality (speech quality) and/or articulation (speech sounds) were deemed by BNH and her colleagues to be grossly defective (designated 'unsatisfactory'). The rationale for this is that the speech of those comprising the 'unsatisfactory' categories in each case, would be universally perceived as bearing some form of speech impediment, whilst the listeners' perceptions of individuals represented in the alternative response categories (indicating no or slight impairment) can be less easily predicted.

The variables pertaining to the assessments have been cross-tabulated with the predisposing factors of sex, age and type of cleft. Reference will be made subsequently to the most notable of the findings, with respect to the objectives of the current follow-up study.

The data indicate that at SAA, when the patients were aged between 54 and 64 months, 'unacceptable' nasality (n=30) was more evident in girls (n=17, 56.7%) than in boys (n=13, 43.3%). Moreover, at the later stage of assessment (LSA), although the overall number of those displaying 'unacceptable' nasality had reduced (n=21), the majority was still female (n=13, 61.9%; males, n=8, 38.1%).

It is notable that when the proportion of individuals exhibiting 'unacceptable' articulation at SAA (n=65) and LSA (n=33) is cross-tabulated with gender, more males than females were incorporated into this category on both occasions (n=38, 58.5% and n=22, 66.7% respectively).

Regarding the association between 'unacceptable' speech and type of cleft, with one exception 'unacceptable' nasality (SAA) and articulation (SAA and LSA) was most apparent in patients with a complete cleft of the lip and palate (unilateral or bilateral). That is, of those presenting with 'unacceptable' nasality at SAA, 56.7% (n=17) had a complete cleft. Similarly, regarding 'unacceptable' articulation at SAA and LSA, 67.7% (n=44) and 66.7% (n=22) respectively, of the patients were born with a complete cleft. The one exception to this tendency refers to nasality at LSA, when the preponderance of individuals displaying 'unacceptable' nasality had a cleft of the soft and hard palate only (n=12, 57.2%). Needless to say, a complexity of different factors determine the relationship between perceived speech impairment and the extent of anatomical dysfunction, not least individual differences.

Concerning the affiliation between nasality and articulation at SAA and at LSA, interest is focused upon the persistence of each type of speech impairment over time. Consequently, comparisons are made between nasality at SAA and at LSA, and of articulation at SAA and at LSA.

Table 4.16
Nasality at SAA and nasality at LSA

Nasality at LSA	Nasality at SAA		
	None/slight nasality considered acceptable	Unaccep- table	Total
None/slight nasality considered acceptable	177	19	196
Unacceptable	10	11	21
Total	187	30	217

NB: $p < 0.01$

Table 4.16 shows the extent to which instances of 'unacceptable' nasality at SAA were still evident at LSA. It appears that over one half of the 'unacceptably' nasal speakers at LSA (n=11, 55.0%), had been assessed as such at their school-age evaluation (SAA). By implication, the majority of 'unacceptably' nasal speakers at LSA, had to contend with the stigma of having an obvious audible defect for most (if not all) of their school years.

Table 4.17
Articulation at SAA and articulation at LSA

Articulation at LSA   Articulation at SAA

	Normal / slight defect within acceptable limit	Unacceptably defective	Total
Normal / slight defect within acceptable limit	142	42	184
Unacceptably defective	10	23	33
Total	152	65	217

NB: p < 0.01

According to Table 4.17 above, 69.7% (n=23) of patients with 'unacceptable' articulation at LSA, had presented with 'unacceptable' articulation at SAA. In interpreting this particular finding, one must remember that a speech impairment of this severity threatens not only effective communication, but also the perception of the speaker as a 'successful' communicator. Therefore, similar to 'unacceptable' nasality, where 'unacceptable' articulation is not assuaged by LSA, the quality of the individuals' everyday personal and social interactions (especially with peers), may have been tarnished by the effects of impaired speech. Whether or not these audible defects were tolerated by the perceivers, was a cause of considerable anxiety to some patients with hindsight.

As anticipated, data analysis relating to nasality and articulation at SAA and LSA, show that patients with 'unacceptable' nasality and/or articulation, were given priority and access to regular periods of speech therapy intervention, over the less severe speech impairments. However, the association between these variables is not statistically significant.

Manifestations of cleft lip affecting the patients' appearance In similar vein to the assessment of speech, aspects of the patients' appearance were also appraised at SAA and LSA by BNH and her colleagues.

The two concerns related to the appearance and/or function of the lip and/or nose, and of the skeletal and dental aspect. Whilst the obvious visibility of the lip and nose is self-evident, the less visible skeletal structure of the maxillary arch and dentition can also affect the individuals' facial appearance.

As with gross speech impairment, the data relating to 'unsatisfactory' appearance at SAA and LSA compel further interpretation. Regarding the relationships between appearance and the three predisposing factors of sex, age and type of cleft, reference is made to the first of these only, as the patients' age is inconsequential on this occasion, and considerations of appearance are generally not applicable to those with cleft palate only.

With reference to the patients whose lip and/or nose was judged to be 'unsatisfactory' at SAA (n=97) and LSA (n=40), there was a preponderance of males (n=57, 58.8% and n=25, 62.5% respectively). A comparable result was found regarding the assessment of skeletal and dental aspect at SAA (n=146) with 86 males (58.9%), although there is no corresponding category designating 'unsatisfactory' progress of skeletal and dental aspect at LSA.

Table 4.18
Lip and/or nose at SAA and lip and/or nose at LSA

Lip and/or nose at LSA	Lip and/or nose at SAA			
	Satis-factory	Unsatis-factory	Awaiting report	Total
Good, or at least adequate	33	56	1	90
Unsatisfactory	0	40	0	40
Awaiting report	0	1	0	1
Total	33	97	1	131

The extent to which the appearance and/or function of the patients' lip and/or nose remained 'unsatisfactory', can be seen by comparing the data pertaining to assessment of these features at SAA and at LSA in Table 4.18. In instances where these assessments were not applicable to patients with cleft palate only (n=86), the data have been omitted.

With respect to the proportion of patients whose lip and/or nose were assessed as 'unsatisfactory' at LSA, 100.0% (n=40) of individuals were considered to have also been 'unsatisfactory' at SAA. The implication of this result is similar to that expounded in relation to impaired speech above, in that the persistence of the disfigurement demands endurance on the part of the patients concerned. The extent to which this endurance challenges or facilitates the development of coping skills, is a matter of fundamental significance to the outcome of the present study, and will be discussed again in due course.

In view of the large proportion of individuals (n=93) who were assessed as either awaiting the optimal time for treatment, or awaiting a progress report, it is regrettable that a direct comparison cannot be made between data relating to the assessment of skeletal and dental aspect at SAA and at LSA. In broad terms, it could be argued that if the skeletal and dental aspect of patients was considered to have been 'satisfactory', the latter would not require active intervention at all. Although speculative, one implication of this reasoning is that for 60.3% (n=88) of those assessed as 'unsatisfactory' at SAA, treatment was still indicated at LSA.

As discussed on an earlier occasion, skeletal and dental intervention is not usually commenced until the patient's natural physical growth has reached a particular stage. Therefore, although the need for treatment implicates the possibility of some degree of visible defect, one should not be surprised by the relatively high proportion of participants awaiting treatment for skeletal and/or dental anomalies. Where these assessments were not applicable to patients due to the extent of clefting (n=61), reference to them has been omitted from the table below.

Table 4.19
Skeletal and dental aspect at SAA
and skeletal and dental aspect at LSA

Skeletal and dental aspect at LSA	Skeletal and dental aspect at SAA		
	Satis-factory	Unsatis-factory	Total
Satisfactory	8	43	51
Wearing denture	0	12	12
Awaiting optimal time to begin treatment	2	88	90
Awaiting report	0	3	3
Total	10	146	156

In view of the need to substantiate the findings of this section with other data, discussion regarding their implications for the patients' psychosocial development and functioning, is preserved for the comparison of data in subsequent chapters. Particular emphasis will then be given to examining the extent to which aspects of personal and environmental disadvantage, are associated with impaired speech and/or appearance. Closely allied to these considerations, is the question as to whether advantageous circumstances actually equip the individual with a psychological 'survival' kit for dealing with cleft-related problems.

Examination of hospital records - Results II

The elicitation of data from the Odstock Hospital records relating to the 217 participants in the study, marks the stage at which the two researchers (namely, BNH and the writer) 'overlap'. That is, whilst BNH gathered information relating to the patients' pre-school years, childhood and adolescence (in some instances), the current researcher has supplemented these data by referring to hospital documentation. Accordingly, the data provide a framework against which the later psychosocial functioning of the participants can be appraised.

Source of information

Since the researcher had access to two independent sources of data held at

Odstock Hospital (plastic surgery and speech therapy), it is necessary to identify the extent to which each of the sources was tapped. That is, although at the time of treatment, the treatment of each patient with a cleft was noted in both speech therapy and plastic surgery records, there was no guarantee that both sets of documents would be available for the purposes of the current data collection.

In searching for the information, both speech therapy and plastic surgery records were found for 85.3% (n=185) of the 217 participants in the study. However, for the remainder of the group, only one set of the documents was located, comprising 12.9% (n=28) speech therapy records, and 1.8% (n=4) plastic surgery records. Further attempts were made to discover the whereabouts of these notes, using the hospital computer data base. With respect to the twenty-eight sets of untraced plastic surgery records, it transpired that in six instances the documents had been transferred onto microfilm. The records of a further ten individuals were classified as 'current', whilst the remainder had been apparently archived. Regarding the four sets of untraced speech therapy notes, the patients concerned had been discharged from treatment. Regrettably, the continued efforts on the part of the researcher, to procure the required data proved to be abortive.

In the instances of access to only one set of records, the reader is reminded that it is the policy to incorporate the speech therapist's comments onto the plastic surgery notes and vice versa. Therefore, although both documents were not located in 14.7% (n=32) of cases, the information held in the available records is expected to be largely duplicated in the absent set of notes.

The sex and age of the patients

As anticipated, details of the patients' gender and age in the hospital records, correlate exactly with those cited by BNH in her survey of the same individuals. In view of this, the reader is referred to Table 4.7 (sex and age (year of birth) of participants).

Home area

At the time of the study, the Wessex regional plastic surgery unit was based at Odstock Hospital in Salisbury. Other hospital clinics situated within the Wessex region were termed peripheral sites, since they were served by the regional unit for the management of the cleft population. The reader is reminded that Odstock Hospital has now been replaced by Salisbury District Hospital, and the Wessex Centre by the Odstock Centre for Burns, Plastic and Maxillo-Facial Surgery. The unit is still run on a regional basis. As in BNH's time, with the exception of patients living in and around Salisbury, the Cleft Palate Team visits the peripheral hospitals and clinics on a regular basis to conduct review/follow-up clinics. Where surgery or intensive speech therapy is indicated, the patient is generally invited to the former Odstock Hospital.

The analysis of hospital records data

This section is concerned with the cross-tabulation of core variables within the second data set relating to the hospital records (Results II). The cross-tabulation of variables across the three quantitative data sets (Results I-III), is preserved for chapter six.

The primary objective of consulting the participants' hospital records, has been to glean further details concerning the individuals' psychosocial histories. As expected, the heavy emphasis placed upon the medical aspects of cleft-related treatment, is reflected by the comparatively little reference made to the patients' psychosocial development and functioning. Therefore, with respect to extracting pertinent variables for further scrutiny, the amount of information available is notably limited. The core variables which have been selected will be subsequently discussed under the following subheadings.

• Parental and family influences upon the patients' psychosocial development and cleft-related treatment.

• Indicators of the patients' psychosocial functioning at various stages of development.

Parental and family influences upon the patients' psychosocial development and cleft-related treatment

Since details of sex, age and type of cleft are the only variables to be defined from birth, they beg further investigation in association with the data collected from the hospital records. However, in cross-tabulating these particulars with variables relating to the patients' psychosocial development and cleft-related treatment, a similar picture emerges to that reported earlier in this chapter. That is, type of cleft appears to exert more influence in relation to the variables than does either the patients' sex or age. In view of the data analysis, no further mention will be made of the respondents' age in this chapter.

Within the developmental paradigm, the first environmental influences to affect the individual are those to which he/she is exposed at home. It is for this reason, that consideration is given to the way in which these influences may not only shape the patients' psychosocial development from birth, but also the course of his/her cleft-related treatment. Although evidence to substantiate these claims is relatively scarce with respect to the details available in the hospital records, two core variables have been pin-pointed which can at least initiate discussion of the significance of the home environment to the cleft-impaired.

The first of the key variables concerns the patient's family environment. In cross-tabulating the data with gender, it appears that 44.0% (n=51) of male patients, and 41.6% (n=42) of female patients were raised in 'unfavourable' circumstances. The close correspondence between the proportion of the two sexes is notable, as is the observation that almost one half of the participants in the study fall into the category of 'unfavourable' home environment.

Further insight can be gained into the characteristics of the disadvantaged patients, by considering the relationship between home environment and type of cleft according to the visibility of the defect in Table 4.20 below. In examining the degree to which the patients' domestic circumstances and type of cleft are associated, it is unfortunate that the relevant details are available for a reduced number of individuals (n=135). The reason for this is attributable to the relatively large number of hospital records which made no reference to the disposition of parents and family (n=80). A further omission related to two individuals with cleft lip and palate, whose home situations were identified by the writer as having both 'favourable' and 'unfavourable' aspects.

Table 4.20
Family environment and type of cleft
according to visibility of the defect

Type of cleft	Family environment		
	Favourable	Unfavourable	Total
Non-visible (cleft of the palate only)	18	26	44
Visible (cleft of the lip and palate)	35	56	91
Total	53	82	135

Although the correlation between the variables presented in Table 4.20 is statistically non-significant, of those who were raised in an 'unfavourable' home environment (n=82), there were comparably more patients with a visible defect (n=56, 68.3% with cleft lip and palate), than with a non-visible cleft (n=26, 31.7% with cleft palate only). At this stage, it is difficult to speculate upon the extent to which the visibility of the cleft actually affects the dynamics of the home, since further data is required for its substantiation. This will be given in subsequent chapters.

The second core variable comprising the patients' attendance at hospital clinics, is of fundamental importance in reflecting parental attitudes towards both the patient and his/her treatment. In many respects, attendance at the necessary clinics is equated by the Cleft Palate Team with commitment to the intervention, whilst non-attendance infers indifference to treatment aims. Having said this, one is aware that there may be diverse reasons for non-attendance. In view of this, the focus of concern rests upon the extent to which non-attendance is explained by the patient or his/her parents.

In considering the possible contributory factors, data relating to non-attendance at out-patient clinics have been cross-tabulated with those of family environment, as evidenced by Table 4.21. With respect to the individuals whose family environment was deemed to be 'unfavourable', 80.2% (n=73) of them proffered no, or only partial explanation for non-attendance at hospital appointments with the Cleft Palate Team. This majority compares with 59.1% (n=26) of patients incorporated into the 'favourable' group, who were inclined to give intermittent or no explanation. Data analysis shows a statistically significant relationship (at the 5% level), between an 'unfavourable' home environment and non-attendance at the requisite hospital clinics.

The implications of this association are far-reaching. Whilst non-attendance may be due to forgetfulness, inconvenience, fear of hospitals and/or the professionals and so forth, one could argue that some explanation is still warranted. Moreover, the decision as to whether or not the appointments are attended, tends to rest with the parents in the early years of treatment. In this way, the chosen course of action may be interpreted by the Cleft Palate Team as reflecting the parents' attitude towards cleft-related treatment. That is, where intervention is perceived as a priority area, non-attendance (where unavoidable) will be at least explained. On the contrary, if regarded with indifference, lack of explanation for non-attendance may indicate the low priority given not only to treatment, but also to the needs of the patient.

Table 4.21
Family environment and explanation by the patient
(or the patient's parents) relating to non-attendance at clinics

Explanation for non-attendance	Family environment		
	Favou-rable	Unfavou-rable	Total
No non-attendance / all non-attendance accounted for	18	18	36
Combination of explanation & no explanation given for non-attendance	19	55	74
No explanation given for non-attendance	7	18	25
Total	44	91	135

NB: p < 0.05

Attention is turned now to elucidating the sex and type of defect associated with those whose treatment was interrupted by non-attendance at hospital clinics. In doing so, no statistically significant correlations emerge. Indeed, there appear to be negligible differences between the proportion of males (n=83, 71.6% of males) and females (n=76, 75.2% of females), whose non-attendance as out-patients was either sporadic or not accounted for.

Further data analysis suggests that visibly-impaired individuals (n=102, 77.9% with cleft lip and palate), were more likely to afford no or partial explanation for non-attendance at hospital, compared with those with non-visible clefts (n=57, 66.3% with cleft palate only).

The core variables delineated above, will be now discussed in relation to the patients' psychosocial functioning at different stages of development.

Indicators of the patients' psychosocial functioning at various stages of development

Further insight into the potential influence of the family environment upon the patients' psychosocial functioning, can be derived from considering the association between family environment and functioning at different stages of development. It is regrettable that limited details are available in the hospital records. Where no reference is made to a particular stage of psychosocial functioning, or a combination of no evidence with potential for psychosocial problems, the total number of responses has been adjusted to represent elicited data, as indicated in the following tables. Particular attention is subsequently paid to instances of an 'unfavourable' family environment coupled with the potential for psychosocial problems.

Table 4.22 below shows that the majority of patients having an 'unfavourable' home environment also had potential for psychosocial problems (n=32, 65.3% of the 'unfavourable' group). Similarly, most of those with potential problems had an 'unfavourable' home background (n=32, 78.0%). At the same time, 'favourable' family circumstances are most apparent where there is no evidence of psychosocial problems (n=11, 55.0% of the 'favourable' group). However, an 'unfavourable' home environment cannot be directly equated with potential psychosocial difficulties, since Table 4.22 shows that the majority of those evidencing no problems were associated with an 'unfavourable' home background (n=17, 60.7% of the 'no evidence' group).

Table 4.22
Family environment and pre-school years (0-about 5 years old)

Pre-school years	Family environment		
	Favourable	Unfavourable	Total
No evidence of psychosocial problems	11	17	28
Potential for psychosocial problems (adverse circumstances / experiences)	9	32	41
Total	20	49	69

It should be stressed that problems displayed may be developmental in nature, and therefore reflect a transient phase in the patients' lives. In view of this possibility, attention is turned to the detection of difficulties during the later pre-teenage years for evidence of persistent problems.

Before doing so, however, mention is made of the relationship between type of cleft and the potential for psychosocial problems at this stage. It transpires that over half of the potential problems group has a non-visible cleft of the palate (n=28, 56.0% of the potential problem group). This correlation reaches the 5% level of statistical significance. Thus, during the pre-school years there does not seem to be a marked association between the visibility of the cleft and psychosocial difficulties.

Concerning the individuals whose home situation was observed to be 'unfavourable', Table 4.23 below shows that a comparatively high percentage of them displayed the potential for psychosocial problems (n=48, 81.4% of the 'unfavourable' group). This figure compares with 56.0% (n=14) of the 'favourable' category who evidenced potential problems, and 50.0% (n=11) of the 'no evidence' group with an 'unfavourable' home background. The correlation reaches statistical significance at the 5% level. The implications of this finding will be discussed at a later stage, as the data suggest that patients may be especially at risk for developmental dysfunction during their pre-teenage years.

Table 4.23
Family environment and pre-teenage years (5-12 years old)

Pre-teenage years	Family environment		
NB: $p < 0.05$	Favourable	Unfavourable	Total
No evidence of psychosocial problems	11	11	22
Potential for psychosocial problems (adverse circumstances / experiences)	14	48	62
Total	25	59	84

When the data relating to potential psychosocial problems is cross-tabulated with type of cleft, it transpires that, unlike the previous stage of development slightly more patients presenting with problems had a visible defect (cleft lip and palate; n=51, 62.2% of those with problems). This finding needs to be borne in mind in considering supplementary data relating to the patients' childhood experiences, especially socialization with peers.

The quantity of data available which pertains to family environment and adolescence is notably scarce (n=37). Whilst one could propose that this factor reflects the absence of adverse circumstances and professional causes for concern, it could be equally argued that specific mention is made of propitious development.

Despite the paucity of data presented in Table 4.24, the tendency remains for potential psychosocial problems to be associated with an 'unfavourable' environment. That is, the majority of patients showing potential problems had a disadvantaged home environment (n=20, 76.9% of the problem group). Similarly, 69.0% (n=20) of the 'unfavourable' category were considered to be susceptible to psychosocial problems. However, as suggested earlier, these two factors cannot be directly equated since it transpires that 81.8% of the 'no evidence' group (n=9), were raised in 'unfavourable' conditions. The implications of these findings will be discussed in later chapters. Whilst not reaching statistical significance, it appears that the majority of teenagers with problematic circumstances had a visible cleft (n=27, 79.4% of the problem group). As with the previous findings, this tendency may be of fundamental import in understanding the personal experiences of those born with a cleft.

Table 4.24
Family environment and teenage years (13-17 years old)

Teenage years	Family environment		
	Favourable	Unfavourable	Total
No evidence of psychosocial problems	2	9	11
Potential for psychosocial problems (adverse circumstances / experiences)	6	20	26
Total	8	29	37

Table 4.25
Family environment and adulthood: (18 years old and above)

Adulthood	Family environment		
	Favourable	Unfavourable	Total
No evidence of psychosocial problems	3	2	5
Potential for psychosocial problems (adverse circumstances / experiences)	10	16	26
Total	13	18	31

It might be anticipated that by adulthood, the transient developmental phases which typify childhood and adolescence concede to more consistent patterns of psychosocial functioning. In view of this expectation, problems which persist into adulthood may be resistant to change. It is with this possibility in mind, that the close association between 'unfavourable' home circumstances and psychosocial problems is highlighted. Concerning the patients whose earlier family environment was identified as 'unfavourable', almost all of them were additionally considered to be prone to psychosocial dysfunction (n=16, 88.9% of the 'unfavourable group'). Likewise, the majority of the potential problem group (n=16, 61.5%) were incorporated into the 'unfavourable' category. The extent to which their adverse disposition is still apparent after discharge by the Cleft Palate Team, is investigated in the light of recent data elicited by postal questionnaire (chapter five).

Further analysis of the data shows that the most common form of clefting presented by those with psychosocial difficulties, again proves to be a visible cleft of the lip and palate (n=37, 86% of those with problems). Moreover, in comparing the proportion of those incorporated into the psychosocial dysfunction category at different developmental stages, with the exception of the initial pre-school phase (Tables 4.22-25), it is notable that there is a gradual increase over time, such that the association between problems and visibility of the cleft is most apparent in adulthood. The implications of this finding will be addressed alongside data gathered from the adult participants (chapter six).

In summary, there is evidence that the psychosocial development and functioning of the participants in the study, are influenced by the climate of the home environment (nurture), and the type of cleft with which they are born (nature). The extent to which potential problem areas are assuaged or persist over time, is a matter of fundamental consequence to the well-being of the individuals in adult life. The following chapter relates the present perceptions and disposition of the participants from an adult perspective.

5 The adult years

Introduction

The discussion of the third and fourth data sets, elicited by postal questionnaire and personal interviews (Results III and IV respectively), marks a significant departure from the perspective adopted in the first two data sets (BNH and hospital records). The essence of the former data (Results I and II), is the accumulation of information relating to the nature and progress of the individuals' cleft-related hospital treatment. Whilst BNH has recorded the outcome of various assessments made by the Cleft Palate Team, the writer's examination of the participants' hospital records, has elicited supplementary details on their hospital management. Consequently, a comprehensive profile has been obtained of the treatment implications for each of the individuals, and their involvement with the Cleft Palate Team.

The objectives of the subsequent two data sets (Results III and IV), necessitate a fundamentally different approach to data collection, since they directly emanate from the (ex-)patients themselves. Unlike the preceding methods, the satisfactory execution of the postal questionnaire and the personal interviews, is largely dependent upon the willingness of those approached to participate in the investigation.

The following data analysis focuses upon cross-tabulating variables pertaining to the postal questionnaire. The reader's attention is drawn to chapter six for the cross-referencing of these data with the two previous data sets (BNH's data and the hospital records).

The presentation of postal questionnaire data - Results III

The sex and age of the respondents

The data relating to the respondents' sex and age, has been detailed already in chapter four (Table 4.7). On this occasion, the reader is reminded that the participants in the study comprised 116 males (53.5%), and 101 females (46.5%). With respect to the age range of the respondents on the 31st December 1991, most individuals were in their twenties (59.0%, n=128), 37.2% (n=81) were in their thirties, and the remaining 3.7% (n=8) of the sample were aged forty years or over.

The marital status of the respondents

It is notable that almost one half of the respondents (49.8%, n=108) were single at the time of questionnaire completion. This figure compares with 41.5% (n=90) of those who stated that they were married. A minority of 6.0% (n=13) of individuals identified their circumstances as 'other', with some explanation given. Into this category, the researcher placed those who were either engaged to be married, or were living with a partner. Common-law spouses were incorporated into the 'married' group. The residual 2.8% (n=6) of participants were divorced.

Children of the respondents

With respect to whether or not the respondents had produced children of their own, the majority of them (63.1%, n=137) were not parents. A smaller proportion of participants (36.9%, n=80) indicated that they did have children, but no further details were provided.

In examining these findings, the influence of hereditary factors should be borne in mind. That is, individuals born with a cleft who are aware of its familial associations, may be reluctant to have their own children if they believe that the cleft defect might recur in their offspring. Some of the respondents had already consulted a genetic counsellor regarding the probability of such an event. Others took the opportunity on receiving the postal questionnaire, to request information from the researcher concerning how to approach a genetic counsellor for advice on this matter. Whilst the idea of having a child with a cleft was clearly distressing to a small proportion of the participants, other respondents appeared to be more prepared to cope with such a possibility.

Family history of the cleft

Although cleft lip and/or palate is known to be inherited, the extent to which it recurs from one generation to another tends to vary. Concerning the data, 83.9% (n=182) of those asked indicated that, as far as they were aware they were the only members of their family to have the congenital deformity. A much smaller proportion (16.1%, n=35) of respondents stated that there was a history of cleft impairment in their family.

It transpires that 1.4% (n=3) of the respondents' parents also had a cleft. The implication of this is that when the patient was born with the defect, the parents would presumably be more familiar with the nature of clefts, compared with parents who had not experienced such an impairment themselves. It is imprudent to assume, however, that because of one parent's personal knowledge of having a cleft, that the birth of a child with a cleft would be any less traumatic for them.

With respect to siblings with a cleft, the data show that a total of 4.6% (n=10) of the participants had either a brother or a sister, who was born with a cleft. Unfortunately, the responses do not infer whether the siblings were older or younger than the patient. Similar to a parent having a cleft, if the affected sibling was older than the respondent, it is presumed that the parents would be already familiar with the possible implications of the congenital impairment when the patient was born. This would obviously not be the case if the sibling was younger than the patient concerned. In two further instances (0.9%), the respondents were parents of cleft-impaired children.

Age on leaving full-time education

Table 5.1
Age respondents left full-time education

Age left full-time education	n	%
15-16 years old	143	65.9
17-18 years old	40	18.5
19-20 years old	8	3.7
21-22 years old	12	5.5
23-24 years old	5	2.3
25-26 years old	1	0.5
27-28 years old	1	0.5
Returned to college	7	3.2
Total	217	100.1

In Table 5.1 above the reader's attention is drawn to the customs of the British education system. That is, the individuals who left full-time education at the age of 15 or 16 years, had either decided not to take 'Ordinary' level examinations (or the alternative options), or had only recently completed these examinations. Thus, according to the findings a predominance of 65.9% (n=143) respondents left full-time education at the earliest opportunity.

In contrast, those remaining in the education system until their late teenage years, may have either stayed on to re-take their 'Ordinary' level examinations (or the alternative options), or completed a further set of examinations, such as 'Advanced' level examinations. In addition, those with special learning difficulties tend to continue their education until aged nineteen years. Given that higher education courses (for example, undergraduate courses at University or the now superseded Polytechnic) do not tend to commence until the age of eighteen years, it appears that at least 18.5% (n=40) of the individuals involved left before pursuing higher education. Table 5.1 indicates that 12.5% (n=27) of the participants left full-time education between the ages of 19 and 28 years, whilst 3.2% (n=7) of individuals decided to return to full-time study, having left the education system at an earlier age.

Table 5.2
Type of employment according to socio-economic grouping

Type of employment according to socio-economic grouping	n	%
I - Professional	14	6.5
II - Intermediate occupations	28	12.9
III - Skilled non-manual occupations	30	13.8
III - Skilled manual occupations	31	14.3
I - Semi-skilled occupations	25	11.5
V - Unskilled manual occupations	6	2.8
Unclear (including self-employed)	32	14.7
Not applicable	48	22.1
No response	3	1.4
Total	217	100.0

Table 5.2 shows the classification of occupations according to socio-economic groups, as specified by the Office of Population Censuses and Surveys (HMSO, 1980). There is a preponderance of economically active employees working in socio-economic group III, denoting either non-manual (13.8%, n=30), or manual (14.3%, n=31) skilled occupations (a combined total of 28.1%, n=61). A further 11.5% (n=25) of respondents had semi-skilled occupations (socio-economic group IV). Unfortunately, the socio-economic status of the employment being undertaken by 14.7% (n=32) of the group, could not be classified from the responses given in the questionnaire. The participants (22.1%, n=48) who considered this question inapplicable, were economically inactive at the time.

Speech therapy intervention

It is noteworthy that whilst the speech and language progress of all the patients would have been monitored and assessed on a regular basis (in conjunction with the follow-up clinics), only 88.9% (n=193) of the respondents recognized that they had received speech therapy at some stage of their treatment.

Having said this, the total of 10.1% (n=22) of individuals who did not know (2.3%, n=5), or who claimed that they had not received any speech therapy (7.8%, n=17), may have been discharged early by the speech therapist, and are unable to remember the details of such intervention. Two individuals did not register any response (0.9%). Other possible interpretations of the findings are that the patients' parents may not have reinforced speech therapy aims at home, and the respondents are therefore unaware that the help they received was speech therapy.

Another plausible explanation for the relatively high percentage who were either unsure, or indicated that they did not receive speech therapy, is that these individuals may equate speech therapy with elocution lessons, rather than therapeutic treatment. Therefore, as in all questions, the responses elicited reflect a presumption on the part of the compiler, that the terms used in presenting the questions are unambiguous and universally understood by the respondent. Needless to say, in postal questionnaires such presumptions may necessarily have to go unchecked.

The participants who indicated that they had received speech therapy were predominantly pleased with the outcome. A total of 65.4% (n=142) of the group were 'satisfied'/'very satisfied' with their therapeutic treatment, with a further 10.6% (n=23) of the respondents reporting to be 'somewhat satisfied'. These figures compare favourably with the smaller proportion of individuals (8.7%, n=19), who indicated that they were 'dissatisfied/very dissatisfied' with speech therapy. The minority group who considered this item 'not applicable' (10.1%, n=22) to their situation, represent those who responded in the negative ('no'), or with uncertainty ('don't know') to the previous question concerning whether or not speech therapy had been undertaken.

When the participants' levels of satisfaction with current speech and appearance are cross-tabulated, a high degree of overall optimism exists (Table 5.3 below). For example, 78.3% (n=170) of the sample expressed some measure of satisfaction with both speech and appearance. This proportion compares favourably with the 3.7% (n=8) of individuals reporting some form of dissatisfaction with the two aspects concerned.

Although all of the patients underwent surgery at some stage, only a total of 85.7% (n=186) of the sample required orthodontic intervention. More respondents appear to be 'satisfied' or 'very satisfied' with their surgery (a total 75.5%, n=164), than with their orthodontic treatment (60.8%, n=132). Similarly, slightly more of the individuals were generally dissatisfied with their orthodontic management (a total of 8.8%, n=19), than were with their surgical results (4.6%, n=10). Nevertheless, 69.6% (n=151) of the sample expressed some degree of optimism about the outcome of both surgical and orthodontic treatment, whilst only 2.3% (n=5) of the group were pessimistic in this respect (Table 5.4 below).

Table 5.3
Current satisfaction with speech and appearance

Satisfaction with appearance

Satisfaction with speech

	Very Satis-fied	Satis-fied	Some-what satis-fied	Dissatis-fied	Very dissatis-fied	No Resp-onse	Total
Very satisfied	27	11	5	1	0	0	44
Satisfied	19	42	14	3	1	1	80
Somewhat satisfied	6	21	25	3	2	0	57
Dissatisfied	1	7	3	6	0	0	17
Very dissatisfied	2	3	2	2	0	0	9
No response	2	1	4	1	0	2	10
Total	57	85	53	16	3	3	217

Table 5.4
Satisfaction with surgery and orthodontic treatment

Satisfaction with orthodontics

Satisfaction with surgery

	Very satis-fied	Satis-fied	Some-what satis-fied	Dissatis-fied	Very dissatis-fied	No resp-onse	Total
Very satisfied	53	9	3	0	0	1	66
Satisfied	17	33	12	2	0	1	66
Somewhat satisfied	10	59	1	0	0	0	25
Dissatisfied	5	4	4	3	0	0	16
Very dissatisfied	0	0	1	0	2	0	3
No orthodontic treatment received	17	5	5	2	0	0	31
Undecided	1	1	0	0	0	0	2
No response	1	3	1	0	0	3	8
Total	104	60	35	8	2	5	217

Estimating satisfaction with hospital treatment is always hazardous, because it involves balancing one's pre-treatment expectations, with the reality of the post-treatment outcome. Thus, a patient with low expectations concerning the potential of surgery or orthodontic treatment (such as the straightening of crowded teeth), may express greater satisfaction with a minor post-treatment improvement, compared to a patient whose unrealistic hopes for post-treatment miracles are severely dashed. Therefore, estimations of satisfaction must be viewed with caution, as they are founded on personal expectations. At the same time, one must not overlook the implications for the professionals involved, to encourage realistic expectations by explaining the procedures to the patients in sufficient detail.

Furthermore, the results elicited reflect the participants' evaluations from their current adult perspective. In view of this, although the findings do not necessarily represent initial reactions to treatment, it is the individuals' prevailing perceptions which are of most significance to the retrospective follow-up study on this occasion.

Experience of teasing

One of the most dramatic findings relating to the questionnaire, concerns the respondents' experiences of being teased about having a cleft. The vast majority (80.2%, n=174) of those asked reported to have been teased, compared with a minority group (15.2%, n=33) who had not been subjected to teasing. The residual 4.6% (n=10) of participants did not indicate either way.

The data can be compared with Noar's (1991) finding that 75% of his sample of 28 patients with unilateral cleft lip and palate had been teased. It is notable that these postal questionnaire respondents were adolescents and adults (16-25 years old).

The implications of such a preponderance of individuals being teased about their defect, will be addressed on subsequent occasions, especially in the cross-tabulating of these data with other pertinent areas of investigation. It is useful at this stage to define the terminology to be used in relation to this aspect of the respondents' experiences.

In May 1992, a national Anti-Bullying Campaign was launched to raise awareness of the prevalent problem of bullying, especially in schools, and to address how such a problem could be effectively tackled by those concerned. Pertinent literature has been published in association with the campaign, to advise the victims of bullying and their parents, as well as offering guidance to schools and teachers. Emanating from the literature available, comes an eloquent exposition (cited below), which explains the relationship between 'teasing' and 'bullying', and the nature of the problem (Tattum and Herbert, 1990, p.1).

> Sadly, bullying is a form of cruelty which is widely practised in our schools and has received little attention from national and local authorities. Nonetheless, most who work in education will agree that it is widespread and persistent. The bullies are to be found in nursery classes, infant, junior and secondary schools. Their behaviour encompasses conduct which includes name-calling and teasing, jostling and punching, intimidation and extortion, assault, and occasionally maiming and murder.

The victims for their part suffer the physical and psychological abuse of their persons, isolation and loneliness, insecurity, anxiety, and fear arising from the threatening atmosphere which surrounds them. At its most insidious bullying focuses on vulnerable children who are regarded as being different because of their ethnic origins, class and sexual inclinations or physical and mental disabilities. It is difficult to understand why bullying has not been taken seriously. Can it be that it is thought to be an inevitable part of school life, or that it is a necessary part of growing up, or that it is so secretive that it defies the vigilance of teachers or other adults working in schools?

Tattum and Herbert (1990, p.3) define bullying as: 'the wilful, conscious desire to hurt, threaten or frighten someone.' In the context of the current study, teasing is perceived as one form of bullying, rather than its alternative, but inappropriate definition to 'make fun of playfully' *(The Concise Oxford Dictionary)*. In subsequent references, the terms 'teasing' and 'bullying' will be used interchangeably. That is, although teasing may be equated with verbal taunting, and bullying with physical intimidation and abuse, the questionnaire respondents themselves appeared to use the two terms without discrimination.

Regarding the incidence of bullying, Tattum and Herbert (1990) suggest that the most reliable source of data emerges from Scandinavia. They refer to a national study of 140,000 pupils in Norwegian junior and senior high schools, which showed the involvement of 15% of the pupils in regular episodes of bullying. This percentage comprises 6% of bullies and 9% of victims who were subjected to bullying. In interpreting this finding, the authors are keen to distinguish between 'direct' and 'indirect' bullying. Whilst the former allude to the bullies and the victims, the latter concern the larger group of pupil onlookers.

An even more disturbing picture, is portrayed in a study undertaken in Britain, between 1984 and 1986 by Elliott (Kidscape literature). In the pilot study concerning children's safety, a total of 4,000 children (aged 5-16 years), were asked about their particular anxieties. One unanticipated finding was that 68% (n=2720) of the sample claimed to have been bullied at some stage. Most bullying occurred when the subjects were travelling to or from school or in school itself, and in the absence of adults.

The discrepancy between the incidences of bullying cited in the two surveys warrants some explanation. Unfortunately, Tattum and Herbert (1990) do not offer further insight into what constituted bullying 'on a regular basis' in the Norwegian research. In contrast, Elliott elucidates that 38% of her sample had been 'more seriously' bullied. This group comprised those who had been abused on more than one occasion, or had been subjected to a particularly frightening bullying incident.

With regard to the data of the present study, the implications of the notably higher incidence of bullying by teasing (80.2%, n=174), in the cleft

112

population will be addressed in conjunction with subsequent findings, relating to the circumstances in which the derision took place. Since these data reflect the respondents' experiences which took place over twenty years ago, comparison of incidence of teasing with the above studies should acknowledge the inherent time difference. Needless to say, whenever victimization occurred, one should be mindful of its potential consequences for the individuals concerned. As Tattum and Herbert (1990, p.19) relate: 'Few memories of childhood may be as powerful as that of the school bully lurking, teasing, threatening - never missing a chance to harass a victim.' The extent to which such memories can be blocked out in adulthood may be a factor of individual coping mechanisms, a consideration which is discussed in chapter seven.

Advice offered by the respondents to parents of a newborn baby with a cleft

In asking the respondents about the advice they would give to parents of a newborn baby with a cleft, the objective was to ascertain the extent to which the participants would project their own experiences of living with a cleft. In doing so, it was anticipated that the responses would suggest how far the cleft-impaired adults had resolved their own situation, in adjusting to the impairment. In the event, a total of 20.3% (n=44) of the sample did not tender any advice.

However, in contrast to the total of 5.6% (n=12) of individuals who mentioned the negative aspects of having a cleft, or identified particular problem areas, most respondents (a total of 74.2%, n=161) focused upon more positive factors. These considerations include advice regarding the use of effective coping strategies (26.7%, n=58), and the need for confidence in the Cleft Palate Team (1.8%, n=4). Further reference to coping strategies was combined with confidence in treatment (35.0%, n=76), emphasis upon positive aspects (7.4%, n=16) and no problems encountered (0.5%, n=1). An additional 2.8% (n=6) of the group reported that they had not experienced any cleft-related problems.

The extent to which the advice offered to parents reflects the respondents' own experiences of having a cleft, will be discussed further in the cross-tabulation of data later in this chapter.

The analysis of postal questionnaire data

The opportunity now arises to investigate the relationship between the respondents' past experiences and their present perceptions of living with a cleft, and to consider what determines their perceptions. The writer has identified the relevant core variables from the wealth of data from the postal questionnaire, which will be discussed under the following subheadings.

113

- The past experiences of the respondents

- The present perceptions of the respondents

The past experiences of the respondents

In presenting the findings in the previous section, it transpired that in some instances the respondents held fundamentally different perceptions of similar experiences. More precisely, with hindsight, whilst a particular experience (such as schooling) was perceived positively by some individuals, others perceived it in clearly negative terms. Although this diversity is anticipated to a certain extent, core variables which reflect the broad distinction between an essentially positive and negative outlook upon earlier life events, merit further investigation in a retrospective follow-up study.

The two core variables concerned, pertain to respondents' perceptions of having a cleft at school, and to the closely related experience of being subjected to teasing by peers. These variables have been cross-tabulated with a wide range of data emanating from the questionnaire, the most notable will be now reported. It should be noted that in attempting to define the circumstances and experiences of the most disadvantaged, particular emphasis is placed upon negative perceptions of school and experiences of being teased. Although the data reflect retrospective accounts of the experiences concerned, the writer is especially interested in the long term impact of the experiences upon the participants.

Attention is paid first to elucidating the association between the key variables and respondents' gender. Although the relationships are not statistically significant, there is negligible difference between the proportion of males (49.2%, n=64) and females (50.8%, n=66), who hold negative perceptions of their school days. However, regarding experiences of being teased, more males (52.9%, n=92) than females (47.1%, n=82) are implicated. The overall similarity in the percentages relating adverse reports, in itself, is noteworthy.

Reference to the predisposing factor of type of cleft will not be made in this section, as this information was not sought in the questionnaire.

Before investigating the strength of the relationships between the two core variables and other pertinent factors, consideration is given to the statistically significant correlation ($p < 0.01$), which exists between the core variables themselves, as indicated in Table 5.5 below. In all of the succeeding references to data, instances have been omitted from the cross-tabulations where the respondents denoted that a question was not applicable to them, or chose not to respond.

A clear relationship is evidenced between experience of being teased and negative perceptions of school (Table 5.5). The implication of this finding is twofold. Firstly, the data show that the majority of those responding to this item, hold negative impressions of their school days (n=128, 59.5% of the total number of respondents). Secondly, the vast majority of participants harbouring these negative perceptions were also teased by their peers (n=126, 98.4% of those expressing negative perceptions). These findings are strengthened by the fact 93.9% (n=31) of those not teased, held positive school perceptions. Thus, it appears that memories of school are highly influenced by experiences of being teased. Indeed, with hindsight some respondents associate their schooling with being hounded by bullies, and being subjected to merciless teasing.

Table 5.5
Perception of being at school with a cleft
and experience of teasing

Perception of school	Experience of teasing		
	Yes	No	Total
Positive perceptions	46	31	77
Negative perceptions	126	2	128
Total	172	33	205

NB: $p < 0.01$

In view of these data, the potential impact of adverse experiences upon the individuals' education and subsequent career choices warrants examination. It is conceivable that on leaving school, further and/or higher education options were rejected, if education per se was equated with negative perceptions of school (including teasing). The data relating to experiences on leaving school (aged fifteen or sixteen) and the two core variables, are presented in Tables 5.6 and 5.7 below.

Table 5.6
Perception of being at school with a cleft
and situation on leaving school

On leaving school	Perception of school		
	Positive	Negative	Total
Employment (including YTS scheme, trainee and apprenticeship)	61	85	146
Continued education (vocational / Further and/or Higher Education)	23	40	63
Other (special needs / unemployed	1	4	5
Total	85	129	214

Table 5.6 suggests that of the respondents expressing negative feelings about their school days, the majority entered employment on leaving school (n=85, 65.9% of the negative perception group). Having said this, proportionately more of this group continued their education (n=40, 31% of the negative perception group), than did those with positive impressions (n=23, 27.1%). Further evidence of these tendencies are apparent in cross-tabulating the variables corresponding to experience of teasing with the situation on leaving school (Table 5.7).

Table 5.7
Experience of teasing and situation on leaving school

On leaving school	Experience of teasing		
	Yes	No	Total
Employment (including YTS scheme, trainee and apprenticeship)	116	24	140
Continued education (vocational / Further and/or Higher Education)	51	9	60
Other (special needs / unemployed)	6	0	6
Total	173	33	206

According to Table 5.7, a preponderance of individuals who were teased, obtained employment at the first opportunity (n=116, 67.1% of those teased). However, when these data are compared with those not teased, a higher percentage of the teased group continued their education (n=51, 29.5% of those teased as opposed to n=9, 27.3% of those not teased). These findings suggest that neither negative school perceptions nor experiences of being teased, are significantly related to activity on leaving school. Therefore, it is tentatively advocated that adverse experiences alone, do not appear to have dissuaded those encountering them from extending their education following school.

Regarding the connection between the two core variables and socio-economic grouping, whilst the previous cross-tabulations required retrospective reporting in the questionnaire, those pertaining to socio-economic status reflect current circumstances. It is regrettable that data indicating the specific type of employment in socio-economic terms, is available for only 61.8% (n=134) of the respondents. In the residual group, reference to type of occupation was unclear from the responses given, not applicable or absent altogether. In two instances no data was provided concerning school perceptions. The relevant cross-tabulations are presented in Tables 5.8 and 5.9.

In examining Table 5.8 below, it transpires that of those incorporated into the 'negative' perception category, most of the respondents were employed in skilled or semi-skilled occupations when completing the questionnaire (n=56, 70.9% of the 'negative' perception group). This finding corresponds with the earlier observation that the majority of respondents with negative impressions of school did not pursue Further or Higher Education after school (Table 5.6). Supplementary information emerges in cross-tabulating employment with teasing (Table 5.9 below).

Table 5.8
Perception of being at school with a cleft and employment according to socio-economic grouping

Type of employment according to socio-economic grouping	Perception of school		
	Positive	Negative	Total
I - Professional	8	6	14
II - Intermediate Occupations	15	13	28
III - Skilled occupation (non-manual and manual)	20	41	61
IV - Semi-Skilled Occupations	9	15	24
V - Unskilled Manual Occupations	2	4	6
Total	54	79	133

With respect to the association between experiences of teasing and current employment, the trend identified in Table 5.8 is reinforced. That is, the majority of the respondents who were victimized are presently engaged in skilled or semi-skilled occupations (n=70, 68.0% of those teased). Thus, it could be suggested that adverse past experiences may influence the nature of the subsequent occupations of those encountering them. An alternative explanation might be that those undertaking skilled or semi-skilled occupations were more susceptible to earlier tribulation.

Table 5.9
Experience of teasing and employment according to socio-economic grouping

Type of employment according to socio-economic grouping	Experience of teasing		
	Yes	No	Total
I - Professional	11	3	14
II - Intermediate occupations	17	9	26
III - Skilled occupation (non-manual and manual)	50	5	55
IV - Semi-skilled occupations	20	4	24
V - Unskilled manual occupations	5	1	6
Total	103	22	125

117

The variable regarding respondents' future career aspirations was isolated as having potential significance. On subsequent analysis, however, no notable findings were yielded.

Having identified some of the factors upon which the adverse experiences seem to impinge, attention is turned now to considering the extent to which they have infiltrated the adult lives of those concerned.

The present perceptions of the respondents

In the questionnaire, the recipients were asked to evaluate the extent to which their perceptions of past experiences had changed with life experience and maturation. They were also invited to estimate the influence their cleft had exerted upon certain aspects of their life, such as education and dating. In order to gain maximum insight into the nature and the extent of change over time, the core variables have been cross-tabulated with the cluster of variables which encompass this information.

Attention is initially given to the statistically significant relationship at the 1% level between negative perceptions of school, and identified changes in those perceptions over time (Table 5.10 below).

Table 5.10
Perception of being at school with a cleft
and identified change since school days

Identified change since school days	Perception of school		
	Positive	Negative	Total
Increased self-confidence	11	80	91
Lack of self-confidence	5	15	20
Not applicable (no change) or no problems experienced	67	30	97
Total	83	125	208

NB: p < 0.01

When the data relating to those who hold negative impressions of their past school days, are cross-tabulated with identified changes in outlook since then, it transpires that 64.0% (n=80) of respondents perceive an increase in their self-confidence. The finding is strengthened by the fact that 87.9% (n=80) of those reporting raised self-esteem indicated negative school perceptions. This suggests that the school environment of the individuals concerned, may have exerted a deleterious impact upon their social functioning, since self-confidence burgeoned on leaving that environment. Although many non-affected adolescents become more self-assured with

118

maturation, it is notable that only 12.1% (n=11) of those with positive school perceptions, reported raised self-confidence with hindsight. The extent to which their enhanced self-confidence is related to the cleft, will be addressed again in subsequent chapters.

Table 5.11
Experience of teasing and identified change since school days

Identified change since school days	Experience of teasing		
	Yes	No	Total
Increased self-confidence	85	3	88
Lack of self-confidence	20	0	20
Not applicable (no change) or no problems experienced	63	29	92
Total	168	32	200

It might be anticipated that on leaving the school environment, those subjected to teasing would be comparatively happier and appeased. Table 5.11 above suggests that some respondents experienced increased self-confidence (n=85, 50.6% of those teased). Since 96.6% (n=85) of those with raised self-confidence had been teased, their self-confidence may have been damaged by teasing in the past. A minority of individuals, however, continued to lack self-confidence (n=20, 11.9% of those teased), or did not identify changed perceptions (n=63, 37.5% of those teased).

The potential trauma of stigmatizing school experiences is reflected in perceptions of the cleft's influence upon other aspects of life. Evidence for this emerges from respondents' evaluations of the effect their cleft has exerted upon education, dating, teasing, occupation and appearance. Tables 5.12-5.16 show a cluster of significant results ($p < 0.01$), when data indicating a 'high'/'very high' influence are cross-tabulated with negative perceptions of school.

Table 5.12
Perception of being at school with a cleft and
perceived influence of cleft upon education

Influence of cleft upon education	Perception of school		
NB: $p < 0.01$	Positive	Negative	Total
Very high / high	10	41	51
Low / very low	60	44	104
Total	70	85	155

Table 5.13
Perception of being at school with a cleft and perceived influence of cleft upon dating

Influence of cleft upon dating	Perception of school		
	Positive	Negative	Total
Very high / high	16	71	87
Low / very low	49	20	69
Total	65	91	156

NB: p < 0.01

Table 5.14
Perception of being at school with a cleft and perceived influence of cleft upon teasing

Influence of cleft upon teasing	Perception of school		
	Positive	Negative	Total
Very high / high	21	95	116
Low / very low	45	11	56
Total	66	106	172

NB: p < 0.01

Table 5.15
Perception of being at school with a cleft and perceived influence of cleft upon occupation

Influence of cleft upon occupation	Perception of school		
	Positive	Negative	Total
Very high / high	8	26	34
Low / very low	67	69	136
Total	75	95	170

NB: p < 0.01

Table 5.16
Perception of being at school with a cleft and
perceived influence of cleft upon appearance

Influence of cleft upon appearance	Perception of school		
	Positive	Negative	Total
Very high / high	16	62	78
Low / very low	57	32	89
Total	73	94	167

NB: p < 0.01

Tables 5.17-5.19 show cross-referencing of the data on the perceived influence of the cleft with experience of teasing. Statistically significant results are obtained for the aspects of education, dating and appearance.

Table 5.17
Experience of teasing and
perceived influence of cleft upon education

Influence of cleft upon education	Experience of teasing		
	Yes	No	Total
Very high / high	50	2	52
Low / very low	73	28	101
Total	123	30	153

NB: p < 0.01

Table 5.18
Experience of teasing and
perceived influence of cleft upon dating

Influence of cleft upon dating	Experience of teasing		
	Yes	No	Total
Very high / high	83	1	84
Low / very low	40	27	67
Total	123	28	151

NB: p < 0.01

121

Table 5.19
Experience of teasing and
perceived influence of cleft upon appearance

Influence of cleft upon appearance   Experience of teasing

	Yes	No	Total
Very high / high	77	1	78
Low / very low	53	30	83
Total	130	31	161

NB: p < 0.01

The impact of the participants' past untoward experiences, can be further investigated according to the type of advice offered to parents of a cleft-impaired baby (Table 5.20).

Table 5.20
Perception of being at school with a cleft
and advice to parents

Advice to parents   Perception of School

	Positive	Negative	Total
Adverse aspects of being born with a cleft highlighted	2	11	13
Positive outlook and/or advice on coping	57	101	158
Total	59	112	171

The fact that the majority of the negative school perceptions group is able to offer positive advice (n=101, 59.% of those with negative perceptions) invites explanation. In similar vein, 63.9% (n=101) of the respondents offering positive advice harboured negative school perceptions.

Whilst speculative at this stage, one interpretation of the findings is that life is comparatively more optimistic from an adult perspective. The shift in perceptions may be attributable to maturation per se, and/or to the development of effective coping mechanisms with which to counter residual problem areas. Further evidence of the changed outlook can be gleaned from cross-tabulating data pertaining to the experience of teasing with advice given to parents (Table 5.21).

Table 5.21
Experience of teasing and
advice to parents

Advice to parents	Experience of teasing		
	Yes	No	Total
Adverse aspects of being born with a cleft highlighted	14	0	14
Positive outlook and/or advice on coping	132	31	163
Total	146	31	177

When the relationship between experiences of teasing and advice rendered to parents is examined in conjunction with the relevant data, the findings of the previous table are clearly reinforced. That is, despite the distressing victimization to which a large proportion of the participants was subjected, most individuals elect to emphasize the positive aspects of their personal experiences (n=132, 90.4% of those teased). This result is contrasted with the finding that 100.0% (n=31) of the respondents not teased gave positive advice. Overall, the data intimate that the adverse experiences of youth do not necessarily wield irreversible damage upon the subjects' psychosocial functioning. Indeed, with reference to additional data it may even transpire that such experiences actively facilitate a positive outcome, but exploration of this notion must await discussion in later chapters.

The role of personality (including self-esteem) should not be underestimated in defining the relationship between past and present life experiences and perceptions. Having said this, no further mention will be made of this crucial dimension in this section, as elucidation necessitates reference to data which is not exclusive to the postal questionnaire. For this reason, discussion is deferred until the next chapter, which seeks to integrate all of the core variables identified previously, before addressing their implications in chapter eight.

6 Making connections: from birth to adulthood

Introduction

The findings relating to the first three data sets have been reported in the previous two chapters (chapters four and five). Where data have not been incorporated into the cluster of key variables, their exclusion reflects the need to impose stringent boundaries upon the potentially extensive scope of the study. Indeed, as the wealth of data collected affords examination of multifarious 'themes', the process of paring the variables necessitates sacrificing other avenues of interest. Reference to the data base can be found in Nash (1993).

The opportunity now arises for further analysis of the key issues emerging from the data, by means of cross-tabulating the core variables emanating from different data sets. The reader is reminded that the information gathered by BNH (Results I), and the writer's inspection of the hospital records (Results II), provides insight into the participants' formative years from a professional stance. The data elicited by postal questionnaire (Results III), reflect the implications of being born with a cleft from the respondents' adult perspective. The different concerns of the data sets are evident in shifting reference to the participants from 'patients' to 'respondents'. Areas to be discussed in this chapter are incorporated under the following subheadings.

- Factors defining the participants' life history: circumstances and experiences encountered during the developmental years.

- The private and public persona of the participants in the study.

- A longitudinal perspective: the impact of aspects of the participants' past life history upon their present perceptions.

Factors defining the participants' life history: circumstances and experiences encountered during the developmental years

It has been established that psychosocial development is fundamentally influenced by two predominant environments, namely, the home and school. Whilst the pre-school child spends most of his/her time with the primary caregiver, much of the school child's time is devoted to school, and by implication, in the company of peers. Since the quality, as well as the quantity of experiences encountered in these two environments wield such import, the data relating to each of them will be examined separately, before being amalgamated.

Factors relating to the home environment of the participants

Since the current chapter offers the first opportunity for the comparison of data sets, attention is drawn to the close correspondence between the core variables of 'environmental aspect' delineated by BNH (Results I), and that of 'family environment' (Results II) deriving from inspection of the hospital records ($p < 0.01$).

As anticipated, the findings evidence the high level of agreement between the writer and BNH, which has been obtained throughout the process of data analysis. It could be argued that information relating to 'environmental aspect', which was based on BNH's perception and personal acquaintance with the individuals concerned, is fundamentally different to that of 'family environment' gathered by the writer from documentary evidence. However, one could equally advocate that this difference serves to strengthen, rather than weaken the association between the two variables in question.

Although the two variables are concerned with denoting the climate of the environment in which the patient is raised, 'family environment' incorporates comparatively more detailed information than the bipolar assessment of 'environmental aspect' (either 'satisfactory/co-operative' or 'detrimental'). Moreover, whilst the former ('family environment') encompasses factors associated with family dynamics, including parental influence, the latter ('environmental aspect') is more concerned with parental attitude towards the cleft-impaired patient, which reflects BNH's particular interest in this area.

With respect to the outcome of the cross-tabulation of 'environmental aspect' and 'family environment', 89.7% (n=26) of those falling into the 'detrimental' parental attitude group, had to contend with an 'unfavourable'

126

family environment. In stark contrast, 93.5% (n=43) of individuals who experienced a 'favourable' family situation, had parents who displayed a 'satisfactory' attitude towards them. In discussing these and other results, it is regrettable that the amount of data available in each instance, depends upon the extent to which reference is made to the various factors by BNH and her colleagues. Thus, in the case of the above cross-tabulation, instances where no reference was made to both variables have been omitted from the calculations.

The plight of those with adverse personal circumstances, can be seen in terms of perpetuated deprivation when considering other data emerging from the hospital records. In one notable instance, the deprivation takes the form of missed opportunities for optimum treatment through non-attendance at out-patient clinics. Within a cycle of disadvantage, it would be anticipated that those reared in unfavourable circumstances, may be the most vulnerable regarding sporadic hospital attendance due to its seemingly low priority.

Whilst data relating to the frequency of attendance at hospital clinics would assist on this occasion, the extent to which non-attendance is perceived as regrettable (and therefore warranting explanation), is perhaps of greater significance in reflecting parental attitudes towards the patient and his/her necessary treatment. As described in chapter four (the developmental years), the constitution of the patients' family environment is significantly correlated with the extent to which his/her non-attendance (if any) at hospital clinics was accounted for ($p < 0.05$). It transpires that the preponderance of individuals with an 'unfavourable' family situation provided no, or only partial explanation for their non-attendance at clinics. The incidence of no or sporadic accountability was considerably reduced for those coming from a 'favourable' family background.

With respect to the association between 'environmental aspect' and explanation for non-attendance at hospital clinics, the vast majority (85.3%, n=29) of the 'detrimental' parental attitude group, proffered intermittent or no explanation for the non-attendance of hospital appointments. In comparison, participants whose parents demonstrated a 'satisfactory' attitude towards them generally attended all the required clinics, or accounted for all instances of absenteeism (91.4% of the 'satisfactory' parental attitude group, n=53).

In interpreting the results, caution must be taken in attributing cause and effect and making value judgements. For example, the findings do show a strong (but statistically non-significant) relationship between the perceived quality of home environment or parental attitude, and inclination to account for non-attendance. However, they provide less convincing evidence of the extent to which failure to explain non-attendance of hospital appointments, is indicative of the patients' home environment and parental concern. Nevertheless, in speculating upon the extent to which the cleft affected the child-parent relationship and family dynamics (and vice-versa), the probability stakes for being 'at risk' in psychosocial terms, are at a premium where a patient had a visible cleft, an 'unfavourable' home background and whose parents demonstrated a 'detrimental' attitude towards him or her.

Therefore, there appears to be evidence of a minority subgroup whose personal circumstances may have exerted a deleterious effect upon their development. However, this advocation needs to be substantiated by further data. For this reason, consideration will be now given to the school environment, with particular emphasis upon those considered to be at a disadvantage.

Factors relating to the school environment of the participants

In addition to the respondents' perceptions of school, another key factor to emerge from the postal questionnaire is the experience of being teased. The close correlation between these two core variables has been already established ($p < 0.01$, Results III). Since most of the victimization occurred within the school context, this section considers the evidence for an 'at risk' subgroup of participants. As the cleft defect is more detectable in some individuals than others, cross-tabulation of the two core variables with type of cleft has been undertaken.

Data analysis indicates that a statistically significant relationship (at the 1% level) exists between the two variables, with 73.8% (n=96) of visibly-impaired individuals holding negative perceptions of their school days. This figure compares with 40% (n=34) of the non-visible cleft group (cleft palate only), who expressed negative feelings about having a cleft at school. Thus, it seems that patients with visible evidence of clefting are more vulnerable to adverse school experiences, than those with non-visible scarring.

If data relating to type of cleft is cross-tabulated with experience of teasing, an even more dramatic picture is obtained ($p < 0.01$). It transpires that 95.2% (n=120) of patients with a visible cleft were subjected to teasing, which contrasts with 66.7% (n=54) of the non-visible group who were teased. On the basis of these findings, it would appear that those born with a visible cleft (cleft lip and palate), are not only more at risk for having unhappy and adverse experiences at school, but also for being victimized by peers. Since most of the teasing occurred within the confines of the school environment, it could be postulated that individuals with cleft lip and palate are likely to be teased at school, and that such experiences may actually determine their long term impressions of their school days.

The association between factors relating to the home and the school environments of the participants

Having established that the visibility of the cleft is associated with negative perceptions of school, especially the experience of being teased, the relationship between home circumstances and school experiences warrants investigation. The purpose of doing so, is to attempt to define the extent to which individuals with disadvantageous personal circumstances (at home), also had to contend with untoward social circumstances (at school).

In profiling the vulnerable minority mentioned above, one should note the evident relationship which exists between family environment and perceptions of school. A statistically significant relationship at the 5% level is obtained, with 60.5% (n=52) of those in the 'unfavourable' family environment category expressing negative feelings about their schooling. However, of more import on this occasion, is the high percentage of individuals with a 'favourable' home background, who also held negative impressions of their school days (78.8% of the 'favourable' environment group, n=41).

The predicament of the minority group is reinforced by data pertaining to a 'detrimental' parental attitude towards the patient and negative perceptions of school (p < 0.05). To clarify further, it transpires that 79.4% (n=27) of individuals whose parents exerted a 'detrimental' influence also held adverse impressions of their school days. This figure compares with 56.9% (n=103) of those whose parents were assessed as displaying a 'satisfactory' attitude, who expressed negative feelings about having a cleft at school. It would seem that the preponderance of those with deleterious personal circumstances, also encountered unrewarding circumstances when at school. Thus, for this subgroup neither their home nor school life appeared to offer them the necessary self-affirming experiences.

One could speculate that where parental attitude towards the patient with a cleft was 'detrimental', the majority of individuals would perceive their school days in negative terms. However, there is a less clear-cut relationship between 'unfavourable' home circumstances and adverse impressions of school, since a relatively high proportion of respondents with favourable circumstances also reported pessimistic accounts of their school days.

In contemplating the implications for those most at risk, the focus of attention must rest upon instances where negative experiences at school are coupled with negative circumstances at home. Thus, it is plausible that as parental attitude toward the patient is inextricably linked with parenting style, where a 'detrimental' attitude is identified the individual lacked parental support. Consequently, when this disadvantaged subgroup encountered more negativism at school, the potentially damaging effects of the experiences such as being victimized by peers were heightened, since they were not necessarily quelled at home. Therefore, it is feasible to suggest that the most potent influence regarding the patients' home environment upon his or her formative years, is the nature of parental attitude shown towards him or her.

With respect to the association between 'favourable' home circumstances and adverse impressions of school, the findings infer that even if the latter proved to be unrewarding, the experiences were more likely to be balanced with an affirming home situation.

The existence of a vulnerable and disadvantaged subgroup, becomes increasingly apparent when consulting the data relating to teasing and personal circumstances. For example, a high proportion of individuals with an 'unfavourable' family situation were teased (86.7%, n=78). Mention must be made also of the 67.7% (n=78) of respondents who reported teasing and also fell into the 'unfavourable' category. However, the experience of being teased appears to be slightly more prevalent amongst those with a 'favourable', than an 'unfavourable'' home disposition (88.6%, n=39). In view of these findings, it could be argued that although teasing is not exclusively associated with a deleterious family background, individuals who are victimized are more likely to have an 'unfavourable' than in a 'favourable' home background.

Consistent with previous findings relating to the participants' home environment, the results pertaining to teasing are especially notable in instances of a 'detrimental' parental attitude. That is, a striking 97.0% (n=32) of those whose parents' attitude towards them was considered to be 'detrimental', were subjected to teasing (p < 0.05). This figure compares with 81.7% (n=142) of patients with 'encouraging' parents, who were also victimized, and 97.0% (n=32) of the group with no experience of teasing whose parents displayed a 'satisfactory' disposition.

Whilst it is tempting to extrapolate that those with a deleterious home environment are likely to suffer further at school, at this stage it would be more feasible to advocate that such individuals are most at risk for encountering further deprivation at school. That is, deprivation in its literal sense of suffering from the effects of not having access to, or being excluded from the type of personal and social interaction which expedites psychosocial maturation. The strong relationship between adverse parental attitude or home circumstances and the social stigma of being teased, suggests that such impoverishment of formative experiences has the potential to cause long term psychosocial dysfunction.

The two subsequent sections examine the degree to which the potential for dysfunction is realized in the respondents' adult lives. Consideration is given to the way in which the participants see themselves and are seen by others, prior to investigating the impact of the individuals' past personal and social histories upon their present perceptions.

The private and public personae of the participants in the study

The term 'persona' has been defined as: 'an aspect of the personality as shown to or perceived by others' (*The Concise Oxford Dictionary*). As such, it is particularly apposite in discussing the participants, since the data in this section reflect how the individuals perceive/perceived themselves (self-perception), and how they were perceived by others (peer perception). On 'private' and 'public' personae refer to the differing identities or roles played in private (personal) and public (social) contexts.

Definition of the participants' private persona in conjunction with factors relating to personal circumstances (type of cleft and home environment)

In pursuing a broadly developmental paradigm, the earliest data to relate to the patients' private persona, are those relating to their personal adjustment to the cleft during childhood (Results I). With reference to BNH's data, the reader is reminded that a statistically significant relationship at the 1% level, was found to exist between 'environmental aspect' and 'personal aspect'. This cross-tabulation indicated that patients whose parents exhibited a 'satisfactory' attitude, were generally perceived by BNH and her colleagues to be well adjusted and 'co-operative'. In contrast, the majority of those whose parents' attitude was deemed to be 'detrimental', displayed some form of personal maladjustment to the cleft.

Whilst it is hazardous to interpret these findings in terms of cause and effect, the potency of a deleterious relationship between the patient and his/her parents, upon the former's psychosocial development and functioning is becoming increasingly apparent. Again, one should be aware of making value judgements.

When details relating to the patients' adjustment to the cleft and family environment are combined, a similar picture of impoverishment is obtained. Although statistically non-significant, it transpires that 79.1% (n=34) of those who experienced some degree of personal maladjustment in their youth, were being raised in 'unfavourable' family circumstances. This proportion compares with 63.6% (n=42) of individuals who were apparently 'well-adjusted', but had to cope with an 'unfavourable' family situation. Moreover, those with a 'favourable' environment tended to have no adjustment problems (72.7% of the 'favourable' group, n=24), with only 27.3% (n=9) of this group displaying personal difficulties.

The emerging labyrinth of disadvantage with which a notable proportion of the participants were entangled, is reinforced by data corresponding to personal problems and explanation of non-attendance at hospital clinics. Regarding those who had personal problems, 84.5% (n=49) gave no or only partial explanation for their absence at hospital clinics.

This proportion, however, should be considered alongside the majority of 'well-adjusted' patients whose explanation for non-attendance was also sporadic or non-existent (75% of the 'well-adjusted' group, n=81). Having said this, there is a tendency for the 'well-adjusted' participants to account for all instances of non-attendance, if indeed, they were absent at all (75% of the no non-attendance or all explained group, n=27).

With the benefit of more recent information (Results III), insight is gained into the personal profiles of the adult respondents, by data deriving from measures of self-esteem and personality. Whilst measures of self-esteem reflect the extent to which an individual values him or herself (private persona), personality characteristics are indicative of one's self-perceived behaviour in both private and public arenas of life. These two domains are integral to the individual's response to being born with a cleft, and largely determine how the developing child and adolescent copes (or fails to cope), with untoward home circumstances and unrewarding experiences at school.

The measures of self-esteem and personality obtained for the study, reflect the participants' disposition when completing the questionnaire, and therefore, are not necessarily indicative of the individuals' early psychosocial development. Although this factor must be borne in mind on examining the data, the findings can be seen as highlighting the impact of earlier circumstances and experiences upon adult psychosocial functioning. With reference to the correspondence between self-esteem and a 'detrimental' parental attitude towards the cleft-impaired patient, there is evidence that the long term effects of the cycle of disadvantage can be reversed.

It is noteworthy that the majority of those whose parents had displayed an unpropitious attitude towards them as children, responded in the direction of high self-esteem as adults. That is, concerning the individuals incorporated into the 'detrimental' parental attitude category, 90.9% (n=20) of them fell into the group indicating highest self-esteem (scores 0 and 1). This outcome compares with 93.5% (n=130) of the 'satisfactory' parental attitude category reflecting high self-esteem. Needless to say, the majority of respondents comprising the two lowest self-esteem groups (81.8%, n=9; scores 5 and 6), were also included in the 'satisfactory' parenting group. As with all cross-tabulations relating to the highest and lowest measures of self-esteem, the small size of the latter group precludes implementation of the Chi Square test of statistical significance. The profile of results to emerge from the cross-tabulation of these core variables (self-esteem and 'environmental aspect'), clearly demonstrates that a 'detrimental' parental attitude per se, does not necessarily exert a deleterious impact upon the self-esteem of the adult offspring of the parents concerned.

A similar trend is seen in cross-tabulating data pertaining to the association between early personal maladjustment to the defect (as perceived by the professionals), and present psychosocial adjustment (as perceived by the respondents themselves). The findings suggest that the potentially damaging effects of early adversity can be reversed in later life. For example, regarding the relationship between current levels of self-esteem and individuals who were deemed to exhibit personal maladjustment during the developmental years, the preponderance of participants responded in the direction of high self-esteem. This pattern mirrors the trend of high self-esteem responses elicited by the majority of those with no documented adjustment problems.

With respect to those assessed as having adjustment problems, 89.5% (n=34) of them show the highest levels of self-esteem (scores 0 and 1). This figure compares with 92.9% (n=79) of respondents considered to display no adjustment difficulties and high self-esteem. In similar vein, the majority of those indicating lowest self-esteem are incorporated into the no adjustment problems category (60%, n=6; scores 5 and 6).

Alongside this optimistic pattern of responses, a remarkably consistent set of results is obtained regarding those who evidence low self-esteem. That is, low self-esteem appears to be more associated with a visible cleft (cleft lip and palate), than a non-visible cleft (cleft palate only). Regarding individuals with a visible cleft, 72.7% (n=8) of the group indicated the lowest levels of self-esteem (scores 5 and 6). A smaller majority of those with a visible defect responded in the direction of highest self-esteem (58.0%, n=87; scores 0 and 1). Although a visible cleft cannot be equated directly with low self-esteem, it does seem that the former predominates in the latter minority group. Moreover, the findings suggest that low self-esteem in adulthood may be associated with visibility of the impairment.

The results implicate that facial disfigurement connected with cleft lip, continues to exert some impact upon the individuals' adult persona. Whilst most of those with a visible cleft demonstrate high self-esteem, there is evidence that a vulnerable, minority subgroup exists during the adult years.

In reviewing the literature (chapter two), reference was made to the controversy surrounding the existence of a 'cleft personality'. The assumption is made by some authorities that individuals who are born with a cleft lip and/or palate, exhibit common personality traits. Whilst the bulk of evidence seems to suggest otherwise, the notion that a physical impairment can influence personality development, warrants some consideration in conjunction with the present study. In the subsequent discussion, personality is initially examined in association with type of cleft.

With respect to the personality measure incorporated into the postal questionnaire, the reader is reminded that it derives from a 'five factor' model of personality (for example, McCrae and Costa, 1987). The findings concerning type of cleft according to the visibility of the defect and personality, will be presented in conjunction with the five factors (Neuroticism (N), Extraversion (E), Openness (O), Agreeableness (A) and Conscientiousness (C)). Since the writer implemented her own shortened version of the inventory, the data cannot be considered in terms of definitive personality test scores. Rather, the adjective pairs have been included in the questionnaire to elicit a broad profile of the respondents involved in the study.

Data analysis shows a remarkably consistent trend across all of the five factors of personality. There appears to be a strong relationship between traits which have negative, or socially undesirable connotations and a visible cleft. For example, concerning the characteristics indicative of Neuroticism, the following pattern of responses was obtained for those with a visible cleft (cleft lip and palate). The letter against each adjective pair denotes its position in the writer's questionnaire.

a) *Calm-Worrying*
64.3% (n=27) of 'worrying'/'very worrying' groups had a visible cleft.
However, 64.9% (n=50) of the visible cleft group was 'calm'/'very calm',
as was 73.7% (n=42) of the non-visile cleft group

f) *Even-Tempered-Temperamental*
62.0% (n=31) of 'temperamental'/'very temperamental' groups had a visible
cleft. However, 64.8% (n=57) of the visible cleft group was apparently 'even-
tempered'/'very even-tempered', as was 66.1% (n=37) of the non-visible cleft
group.

k) *Secure-Insecure*
66.0% (n=31) of 'insecure'/'very insecure' groups had a visible cleft.
However, 63.5% (n=54) of the visible cleft group was apparently
'secure'/'very secure', as was 71.4% (n=40) of the non-visible cleft group.

p) *Comfortable-Self-Conscious*
65.5% (n=57) of 'self-conscious'/'very self-conscious' groups had a visible
cleft (NB: $p < 0.05$). Similarly, 68.7% (n=57) of the visible cleft group was also
'self-conscious'/'very self-conscious', which contrasts with 52.4% (n=33) of
the non-visible cleft group which was 'comfortable'.

Figure 6.1   Opposing pairs of personality traits measuring Neuroticism

Whilst one must be cautious in interpreting the results according to cause
and effect, it appears that the characteristics indicative of neurotic tendencies
are most apparent in respondents with a visible cleft. However, since the
majority of those with a detectable cleft were inclined to respond in the
opposing direction of stability (such as 'calm', 'even-tempered' and 'secure'),
visibility of the defect per se cannot be equated with neurotic traits. Where
there is evidence of neurosis, the individual concerned is more likely to
present with a visible than a non-visible cleft.

The pattern of responses which emerges from the above set of results
pertaining to Neuroticism, is evident throughout the remaining measures of
personality. The most notable findings are presented below in terms of the
relationships which reach statistical significance.

Whilst the emphasis of the following subsection is upon identifying traces
of Extraversion (E), by implication, responses which do not denote this trait
reflect characteristics of introversion. With respect to the cross-tabulated
data, in each instance, the majority of individuals who responded in the
direction of introversion, also had a visible cleft. The most notable example
of this concerns the opposing pair 'reserved-affectionate', for which the
association between visibility of the cleft and a reserved character reaches 1%
level of statistical significance. More specifically, 78.6% (n=44) of the
'reserved' group were born with a cleft lip and palate.

Needless to say, in accordance with the pattern of responses already inferred, the preponderance of respondents with a visible or non-visible defect were reportedly 'affectionate' (55.1% of the visible group, n=54, and 80% of the non-visible group, n=48). A similar, but statistically non-significant trend is detected for the other measures of Extraversion, in that the majority of those who responded in the direction of introversion has a cleft which is visible. In interpreting this finding, one must bear in mind that adverse circumstances and experiences especially subjection to teasing, appear to be more closely associated with having a visible, than a non-visible cleft.

Regarding the other factors tapped by the personality inventory, the items identifying an attitude of Openness (O) to experience, show further demonstration of the trend of results previously established (although statistically non-significant). That is, most of the individuals in both the non-visible and visible cleft groups evidenced traits of Openness ('original', 'imaginative', 'broad interests' and 'daring').

At the same time, however, the majority of those whose responses reflect a closed disposition (opposite of Openness), has a cleft lip and palate. Thus, the most apparent characteristics in the visible cleft group appear to be 'conventional', 'narrow interests', 'down-to-earth', and 'unadventurous'. For example, regarding the 'conventional-original' measure, 63.0% (n=29) of the non-visible cleft group and 57.4% (n=35) of the visible cleft group were reportedly 'original'/'very original'. These figures compare with 60.5% (n=26) of visibly-impaired respondents who considered themselves to be 'conventional'/'very conventional'.

The detection of a distinct subgroup amongst the respondents becomes yet more obvious in consulting data regarding type of cleft and the remaining factors of Agreeableness (A) and Conscientiousness (C). Although most participants responded in the direction of Agreeable and/or Conscientious regardless of their cleft type, an association does appear to exist between their corollaries Antagonism and Undirectedness (respectively), and a visible cleft. In each measure relating to Agreeableness versus Antagonism, the majority of respondents in both the non-visible and visible cleft groups were seemingly, 'trusting', 'flexible', 'cheerful' and 'humble'. In contrast, the responses evidencing Antagonism tend to be associated with individuals born with cleft lip and palate (namely, 'suspicion', 'stubbornness', 'seriousness' and 'proud'). The trend can be shown by data for the 'suspicious-trusting' adjectives.

On this occasion, the majority of participants with either a non-visible or a visible cleft identified with 'trusting' (70.7%, n=41 and 69.3%, n=61 respectively). Although there appears to be a negligible difference between the two groups, further analysis shows that 61.4% (n=27) of those reporting to be 'suspicious' had a visible cleft, compared with 38.7% (n=17) with a non-visible deformity.

Similarly, most of the participants, regardless of their cleft type denoted the socially desirable characteristics associated with Conscientiousness, namely, 'hardworking', 'ambitious', 'emotionally stable' and 'energetic'. On the other hand, those who exhibited their undesirable opposites reflecting Undirectedness (namely, 'lazy', 'aimless', 'emotionally unstable' and 'unenergetic' are more likely to have a visible, than a non-visible cleft. For example, whilst emotional stability is evidenced by 87.5% (n=56) and 89.2% (n=83) of the non-visible and visible cleft groups respectively, 55.6% (n=10) of the 'unstable' category has a visible defect. Attention is drawn to the smaller number of people having a non-visible cleft (44.4%, n=8).

In view of the consistent pattern of results, there is a clear association between type of cleft and personality characteristics. That is, the preponderance of adult respondents appear to have desirable personality traits, regardless of their type of cleft. However, as the data portray, this outcome is not universal, since there is a minority of participants who evidence the opposite, less socially appealing characteristics. In considering the implications of the results, one must be aware of making unwarranted value judgements. Nevertheless, since the traits having negative connotations seem to be most evident in the visible cleft population, it could be postulated that these two factors are, in some way related. For instance, since one is born with a certain type of cleft, it is plausible that an individual's personality develops in response to that condition. However, some protagonists would argue that like the severity of clefting, personality is determined before birth.

Definition of the participants' persona in conjunction with factors relating to childhood and adolescent experiences (perceptions of school and victimization)

In this section, attention is turned to the association between previous circumstances and experiences (especially those related to school), and the way in which the individuals now see themselves. When focusing upon the individuals' own adjustment to the cleft and their perceptions of school, a close association is found between the encountering of personal problems and negative impressions of school. Although the correspondence does not reach statistical significance on this occasion, it is noteworthy that 72.4% (n=42) of patients with unhappy memories of their school days, also suffered some psychological adjustment problems. This figure compares with the minority who perceived school negatively, but appear to have had no adjustment problems (30.2% of the 'well-adjusted' group, n=16). At the same time, however, most participants, regardless of personal problems, held their schooling in positive esteem (62.5% of those with problems, n=70 and 69.8% of the 'well-adjusted" group, n=37).

On the basis of these findings, the prediction is realized that negative perceptions of school are more associated with personal adjustment problems in adjusting to the defect, than with no adjustment problems. What is harder to establish is the extent to which the problems were exacerbated at school or vice versa, as there is evidence to support both of these possibilities. In attempting to unravel the most potent influences upon the individuals' psychosocial development, reference is made to the impact of school-related experiences upon the participants' private persona.

Given that teasing directly impinges upon the victim's private persona, data relating to teasing have been cross-tabulated with those of personal adjustment to the cleft. As anticipated, there is an apparent (although non-significant) correspondence between people who encountered personal problems and those who were teased. More precisely, it transpires that of those displaying some form of psychological maladjustment, 91.1% (n=51) were victimized by peers. Conversely, no experience of being ridiculed appears to be associated with satisfactory adjustment (66.7% of those not teased, n=10). Having said this, 90.3% (n=93) of individuals with no apparent problems were also ridiculed. Needless to say, it is conjectured that personal adjustment difficulties tended to be compounded by additional teasing.

The impact of adversity is also apparent regarding untoward school experiences. Indeed, previous suggestion of a persisting cycle of disadvantage into adulthood gains credence, when the relationship between self-esteem and negative perceptions of school is examined. As the findings indicate, 72.7% (n=8) of the lowest self-esteem groups (scores 5 and 6) held negative perceptions of their schooling.

Alongside this finding, however, are data relating to self-esteem which support the trend that most respondents show resilience in adulthood, despite their earlier circumstances and experiences. That is, the majority of those incorporated into the highest self-esteem categories (55.0%, n=82; scores 0 and 1) also had unhappy memories of their school days.

Although negative school perceptions predominate in the low self-esteem group, most of the participants in both the positive and negative perception categories demonstrate high levels of self-esteem (95.7%, n=67 and 91.1%, n=82 respectively). Indeed, it appears that a greater proportion of respondents with adverse memories of school fall into the high self-esteem category, compared with the positive memories group.

Therefore, it transpires that the majority of respondents with low self-esteem, are characterized by having a visible cleft and negative school perceptions. The findings implicate that whilst the majority of participants can enjoy high levels of self-esteem in their adult years (whatever the nature of their school memories), a small number of them seem to be adversely affected by them, as may be evidenced by a low self-esteem. As the various findings increasingly suggest, a minority subgroup continue to be at a disadvantage on reaching adulthood.

The fundamental issue to emerge from this picture concerns the identification of what can be broadly classified as coping mechanisms. More precisely, one needs to ask what determines the impact of participants' past adversity upon their present psychosocial functioning, since some respondents appear to emerge unscathed, whilst others evidence further tribulation. By way of gathering testimony to these discrepant outcomes, reference is made to supplementary data prior to discussing the implications in chapter eight.

The notion that early adverse experiences do affect the long term psychosocial functioning of those encountering them, is reinforced in consulting the data relating to teasing. The results below are amongst the most striking found in the study, in that they implicate the potentially persistent and psychologically damaging effects of being teased by peers. On analyzing the data, it becomes immediately apparent that all of the respondents indicating the lowest levels of self-esteem, had been subjected to teasing (100.0%, n=10; scores 5 and 6). In contrast, all of those who reported no experience of victimization responded in the direction of highest self-esteem (100.0%, n=29; scores 0 and 1). At the same time, however, the majority of the high self-esteem group were teased in their youth (79.9%, n=115; scores 0 and 1). Therefore, whilst subjection to teasing is not exclusive to the low self-esteem participants, it is evident that the former is a common feature of the latter.

When consulting the data referring to personality traits and adverse experiences, there is further substantiation of a disadvantaged subgroup amongst the participants. That is, the majority of those exhibiting the less socially desirable personality traits of neuroticism, introversion, a closed and antagonistic outlook upon life, and undirectedness report negative perceptions of school and/or experiences of being teased.

It will become immediately apparent to the reader, that it is precisely these characteristics that have been already identified in conjunction with a visible cleft above. Concerning measures of Neuroticism, 72.3% (n=34) of respondents who were reportedly 'insecure'/'very insecure', expressed negative perceptions of school ($p < 0.05$). This percentage is increased to 93.5% (n=44) for the 'insecure' group who had been subjected to teasing ($p < 0.05$). However, as with data concerning type of cleft, there is a trend for the majority of individuals harbouring either positive or negative impressions of school, to be 'secure' (78.0% with positive perceptions, n=46 and 58.5% with negative perceptions, n=48 respectively).

Similarly, the preponderance of respondents perceived themselves to be 'secure', regardless of whether or not they had been teased in their youth (61.6% of those teased, n=69 and 86.4% of those not teased, n=19). However, as is evident in many instances, the effect of adversity may be reflected in the difference between the two proportions elicited for the 'secure' group. For example, there is almost a twenty per cent difference between those with positive (78.0%), or negative (58.5%) school perceptions, who identified themselves as being 'secure' (or 'very secure'). An even greater difference is found for the subsequent results pertaining to teasing and being 'secure' (86.4% and 61.6% respectively). In that the above pattern of responses is evident in nearly all of the remaining measures of personality in association

138

with school perceptions and incidents of teasing, reference is made only to the statistically significant findings.

Although it was established earlier that the personality traits are indicative of the participants' adult functioning, there is some value in considering the way in which the less socially desirable characteristics could have been reinforced by unrewarding personal and social interactions, such as take place at school. Alternatively, since interaction can be defined broadly as the active engagement of personalities, the constellation of an individual's public persona could influence the nature of the interaction. For example, there is evidence of an association between 'self-consciousness' (indicative of Neuroticism), and both negative impressions of school and subjection to teasing. These relationships reach 1% level of statistical significance.

Regarding those who considered themselves 'self-conscious', 74.1% (n=63) held negative school perceptions. In addition, 72.4% (n=63) with negative school perceptions were 'self-conscious'. Moreover, 91.5% (n=75) of the 'self-conscious' group had been subjected to teasing, and the majority of those teased were 'self-conscious' (64.1% of the teased group, n=75). On these occasions, the majority of those with adverse experiences do not display the positive dimension of the measure (that of 'comfortable'). Indeed, only the preponderance of those with optimistic school perceptions and with no experiences of victimization, believe that they are now 'comfortable' (61.4% of the positive perception group, n=35 and 69.6% of those not teased, n=16).

In view of the findings, it could be argued that previous experiences of school (including victimization), were so distressing as to have exerted a long term deleterious effect upon the participants' public persona. On the other hand, it is also plausible that personalities which were perceived by peers to be vulnerable (including self-conscious), were precisely those who became the targets for stigmatization. Whilst it is conceivable that both interpretations are tenable, the extent to which the factors are directly related to the cleft cannot be easily determined. Despite the fact that one has to contend with speculations on this matter, other data elicited by the shortened personality inventory support the notion that those whose earlier experiences were disadvantaged by trauma and tribulation, are the most likely candidates for persistent disadvantage in adulthood. In this instance, the yardstick is defined by the constellation of a socially desirable personality.

With respect to the five factor model of personality, it is notable that all measures of Neuroticism reach statistical significance when compared with data relating to school perceptions. In addition to the two items discussed above ('insecure-secure' and 'comfortable-self-conscious'), there appears to be a close correspondence between the undesirable traits of 'worrying' and 'temperamental' with adverse experiences at school.

Concerning the respondents who identified themselves as 'worrying'/' 'very worrying', 75.0% (n=30) of them carried untoward memories of their schooling (p < 0.01), whilst 85.4% (n=35) of the worriers had been teased

139

(non-significant). As might be anticipated by now, the majority of the respondents was 'calm'/'very calm' irrespective of whether or not their schooling had been happy (82.8%, n=48 and 59.5%, n=44 with positive and negative perceptions respectively), and/or whether or not they had been teased (65.7%, n=67 and 76.9%, n=20 of those teased or not teased respectively).

Further evidence of the neurotic tendencies of the minority subgroup amongst the participants, emanates from the measure of temperament. That is, 70% (n=35) of those claiming to be 'temperamental' harboured pessimistic feelings about school (p < 0.05), and a striking 91.7% (n=44) of them had been subjected to teasing (non-significant). In contrast, of the respondents with positive perceptions of school, 74.6% (n=44) reported to be 'even-tempered', as did the small majority of those with negative impressions of school (57.8% of the negative group, n=48). Similarly, the preponderance of individuals were 'even-tempered' despite the fact that some of them had been victimized (62.1% of those teased, n=72 and 82.6% of those not teased, n=19). Once again, the reader's attention is drawn to the disparity between the findings pertaining to respondents with and without a history of adversity, which suggests that the former does exert some impact upon adult psychosocial functioning.

Therefore, it appears that those whose previous experiences of peer interaction have been impaired to some degree, are most susceptible to a neurotic disposition in adulthood. Neurotic traits are precisely those which can impede effective personal and social relationships. It follows that the cycle of disadvantage, in terms of being deprived of rewarding relationships may persist for this unfortunate minority into adulthood.

In consulting data which measure Extraversion, the plight of those who are by implication introverted, provides further insight into a disadvantaged subgroup amongst the respondents. For example, regarding the item 'retiring-sociable', 73.5% (n=25) of those in the 'retiring'/'very retiring' categories felt negatively about their school experiences (p < 0.05). However, consistent with previous findings, the majority of those with either positive or negative impressions of school considered themselves to be 'sociable' (84.5% of the positive group, n=49 and 67.9% of the negative group, n=53 respectively).

Likewise, the vast majority of respondents who were 'reserved' (as opposed to 'affectionate'), had been subjected to teasing in their youth (96.3% of the 'reserved' group, n=52). This correlation reaches 1% level of statistical significance. Needless to say, most of the individuals evaluated themselves as being 'affectionate', regardless of having been teased (60.0% of those teased, n=78 and 91.3% of those not teased, n=21). On this occasion there is a marked discrepancy between the two scores pertaining to 'affectionate', which suggests that the experience of being teased may have a profound effect upon the victim's public persona in adult life.

The potential association between unsatisfactory social intercourse and socially undesirable personality traits, is strengthened in examining measures reflecting the antithesis of the factors of Openness, Agreeableness and Conscientiousness (namely, a closed, antagonistic and undirected outlook respectively). For instance, the data show a strong correspondence between an 'unadventurous' spirit and negative school perceptions (p < 0.01). That is, of those reporting to be 'unadventurous' or 'very unadventurous', 78.9% (n=30) held adverse impressions of their schooling. This figure compares with the majority of respondents who were 'daring'/'very daring', whatever the nature of their school memories (82.2% with positive perceptions, n=37, and 58.9% with negative perceptions, n=43).

Within the dimension of Extraversion, further substantiation is available of the fundamentally different personality types which seem to typify the majority and minority subgroups amongst the participants. Another statistically significant result (p < 0.05) which points to the existence of these subgroups in adulthood, concerns the finding that a 'conventional' approach to life is more apparent in respondents who were teased, compared with those were not teased (95.1% of those teased, n=39 versus 4.9% of those not teased, n=2). Needless to say, most individuals fell into the 'original' category whether or not they had been victimized (55.2% of the teased group, n=48 and 86.7% of those not teased, n=13).

Since the emerging pattern of responses is common to all measures of Extraversion, it transpires that the participants who veer towards introversion, tend to be those whose school experiences were disadvantageous. Whilst it could be argued that introverts do not necessarily seek, nor need the company of other people compared with more extravert personalities, the issue concerns the quality, rather than the quantity of personal and social relationships.

In examining the factor of Agreeableness versus Antagonism, a similar set of results is discovered regarding perceptions of school and the experience of teasing. For example, although none of the cross-tabulations relating to the respondents' school perceptions reach statistical significance in this dimension, the great majority of those claiming to be 'serious' had been teased (93.5% of those teased, n=29). This high incidence contrasts with the preponderance of individuals who considered themselves 'cheerful', despite victimization in their youth (69.5% of those teased, n=66 and 91.3% of those not teased, n=21). This correlation reaches 1% level of statistical significance.

Thus, whilst socially undesirable traits indicative of Antagonism (namely, 'suspicious', 'stubborn', 'serious' and 'proud') are most apparent in those with adverse school experiences, most participants displayed the socially desirable characteristics associated with its corollary Agreeableness (namely, 'trusting', 'flexible', and 'cheerful'). The only exception to this pattern concerns the opposing pair 'proud-humble', in which the majority of the respondents, regardless of whether or not they had encountered unhappy incidents at school (including teasing), reported to be 'proud', a trait indicative of Antagonism (for example, 82.8% of the positive perception group, n=48 and 74.7% of the negative perception group, n=59).

As with all measures, the responses made in this instance depend upon the respondents' understanding of the terms used. It is therefore conceivable that the adjective 'proud', was equated with feeling unashamed rather than conceited. In this respect, the high incidence of responses incorporated into the 'proud'/'very proud' category can be seen to correspond with the general pattern of results, indicating the socially valued traits exhibited by the majority of participants.

Findings deriving from the fifth factor of Conscientiousness versus Undirectedness, continue the trend identified above. That is, in all measures reflecting the socially unattractive inclination towards Undirectedness, the majority of responses were elicited by those with adverse school memories and/or who had been teased. In contrast, the preponderance of the positive and negative perception groups responded in the direction of Conscientiousness, as did those with or without experience of teasing.

Although none of the cross-tabulations pertaining to this dimension of personality reach statistical significance, the reader's attention is drawn to two particularly notable findings regarding the association between aimlessness and emotional instability, and teasing. Concerning the former, 94.7% (n=18) of those who were reportedly 'aimless' had been teased, compared with most respondents who considered themselves 'ambitious' despite peer victimization (82.4% of those teased, n=84 and 95.2% of those not teased, n=20). Similar proportions are found for the emotionally 'unstable' group (94.1% were teased, n=16), and for individuals with or without experience of being teased, who were 'emotionally stable' (87.0% of those teased, n=107 and 96.2% of those not teased, n=25).

The implications of the findings relating to personality and adverse school experiences, reinforce the notion of a persistently disadvantaged subgroup amongst the participants, which evolved during the individuals' formative years. Overall, the findings appear to point most convincingly towards a compromise position. Just as a visible cleft may predispose the child towards the likelihood of encountering adverse social experiences (such as teasing), the possession of certain personality traits may increase the likelihood of experiencing adversity. One needs only to consider the potentially fated plight of the vulnerable child, whose bullying peers perceive as insecure and self-conscious, and therefore a rewarding target.

In contemplating this scenario, it must be recalled that the majority of those with a visible cleft, negative school perceptions, and/or experience of being teased, are able to project optimism as adults. That is, instead of being stigmatized by their earlier disadvantages, they believe themselves to be free of neurotic tendencies, verging on extraversion, open-minded, agreeable and conscientious. Into this camp, can be placed those participants, who despite being raised in potentially deleterious circumstances, now respond in the direction of high self-esteem.

As yet, discussion has centred upon the connection between aspects of the participants' past and present lives, in terms of psychosocial functioning. The opportunity is now seized to extend the analysis, by considering the way in which the cleft defect was manifested, and thus comprised an integral component of the individuals' public persona. By cross-tabulating the relevant data with perceptions of school and experiences of teasing, one may appreciate more fully, the extent to which adverse experiences can be attributed to the presence of the defect. In doing so, tentative explanations can be proposed to account for the persistence of the cycle of disadvantage in adulthood.

Definition of the participants' public persona in conjunction with factors relating to social interaction (perceptions of school and victimization)

This section focuses upon the way in which the individuals presented themselves to the 'outside' world (public persona). That is, how they appear to their peers, and how peers respond to what they see.

It is anticipated that the extent to which the cleft is visible will affect peer perception of the cleft-impaired person. Consequently, the quality of interaction between the cleft-impaired individual and his orher peers, will be inevitably influenced by the presence of the defect. At the same time, the individual's self-perception and the way in which he or she senses peers to be perceiving him or herself, actively influences the nature of the social intercourse. Thus, the public image which the visibly cleft-impaired portray, and the response it elicits from peers warrants attention, in detecting the existence of an 'at risk' group amongst the participants.

BNH's data concerning the monitoring of speech and appearance at School Age Assessment (SAA) and Latest Speech Assessment (LSA), indicate the extent of the patients' impairment in terms of audible and/or visible defects (chapter four). These data can now be compared with those reflecting instances of social interaction, such as school perceptions, and the experience of teasing. For example, it is expedient to ascertain whether or not 'unacceptable' speech and/or 'unsatisfactory' appearance correlates positively with negative perceptions of school and/or incidents of teasing. Within the developmental framework being pursued, the data relating to School Age Assessment will be examined prior to the later stage regarding Latest Speech Assessment.

School Age Assessment (SAA) School Age Assessment was undertaken by BNH and her colleagues, when the patients were aged between 54 and 64 months (4.5-5.5 years old). Consequently, the results broadly represent the extent of the audible (speech) and/or visible (appearance) impairments evident on commencing school. In view of this, the data have been cross-tabulated with the more recently acquired information regarding the individuals' perceptions of being at school with a cleft, and incidents of teasing. The most notable of the findings will be now discussed.

The following findings pertain to the way in which the young children presented themselves to their peers (in terms of speech and appearance), and the nature of the school-related experiences which they subsequently encountered. Given the small number of patients who were assessed as having 'unacceptable' nasality at SAA (n=30), it is notable that 63.3% (n=19) of them retrospectively perceived their school days in negative terms. This figure, however, contrasts with a similar percentage of children with no or slight nasality who also expressed pessimistic feelings about school (60.0%, n=111). Needless to say, 87.1% (n=74) of those with positive memories of their schooling were deemed to have no, or negligible nasality.

Articulation at SAA evidences similar results, with most of those displaying 'unacceptable' articulation reporting negative impressions of school (70.3% of the 'unacceptable' group, n=45). However, a smaller proportion of participants whose articulation fell within 'acceptable' limits felt adversely about school (56.3%, n=85). Once again, a comparatively strong association exists between a positive perception of school and 'acceptable' speech (77.6% of the positive perception group, n=66).

With respect to appearance at SAA, the relationship between severe impairment and negative school perceptions is even more apparent. Concerning the children with an 'unsatisfactory' lip and/or nose (n=97), the majority of them appeared to have been unhappy at school (76.3% of the 'unsatisfactory' group, n=74), but so too was most of those with 'satisfactory' assessment (68.8% of the 'satisfactory' group, n=22). However, only a minority of patients were happy at school and had 'satisfactory' facial features (30.3% of the positive group, n=10).

Mention must also be made of the assessment of patients' skeletal and dental aspect at SAA. In undertaking the relevant cross-tabulations, there is strong evidence to support the relationship between obvious impairment and pessimism about schooling. For example, of the individuals whose skeletal and dental aspect was deemed to be 'unsatisfactory' (n=145), 69.0% of them perceive their school days in negative terms. Whilst this figure is set alongside the total of 60% (n=6) of patients with a 'satisfactory' assessment who were pessimistic about their schooling, the reader's attention is drawn to the number of participants represented in each case (n=145 and n=6 respectively). Furthermore, it appears that a mere 8.2% (n=4) of those with positive school memories presented with a 'satisfactory' skeletal and dental aspect.

Although the results relating to SAA and school perceptions are statistically non-significant, a consistent picture emerges which suggests that even at the start of schooling, an 'at risk' group of children can be identified. Indeed, the findings infer that where a child begins education with 'unacceptable' speech and/or 'unsatisfactory' physical cleft-related features, he or she is prone to encounter adverse experiences at school. This association is particularly apparent in instances of 'unsatisfactory' appearance. Furthermore, it seems that where the symptoms of clefting are manifestly obvious to peers (whether in audible and/or visible terms), the children concerned are more likely than those with less evident manifestations, to harbour negative impressions of their school days. The extent to which such pessimism may be attributable to peer victimization at school, is the subsequent area of investigation.

In that the act of teasing may be seen in terms of provocation, it is important to attempt to identify what factor(s) may have induced this untoward response. Since most of the teasing reported by participants took place in the school context, the bullies and the bullied were usually school contemporaries. In general, it is plausible, that where the projected image of a person encompasses disfigurement (whether audible and/or visible), the disfigurement acquires disproportionate significance in distinguishing the individual as 'different' by his or her peers. Moreover, being 'different' appears to warrant differential treatment by other people, perhaps to the extent of legitimizing victimization in their eyes.

In comparing the data relating to teasing with aspects of cleft-related speech and appearance, the implications for those with 'unacceptable' features are all too evident. For example, of the patients with 'unacceptable' nasality at SAA, 92.9% (n=26) of them were subjected to teasing. This figure compares with 82.7% (n=148) who exhibited 'acceptable' nasality yet were still teased. The percentage increases to a statistically significant level ($p < 0.01$), for those presenting with 'unacceptable' articulation who were teased (95.0% of the 'unacceptable' group, n=57). However, the majority of children with 'acceptable' articulation were also victimized (79.6% of the 'acceptable' group, n=117).

The trend suggesting differential treatment continues with respect to the association between assessment of physical features and teasing. That is, whilst 95.7% (n=90) of the patients with an 'unsatisfactory' lip and/or nose were apparently teased, so too was 92.0% (n=126) of those with an 'unsatisfactory' skeletal and dental aspect. These high percentages need to be compared alongside the proportion of individuals who presented with 'satisfactory' features who were ridiculed by peers (93.8% of the 'satisfactory' lip and/or nose group, n=30, and 90.0% of the 'satisfactory' skeletal and dental aspect group, n=9).

The implications to emerge from this array of findings, is that teasing is an almost universal experience of those with obvious impairment. At the same time however, it appears that a high proportion of participants with 'acceptable' speech and/or appearance were victimized. The most feasible explanation for this outcome is that whilst the great majority of participants were teased, it is possible that those with 'acceptable' speech (nasality and/or articulation) may have been teased about their 'unacceptable' appearance (lip and/or nose and skeletal and dental aspect), and vice versa.

145

For example, cross-tabulation of details concerning aspects of speech with appearance at SAA, show that 75.9% (n=85) of patients with 'acceptable' nasality had an 'unsatisfactory' lip and/or nose.

Similarly, most of those with 'acceptable' articulation, were perceived to have an 'unsatisfactory' appearance (73.8% of the 'acceptable' articulation group, n=62). On the other hand, only a minority of individuals whose lip and/or nose was considered to be 'satisfactory', displayed 'unacceptable' nasality or articulation (18.2% and 33.3% of the 'satisfactory' group respectively, n=6 and n=11 respectively).

With respect to the results relating to the participants' public persona at SAA, there is evidence that a disadvantaged subgroup exists, whose early psychosocial development is potentially at risk. The fundamental question still to be addressed, is the extent to which individuals are able to avert the potentially damaging consequences of their experiences in later life. Attention is first turned to examining the consistency of results concerning School Age Assessment and Latest Speech Assessment.

Latest Speech Assessment (LSA) As stated previously, the age of the patients at the Latest Speech Assessment, was determined by BNH and her colleagues' decision to cease data collection on 31st December 1975. Consequently, at LSA the patients ranged from five to twenty-six years old. The diversity of the individuals' ages need to be borne in mind in interpreting the subsequent findings.

In perusing the data there is a consistent relationship between 'unacceptable' speech (nasality and/or articulation) or 'unsatisfactory' appearance (lip/nose and skeletal/dental), and negative school perceptions. That is, of the small number of patients displaying 'unacceptable' nasality at LSA (n=21), 71.4% (n=15) held negative impressions of their school days. In comparison, a lower proportion of those with 'acceptable' nasality felt adversely about their schooling (59.3% of the 'acceptable' group, n=115). Similarly, in the case of 'unacceptable' articulation at LSA (n=33), 63.6% expressed negative feelings about school, which contrasts with the slightly diminished figure of 59.9% (n=109) of patients with 'acceptable' articulation who were unhappy at school.

This pattern of responses continues with respect to 'unsatisfactory' appearance of the lip and nose at LSA (n=40), with 70% (n=28) reporting negative perceptions of school. Concerning the assessment of skeletal/dental aspect at LSA, although there is no directly comparable category designating unsatisfactory progress, reference on this occasion is made to the group who were awaiting intervention (n=89). The inference is that these individuals would not be requiring treatment if their features were satisfactory. Needless to say, 65.2% (n=58) of those anticipating further intervention felt negatively about their schooling. However, of those with a 'satisfactory' lip and/or nose, 76.4% (n=68) held their school days in low esteem, as did 60.0% (n=6) with a 'satisfactory' skeletal/dental aspect.

146

Although none of these findings reach statistical significance, it does appear that most of those with 'unacceptable' or 'unsatisfactory' speech and/or appearance (respectively), perceived their school days in a negative way. The data also show that the preponderance of those with an 'acceptable' or 'satisfactory' outcome, also harboured adverse school memories. Whilst these findings implicate that a clear-cut association cannot be detected between severely impaired speech and/or appearance and pessimistic attitudes towards school, two alternative explanations invite consideration.

Firstly, since LSA was undertaken at diverse ages (5-26 years old), the assessment results are not representative of a specific stage of schooling (unlike SAA). The data do not necessarily reflect the way in which the individuals spoke nor appeared to their peers and teachers at school. Secondly, although a patient's speech and/or appearance may have been assessed as within the 'acceptable' limit, this evaluation may not have equated with the individuals' self-perception and peer perception of the features concerned. Thus, if and when the patient perceived him or herself negatively, and/or was treated as such by peers, it is conceivable that his/her memories of school have been coloured by the nature of personal and peer perceptions, rather than those held by the professionals conducting the assessment. This has clear implications for the professionals' role in raising the patients' self-confidence.

Regarding the association between LSA and the participants' experiences of being teased, a close correlation emerges between 'unacceptable' nasality at LSA and teasing ($p < 0.05$). That is, 100% (n=20) of the patients exhibiting 'unacceptable' nasality were teased. There is also evidence of a strong relationship between 'unacceptable' articulation at LSA and victimization ($p < 0.01$). In this instance, 96.7% (n=29) of those with 'unacceptably' defective articulation reported subjection to teasing. Although it is notable that individuals with no or slight (within 'acceptable' limit) nasality or articulation were also teased (82.3%, n=154, and 81.9%, n=145 respectively), it is propounded that teasing is more inevitable where the degree of nasality or articulation is perceived to be 'unacceptable'.

The inclination for 'unacceptable' impairment to provoke ridicule is also reinforced by data pertaining to appearance at LSA, although they do not reach statistical significance. For example, in 97.4% (n=37) of instances where the appearance of the lip and nose was deemed 'unsatisfactory', the individuals concerned had been teased. Likewise, of those awaiting treatment for skeletal/dental anomalies (n=84), the great majority of patients (91.7%, n=74) had been victimized. The findings relating to 'satisfactory' appearance at LSA also show a high correspondence with reported teasing. For instance, of the 'satisfactory' lip and nose group 94.3% (n=87) of the individuals had been teased. Concerning the 'satisfactory' skeletal/dental group, 89.8% (n=44) were apparently teased.

The comparatively high proportion of patients with 'normal' speech and/or appearance who were still teased, requires some explanation. In doing so, reference is made to the suggestion cited above, that instances of perceptually 'normal' speech may have been accompanied by 'unsatisfactory' appearance, and vice versa. By implication, the impairment(s) may have provoked teasing. For example, at LSA, 30.3% (n=37) of patients with 'acceptable' nasality, and 27.1% (n=29) of those with 'acceptable' articulation exhibited 'satisfactory' lip and/or nose features. These figures compare with 5.6% (n=5) and 13.3% (n=12) of individuals with a 'satisfactory' appearance, but who presented with 'unacceptable' nasality or articulation respectively.

Overall, these results suggest that it may be possible to predict the potential victims of teasing. In doing so, one hopes that effective measures can be taken to avert the suffering which such victimization clearly causes. The implications of these findings will be further addressed in chapter eight.

A longitudinal perspective: the impact of aspects of the participants' past life history upon their present perceptions

In view of the discussion so far, one of the most notable findings concerns the identification of a subgroup of participants, whose personal and social development appears to have been hampered by disadvantage. Whereas the previous sections have explored the evidence for a disadvantaged minority, this section investigates the determinants of the persistence of the cycle of disadvantage into adulthood. In doing so, emphasis is placed upon the adult participants' own evaluations concerning the impact the cleft has exerted upon their lives.

It will be recalled that in evaluating the influence of the cleft upon aspects of life (chapter five), most of those registering the defect's 'high'/'very high' impact upon their education, dating, teasing, occupation and/or appearance, harboured negative feelings about school ($p < 0.01$ in each instance). The same trend was evident regarding the defect's impact upon aspects of life and experience of teasing. That is, where the deformity was believed to have wielded a 'high'/'very high' effect in an area of life, the majority of the participants had been teased ($p < 0.01$ pertaining to education, dating, and appearance). On the basis of these data, it seems that adverse school experiences including teasing, may be attributable to the cleft even with the wisdom of hindsight.

In attempting to extrapolate the extent to which the type of cleft determines the perceived influence of the defect upon life, it transpires that a visible cleft (cleft lip and palate) exerts a notably higher influence than a non-visible cleft (cleft palate only) upon all areas of life investigated. As in all discussion regarding type of cleft in the current study, it should be remembered that those with a visible defect (cleft lip), have also had to contend with the problems associated with a non-visible defect (cleft palate), since they have both cleft lip and palate. The reader's attention is drawn to the relevant data below, which for the purposes of clarity are displayed in tabular form (Tables 6.1-6.5).

Table 6.1
Perceived influence of cleft upon education and
type of cleft according to visibility of defect

Type of cleft	Perceived influence of cleft upon education		
	High/ very high	Low/ very low	Total
Non-visible cleft of the palate only	13	39	52
Visible cleft of the lip and palate	52	52	104
Total	65	91	156

NB: $p < 0.01$

Tables 6.1 and 6.2 are concerned with areas of intellectual functioning namely education (Table 6.1), which is superseded in life by occupation (Table 6.2). With respect to type of cleft and the influence of the deformity upon education and occupation, the data intimate a close correspondence between perceptions of a 'high'/'very high' influence and visibility of the cleft. That is, regarding the area of education, the great majority of individuals who perceive the defect to have exerted a 'high'/'very high' impact upon their education, also have a visible cleft (80%, n=52). This finding reaches 1% level of statistical significance.

Similarly (although statistically non-significant), most of those feeling that their occupation has been 'highly'/'very highly' influenced by the defect, have a visible cleft (64.7%, n=22). On the basis of these data, it appears that where the cleft is considered to have been an influential factor regarding education and occupation, the respondents have a visible rather than non-visible cleft.

Table 6.2

**Perceived influence of cleft upon occupation and
type of cleft according to visibility of defect**

Type of cleft	Perceived influence of cleft upon education		
	High/very high	Low/very low	Total
Non-visible cleft of the palate only	12	62	74
Visible cleft of the lip and palate	22	75	97
Total	34	137	171

Table 6.3

**Perceived influence of cleft upon appearance and
type of cleft according to visibility of defect**

Type of cleft	Perceived influence of cleft upon appearance		
	High/very high	Low/very low	Total
Non-visible cleft of the palate only	8	65	73
Visible cleft of the lip and palate	71	24	95
Total	79	89	168

NB: p < 0.01

When contemplating the perceived impact of the cleft upon the physical domain of appearance in relation to type of cleft, one needs only to refer to Table 6.3 to discover that 89.9% (n=71) of those who believed that their appearance had been affected by the cleft to a 'high'/'very high' degree, had a visible deformity (p < 0.01). The implication of this tendency is that the majority of those with a cleft lip and palate were self-conscious about their disfigurement, to the extent that their self-perception seems to have been defined by the presence of the cleft.

The subsequent two tables are concerned with the influence of the cleft upon aspects of psychosocial functioning, namely dating and teasing, and the association with type of cleft. In both instances, most of the individuals presenting with a visible defect, attribute 'high'/'very high' influence to the cleft.

Table 6.4
Perceived influence of cleft upon dating and
type of cleft according to visibility of defect

Type of cleft	Perceived influence of cleft upon dating		
	High/ very high	Low/ very low	Total
Non-visible cleft of the palate only	15	51	66
Visible cleft of the lip and palate	73	19	92
Total	88	70	158

NB: $p < 0.01$

With reference to Table 6.4, 83.0% (n=73) of the individuals who perceived the cleft to have exerted a 'high'/'very high' influence upon dating had a visible impairment. The corresponding figure for these categories regarding teasing is 69.2% (n=81) of respondents (Table 6.5 below). These statistically significant correlations (at the 1% level) reinforce the emerging picture, that the personal and social relationships of respondents with a visible cleft may be particularly vulnerable.

Table 6.5
Perceived influence of cleft upon teasing and
type of cleft according to visibility of defect

Type of cleft	Perceived influence of cleft upon teasing		
	High/ very high	Low/ very low	Total
Non-visible cleft of the palate only	36	38	74
Visible cleft of the lip and palate	81	18	99
Total	117	56	173

NB: $p < 0.01$

In view of the demonstrable relationships between the visibility of the cleft, and the influence attributed to the cleft in intellectual, physical and psychosocial spheres of the participants' lives, it is postulated that those born with a visible cleft are most 'at risk' within the cleft population. To clarify further, the findings relating to the perceived impact of the cleft, consistently suggest that the cleft is considered to have been most stigmatizing, where its existence could not be disguised nor denied.

Moreover, since 'high'/'very high' influence infers that the defect expended a negative, rather than a positive impact upon the stipulated areas of life, these personal evaluations can be seen as reflecting the stigma experienced by the respondents in each instance.

Attention is turned subsequently to the association between areas of life which were evidently influenced by the cleft, and the participants' changed perceptions on reaching adulthood. The reader is reminded that the majority of individuals holding adverse school perceptions reported increased self-confidence since leaving school ($p < 0.01$), as did those who were teased (chapter five). The optimistic outcome which these results infer is reinforced by the finding that even in the face of earlier adversity, most of the adult respondents were able to proffer positive advice to the hypothetical parents of a cleft-impaired infant.

Since type of cleft (visibility of the cleft), has been an instrumental variable in identifying the existence of a cycle of disadvantage, it has been cross-tabulated with the respondents' changed perceptions about school since leaving school. It transpires, that the majority of those reporting increased self-confidence have a visible cleft (cleft lip and palate), compared with those who perceive no change in their outlook, or lack self-confidence (78.0%, n=71 and 52.9%, n=63 respectively). This association between identified change and type of cleft reaches 1% level of statistical significance. Thus, it seems that although individuals with a visible cleft are most prone to negative school perceptions, they are more likely than those with a non-visible cleft to experience increased self-confidence on leaving the school environment.

The statistically non-significant findings regarding the participants' current levels of satisfaction with speech and appearance, show that the great majority of both the visible (cleft lip and palate) and non-visible (cleft palate only) groups are 'satisfied'/'very satisfied' with their speech (89.1%, n=82 and 87.0%, n=60 respectively). Although this trend continues with respect to current appearance, there is a lower incidence of those who are 'satisfied' or 'very satisfied' with their appearance amongst the visible cleft group (75.6% with a visible cleft, n=62). The non-visibility of the defect is reflected in the greater satisfaction reported by the cleft palate only group (91.2%, n=62).

Since 76.9% (n=20) of those 'dissatisfied' or 'very dissatisfied' with appearance has a cleft lip and palate, it appears that the disfigurement associated with cleft lip features strongly in the self-perception of some participants. The set of results reach statistical significance ($p < 0.05$).

These findings reinforce the developing picture that whilst the cycle of disadvantage may derive from the formative years, its potentially deleterious long term effects can be reversed for those entangled in it. Nevertheless, there is accumulative evidence that the cycle persists for a minority of adult participants.

In attempting to elucidate the consequences of past adversity upon present perceptions, reference is made to the advice offered by the respondents to parents of a newborn baby with a cleft. The objective of eliciting advice to parents from the adult respondents was in the expectation that their responses would be a projection of their current perspective. Although one might anticipate that previous tribulations would flavour the advice given, a notable majority of respondents extended an optimistic outlook regardless of their earlier adversities (Results III).

In view of the anticipated findings, the cross-tabulation of data relating to advice to parents with those of type of cleft, renders an ambiguous outcome. That is, whilst, 92.9% (n=13) of respondents who emphasized the negative connotations of being born with a cleft had a visible cleft (cleft lip and palate), 88.3% (n=98) of the visible cleft group highlighted the positive aspects of their lives. Furthermore, 98.4% (n=62) of those with a non-visible cleft (cleft palate only) divulged a positive outlook to the hypothetical parents.

By implication, these statistically significant results (p < 0.05) suggest that although a negative outlook tends to be associated with a visible cleft, being born with a visible cleft per se does not necessarily embitter the individual's attitude towards his or her predicament. Indeed, further data analysis relating to the advice offered to parents in conjunction with other core variables, appears to contradict expectation in highlighting the apparent resilience of those considered to be most at risk in their early years.

A prime example of the apparent reversibility regarding the impact of adversity, is evidenced by the association between advice offered to parents and 'environmental aspect' (chapter four). That is, 95.8% (n=23) of respondents whose parents demonstrated a 'detrimental' attitude towards them in their developmental years, highlighted the positive aspects of their experiences in advice given to parents. This percentage exceeds that representing those with 'satisfactory' parenting, who advanced positive advice (91.3% of the 'satisfactory' parental attitude group, n=136). The implications of this finding are particularly optimistic, since the advice proposed might be expected to directly reflect the quality of parenting received by the respondents themselves.

A similar pattern of responses is detected in the type of advice imparted by respondents raised in an 'unfavourable' family environment (chapter four). For example, 91.7% (n=66) of individuals with an 'unfavourable' home situation advocated the positive aspects of being born with a cleft. Once again, this figure surpasses the 90.5% (n=38) of respondents with a 'favourable' home background who projected a positive outlook in their advice to parents.

The evident resilience of the participants is further attested by the finding that, almost all of those who had experienced personal problems in adjusting to the cleft, were now able to offer affirmative advice to parents (97.7% of the personal problems group, n=42). This proportion compares with 87.2% (n=82) of respondents, who were perceived to be 'well-adjusted' in their youth, and who proffered a positive outlook to parents.

In interpreting these findings, the reader will recall that data relating to advice given to parents, were cross-tabulated with adverse perceptions of school and with experiences of teasing (chapter five). The results elicited support the notion that the effects of earlier disadvantage are reversible. Indeed, in both instances, the vast majority of participants who held negative school perceptions, or who were subjected to teasing, wished to capitalize upon the positive aspects of their experiences.

In summary, a clear yet challenging pattern of findings has been established. In one respect, the data show that by adulthood most participants in the study, appear to be functioning satisfactorily in psychosocial terms, regardless of earlier tribulations. In doing so, they reflect an optimistic outcome in the face of adversity. On the other side of the proverbial 'coin', there is consistent evidence that a minority of participants do not necessarily experience positive consequences in adult life. In contrast, the impact of their disadvantaged youth seems all too apparent in their present functioning, demonstrating a pessimistic outcome in the persistence of adversity. In assimilating these two dimensions of the investigation, reference to a metaphorical 'coin' may be peculiarly apposite. That is, the question still to be addressed is what determines for each individual, on which side of the coin he or she will fall. It is to this end (amongst others), that the discussion will be directed in chapter eight, which incorporates the main findings from all four data sets.

7 Living with disfigurement: personal reflections

Introduction

The qualitative, anecdotal data collected during the interviews, have been arranged in such a way as to correspond, as far as possible, to the quantitative data elicited by postal questionnaire. For this reason, the interview data will be presented according to the section headings ('themes') of the questionnaire, with the addition of the final 'Recommendations' section. As the presentation of all the interview data would be inappropriate on this occasion, some data has had to be sacrificed. In classifying the data to be documented, therefore, careful attention has been given to incorporating excerpts which reflect the diversity of interviewees' perceptions and experiences. At the same time, the objective of balanced representation of 'themes' has been of primary importance in identifying pertinent material. In portraying the implications of being born with a cleft from the participants' perspective, the writer has kept her commentary to a minimum, letting the data speak for themselves.

Regarding the selection of participants for interview, the reader is referred to the criteria stipulated in chapter three (design of the study). Following the systematic elimination of individuals who did not meet the criteria, a total of thirteen potential candidates were invited for interview. As one person expressed a wish not to be involved further in the study, interviews were conducted with twelve participants.

During the investigation, two further interviews took place with members of BNH's original Cleft Palate Team. Reference has been made already to their personal recollections (chapter one).

It should be noted that throughout this chapter the identification of the interviewees will remain anonymous. With the exception of added grammatical punctuation, the editing out of redundant 'filler' speech (such as 'um' and 'you know'), and irrelevant material (where diversions were made by the speaker), the data presented are authentic and verifiable. This is evident in the preservation of colloquial language of some excerpts. Where necessary, the researcher has specified the context of a comment by inserting parentheses within quotations.

The themes to be documented and their correspondence to sections of the postal questionnaire are delineated as follows.

- Section A - Personal details
- Section B - Education
- Section C - Employment
- Section D - Speech and appearance
- Section E - National Health Service treatment for the cleft
- Section F - Experiences and perceptions related to the cleft
- Recommendations

Prior to addressing each of the sections in turn, reference is made to data which indicate the interviewees' reactions on receiving the questionnaire, which are generally positive in their sentiments.

I thought it was quite nice actually because ... when you're small you don't really understand what's going on anyway, but when you get older, and talk to other people who have been to the speech therapist, you begin to appreciate what's actually been done, ... its like a way of paying back really what has been done for me, ... I think its nice ... helping ... you the way ... you've helped me, ... I didn't mind at all.

... it was ... pleasant in a way, it was almost like going back to a very old family, because I've always regarded Odstock as my family up here.

Some interviewees volunteered information regarding the reaction of their parents to the sending of the postal questionnaire, which exhibit mixed responses.

I think quite excited really, ... after all the trouble they went through, and how much I would like to put something back in, ... they were quite surprised actually.

(Regarding mother) ... I didn't get any of the sort of 'ooh, let's have a look see then', ... you know the list of qualities ... she never offered any sort of advice as to what she thought her daughter might be, ... so I'm convinced

now in my own mind, true or otherwise, that we're just trying to pretend it never happened.

Section A - Personal details

In preserving the anonymity of the interviewees, details relating to their personal circumstances are contra-indicated on this occasion. Suffice it to say that the individuals comprised six males and six females, whose ages spanned twenty-one to thirty-eight years. In four instances, the interviewees were married with at least one child, the remaining eight were single.

Section B - Education

In examining interview data relating to the interviewee's education, one particular theme tends to predominate, that of teasing at school. In order to maximize insight into the nature and experiences of the interviewee's school days, this section has been further subdivided into level of schooling and aspects relating to teasing.

Memories and perceptions of primary school

Reference to school work (cognitive functioning) The following excerpts strongly suggest that individual learning abilities were thought to be adversely affected by the cleft, either because of the treatment involved, or because of problems relating to the deformity (especially those of hearing loss and teasing).

> *... missing school through hospital appointments and things ... in junior and infants school, and I missed so much of that ... I was ... put in a lower class at school because I was a little bit behind on my reading.*

> *... not being able to hear in class properly ... set me back I think, ... its only one ear ... partially deaf, ... it wasn't really noticed until quite late on.*

> *... it was just teasing, I never liked to read out loud in class because I knew that at playtime or whatever ... I would be teased.*

Reference to teasing and peers (psychosocial functioning) The extent and suffering caused by teasing at primary school becomes increasingly apparent in the ensuing comments, particularly in contrasting home and school environments, and the experiences of being a 'new' pupil at a school. Some individuals, however, appear to have affirmative impressions.

> *... you come from your mum's wing, and then you go to school and*

suddenly there's cruel kids, ... you've never met cruel people ... because your mother's said you're lovely, and you presume you're like everyone else ... you come up against real cruelty, ... so in some degrees it hurts you deeply.

(Regarding new school) ... whenever we were new, you were always introduced ... the teachers never actually said well X's got a cleft palate or anything like that, they just introduced you ... Sometimes I found that hard because then I would think oh, they don't know, how are they going to react when I talk, so quite often I wouldn't talk for ages, because I was frightened of what they'd think.

... apparently before I came, the headmaster made an announcement that I was coming, ... I had no idea that had happened, it was only mentioned in passing ... afterwards, but I think that's quite a good idea ... he told the whole school.

Reference to cleft-related problems (physical functioning) Insight into the impact of having a cleft upon everyday events at school, and how it could alienate a child is offered by the following contributions.

... we used to have the dreaded milk, ... I could never drink very fast out of a straw ... I would have to ... suck four times as hard as anybody else to get any milk up, ... and I always used to be the last to finish, ... I could manage a straw, it'd just take me that little bit longer ... it was something I actually could do ... with everybody else ... but no, ... I got it in a cup ... about seven or eight then.

One interviewee recalled an incident which occurred at school when aged seven, revolving around her need to leave school early in order to attend a follow-up clinic for her cleft at hospital. Apparently, in front of the whole class the teacher asked her where she was going and why. In view of her self-consciousness she did not respond, and was brought to tears by the teacher's further questioning and reprimanding. Although she did not wish to tell the teacher and her classmates that she was going to hospital, a friend subsequently explained this to all present.

Memories and perceptions of secondary school

Reference to school work (cognitive functioning) Regarding perceptions of secondary schooling, there is some speculation that the cleft had a deleterious effect upon educational achievement, but the results were not always disadvantageous according to the interviewees.

... the only thing that ... could have suffered in any way was probably schooling, possibly my parents ... spoiling me too much ... when I got to college ... I didn't work as hard as I could ... so it sort of carried on, because I

didn't have the discipline in my life, because my parents let me get away with things.

... I actually amazed the school because they thought, oh, she won't do any good, ... and I actually passed eight CSEs (Certificate of Secondary Education) at the end of it, and ... from starting off in the lowest class I've managed to prove myself that I can do it.

Reference to teasing and peers (psychosocial functioning) The increasingly significant role played by peers in adolescence, needs to be borne in mind when studying the comments relating to peer relationships and treatment by peers in the secondary school, since it can greatly influence the individual's emerging self-concept and self-esteem.

... I found it very hard, not to make friends but very hard to trust friends. I used to think that people felt sorry for me, that's why they were my friends.

... I tried to join in as much as I could, ... once you're teased you realize you ... always take a step back, and so therefore you were weak ... there's always a weak, ... like nature ... the weak ones are always hounded out ... and the stronger ones get stronger, ... how does one fight back?

At that age they don't know, they don't understand ... always got the odd question, what happened to your face? ... how did you get that scar? ... what's wrong with your face? ... names and just ... endless names, ... I used to cry and cry and cry.

One person said that her older sister with a cleft probably 'broke the ice' for her, when she joined her sister at the same secondary school.

(Regarding hospitalization and class mates) They knew and they all sent me get well cards ... and also presents, ... when I came back they made me feel quite special which was lovely.

Reference to cleft-related problems (physical functioning) The implications of the hospital treatment for a cleft deformity, appear to be addressed by some parents in selecting a school, and by some school staff.

I went to X School (public school) ... and one of the reasons I went there, was because it was sufficiently near Odstock in case anything happened, and would be brought here rather than anywhere else.

I know when I was leading up to an operation that I had, I did ... get a bit frightened ... and my housemaster, he was very good ... and he did sit me down and listen to me and explain, ... but other than that none of the other ... tended to.

159

Circumstances in which teasing occurred at school

Having elucidated from the interview data that teasing was a common experience for those with clefts at both primary and secondary levels of schooling, it is possible to glean further information regarding the circumstances in which the tormenting was likely to occur. The school playground seemed to be the bully's favoured environment, where he/she could make a hasty retreat following the incident, but this was not necessarily the case at boarding school.

> *... at secondary school, especially in my first year ... I can remember being teased in a lunchtime playground by two fourth year girls, and I was only a first year ... and they would just mimic how I spoke ... sometimes I would be on my own, other times I would have friends with me ... it didn't really happen in the classroom as much as it happened in the playground.*

> *... you went along in a class, ... and that class went with you ... through the school, ... so it was usually the same ... meal times, anywhere ... going to bed at night ... playing a sport or you're walking out to the rugby pitch or football pitch, anywhere ... weekends were always worst because all the boys were bored, nothing else to do ... no specific time, continual harassment really ... there were good days, and there were some bloody awful days as well.*

Identification of those responsible for teasing

Those responsible for teasing at school seem to fall into several different categories of bully, although they are, with hindsight, generally regarded as being deficient in some way by the interviewees describing them.

> *... you've got the children ... going 'you look funny', ... or ... 'you look different to me because you're squidgy' ... and then you've got children that are just being honest and saying ... 'you look different to me', which is perfectly true. The next band is where you get the ones that add that little tiny malicious little sentence on the end of it, ... when you're ten you don't understand that they're probably either inadequate, unloved ... insecure or anything ... When you get older you think oh yes, ... I really ought to have felt sorry for them ... maybe that's the only way they can get people to notice them, ... but when you're ten, that sort of adult logic doesn't come into it.*

> *... its their imagination or their inadequacies that will fire at the one person that they feel is weak.*

Teasing stems from the ignorance of other people

With maturity, many interviewees recognized that the teasing they received may have stemmed from ignorance and unfamiliarity with clefts. When some explanation was offered as to why the person looked and/or spoke in a certain way, the ridicule sometimes ceased altogether.

... I think you'll never ever change it, children are honest which is their biggest problem.

... children ... or even adults don't understand things that people do go through, they think oh you're a freak, there's something wrong with you, and until you actually explain it ... they know different and they know its something that can't be helped.

I think that's mainly the general thing, is ignorance from people, because they don't know, I think that's mainly why people tease.

Telling the school teacher about incidences of teasing

Whilst teasing is a predominant feature of some participants' school days, and undoubtedly caused immense suffering at the time, it is notable that very few of them either told their teachers, or thought that the school staff were in a position to help them. Perceptions concerning the negative impact of peer pressure, and the teachers' own lack of understanding suggest why teachers were not approached.

... you go telling the teacher and there's the bully out there, ... I could have (got) hit or anything in my mouth, ... it would have made it worse for me, ... its helped me to stick up more for myself as well.

.. From my own experiences at school, sometimes if you did tell the teacher ... they would say, oh you go running to teacher ... the teacher sticks up for you.

Not an awful lot. I always think, well, if a boy was crying in the corner, one (a teacher) would always come up and say are you alright, come on, come back in, but I don't think any of them really understood, because on the outside all there is, is a scar, you can't see anything more ... where the problems are is inside ... one's head ... being shy it was hard to talk about it.

Telling parents and/or friends about incidences of teasing at school

Although teachers were not considered to be a source of solace for those who were teased at school, the data show that parents rather than friends were told about incidences of teasing. Some individuals preferred not to share their experiences with anyone, and considered the psychological loads carried by their parents in choosing not to tell them.

161

... a few times it did get to me, ... I didn't really speak much to my parents about that sort of thing, ... they've had enough problems I didn't like to burden them with any of mine, ... I think it was really friends and my sister (also with a cleft) at times, not very often, but I'd usually speak to her when she got upset.

... I felt even more alone ... because I didn't go back to my parents and say look, ... because they gave me so much love ... I couldn't break down the walls between my mum and dad and say look, I'm having a bad time, just couldn't do it.

Only my mother really, ... A lot of it I didn't tell her ... I just kept it inside. I used to ... go out to the woods for half an hour and scream and shout, and jump up and down, and sort of try and get it out of my system.

Coping strategies for teasing

In discussing the nature and impact of being teased with the interviewees, it transpired that the teasing elicited a variety of reactions. Some of the reactions constituted effective methods of coping with the ridicule, in that they deflected the provocation, either actively or passively. Other reactions were less successful, and encouraged further tormenting by the obvious distress caused. It appears to be these latter instances which caused the greatest long term trauma and suffering. Since the coping strategies are self-explanatory, further explanation is not deemed necessary by the writer.

a) *Humour*
   ... humour definitely, I was the life and soul ... it had to be channelled into that, ... then you realize ... its nothing to do with how you look, that's the biggest one, when you actually realize that which takes a long time.

   You have to be either twice as humorous, or twice as intelligent with someone to get through to them sometimes, or you've got to just put so much more effort into trying to fit in ... that's the thing, its getting it into your mind that you're going to do that early on, ... it really is the key thing I think.

   ... I've always been told that I have a sense of humour, ... and always see myself as relying on my sense of humour and my personality ... rather than anything else.

b) *Explanation offered by the victim being teased*
   (At senior school) ... I was at the age when I could explain as well, why I was like it ... and it made it easier for the other children too.

   ... the girl I ... went around with, I know at times she would say ... why is

162

your mouth different to mine? And I would say its just something I've got,
a special feature ... and things like that.

c) *Verbal reciprocation*
   (Regarding older sister who has a cleft and was teased) ... I said it doesn't
   matter, think of one (a name) for them, and we used to sit all evening
   writing these names until we found one ... about ten and twelve (years old),
   ... one that really suited ... that would hurt. I said to her you have to say
   things back, or ... say ... sticks and stones and things like that, but she
   always took it to heart.

   Tell them where to go sometimes ... I can't always hold it in, just can't do
   that.

   Tell you what ... you need a book of sarcastic retorts, ... I've had to work out
   a load ... its the only defence apart from actually whacking somebody that
   you've got.

d) *Active avoidance behaviour*
   ... I would (say) to the ... person who's being bullied ... what are you good
   at? ... What do you enjoy doing most that would take you away from the
   situation?

   ... any people that did feel that they wanted to tease me I would just keep out
   of their way anyway, ... because I had my own friends around me they'd
   just leave it.

   ... had a lot of sport ... I had squash, ... a single sport ... off on one's own ...
   still carry it on, but the only reason is because I enjoy being on my own.

e) *Ignore teasing comments*
   ... I'd either ignore them, because they were obviously looking for some
   sarcastic comment or something to get them into a temper ... so I'd either
   just keep quiet, or just hang about with my friends and they wouldn't
   bother really.

   At secondary level ... I went round with the circle which would have given
   the torments, ... the friends I went with they would pick on the fatties ... I
   wouldn't really say I suffered, I took no notice of it ... I ignored it.

f) *Deriving solace from the fact that others face a worse situation*
   What I've been through is nothing compared to what a lot of people have
   been through, and yet, I think, in one context, your own problems always
   seem greater than anyone else's.

(Regarding seeing other children in worse situation in hospital) I think that's probably one of the things that brought it home to me more than anything else.

g) **Felt protected by family and/or friends**
... I've been lucky because I've got a big family, ... I've been to small schools ... I've been quite lucky with ... friendship really, ... if I didn't have ... that I probably would have been a totally different person.

I think in primary school I coped with it better because I had my brothers and sisters with me.

... although it hurt, and it still hurts now if I think about it, ... I think my family helped me cope, because they would always stick up for me. I knew they were there and that I could always when I was small run to one of them, ... I think it would have been harder probably if I hadn't had a large family.

h) **Teasing perceived as being character building**
I think the person (who's) ... teased often comes out ... a more caring person really, ... if its channelled in the right way.

... I think you come out a very strong person anyway out of it, ... I think I matured quite early on from it, ... the key with me is I just really try not think about things.

... teasing is all part of school life, ... and for blokes I suppose it makes a man out of you at the end of the day, ... instils a little bit of discipline.

i) **Positive outlook**
Knock off the negatives, get rid of them ... concentrate on the positives.

... (I) keep going back to this word confidence, ... confidence ... to stand up and say, this is me, this is what I am, take me ... as I come.

She's (mother) never given me any sort of concession whatsoever in any respect. So its like everybody else ... you have to fight for it, which I think now I'm actually grateful for because ... I know ... how to go out and get it,

its never made me rely on people's pity or whatever to give me my own way.

I was taught ... at a very early age that whatever you do, be good at something.

One participant reported that she resolved that her cleft palate would not adversely affect her life in any way, and that with strong will-power and determination it has not done so.

j)   *Negative outlook and response to teasing*
     The person who's being bullied, if you've got a hare lip ... I was told, you're not allowed to get into a fight for obvious reasons, ... so what does one do? I used to ... burst into tears, and you get hounded even more for crying.

     ... its something I've always lacked really ... a lot of confidence, ... and that's ... held me back from ... certain situations.

     (I've) become more introverted I think, and very suspicious of people ... I often think to myself, I wonder what would have happened if I had tried to fight everybody that had a go at me, but then I realize because of my size ... I think it made me very vulnerable psychologically, ... I was always aware that everybody else was bigger than me, and I just didn't fancy getting beaten up every time. I had a few goes, but invariably lost. And in the end, I decided it just wasn't worth it.

If and how teasing changed on leaving school

     I'm an adult now but ... I still have the mickey took out of me, ... anyone really in the street ... just got to live with it.

     ... once I left school that was the end of it. I found my friends at home were totally different, it wasn't that closed environment.

     ... as an adult it's fine, ... I went to work ... but I had some problems in there with male chefs ... I think personally they were just ... ignorant men, but they mimicked me twice, and the first time I ignored it, the second time I got very upset, and I told the manager, but I never went back after that ... I got angry more than upset, ... he was in his fifties this man, the chef.

Perceived change in the attitudes of other people on leaving school

     ... when I first went to work I was an apprentice ... my first year I was still going to college full-time, ... so that was still continual harassment there ... Then after that, it was day release, and some of the lads that started with me, their attitude changed when we went to day release, and there wasn't so much hurt when I was working in the factory on a machine job, ... I was working with a lot of older blokes, and it never even crossed their mind.

     As an adult, I find people are more embarrassed than I am ... couple on holiday we met (daughter had cleft) ... I knew she (mother) was dying to ask me something, because ... you develop this sixth sense, ... they tend to just

165

fidget a bit ... what she wanted to ask me was ... who operated on you? ... Has it ... affected you sort of emotionally? And is there any chance that you could give me a few pointers for when X grows up? ... and yet it took her so long to get round to it.

I've never really had an adult actually make a comment and ask why ... adults tend to understand more, probably because they've been through childhood as well, and they know what its like.

Section C - Employment

The interviewees were asked by the researcher whether or not they felt that they had been discriminated against regarding their employment opportunities. A variety of responses was elicited, ranging from evidence of a blatant display of negative discrimination (due to cleft-related speech), to the recognition that an unimpaired image is generally desirable.

I've only had that happen to me once and that was as an adult, ... I eventually got my interview ... and when he saw me he asked me if I could work in the kitchen, and I said no because I wanted to waitress, and it was because of my speech he wanted me in the kitchen and not to waitress, ... well I went out of there and cried ... I was so hurt and upset.

I think some jobs are like that actually, where you're working with the public and they want you to look good, ... I didn't come across that, but there are jobs around I think ... you can't judge a book by its cover.

... I don't think I've been discriminated against at all, ... I'm always slightly conscious because I do work which involves some public speaking in Magistrates Courts and County Courts, ... that I may not be heard as well as I might be.

Section D - Speech and appearance

Teasing focused upon speech and/or appearance

Although the contributors of the following two excerpts have both cleft lip and palate, their cleft-impaired speech appears to have provoked greater teasing than their facial appearance.

Scar and speech, ... you ... stand up to read some poetry in front of ... twenty boys, they all pick on it straightaway.

... the main reason for my teasing was my speech ... that's why I couldn't

166

*fight back with it, because as soon as I started saying something back ... I'd
get ... (mimicking) back at me.*

Speech therapy

The extent to which individuals were aware that they had received speech
therapy when they were younger clearly varies. Such awareness may have
contributed to a sense of feeling 'different' to one's peers.

*(Regarding speech therapy) I think really I thought it was just part of
growing up sort of thing, that every child had to go, I didn't realize at the
time it was just me and other children in that situation.*

*(Regarding the value of speech therapy) Oh in a big way, ... I
think that was the best thing of all, coming out of it was the pronouncement
of the speech really.*

Perceptions of what having a cleft must be like for the opposite sex

Consideration was given by some participants as to how the experience of
having a cleft might differ for the opposite sex. These insights were entirely
volunteered, and centred on the implications for physical appearance and
being able to cover up the deformity. In all but one instance, the conclusion
drawn was that males were better off in comparison, which reaffirms the
social stereotype of the importance of female attractiveness.

*... I feel its worse for a woman though than it is for a man, ... a man can
grow a beard or moustache, but ... for a woman ... dab a bit of make-up on ...
but that's it.*

*I often think how lucky I am not to have a hare lip, because ... I think if I had
a hare lip as well it would have been twice as hard, because not only would
you be teased about your speech, you would be teased about your looks. I
think for a chap its easier once they grow up, because they can grow a 'tache
(moustache).*

*... it must ... be awful for a girl to be born with one (a cleft) ... I think a bloke
can usually cope with ..., but ... all girls ... like to be pretty and attractive.*

Section E - National Health Service (NHS) treatment for the cleft

Memories and perceptions of hospital

In order to receive the optimum treatment for a cleft, the patient is required to
countenance the sometimes lengthy treatment programme. This will

necessitate hospital admission(s) as an in-patient, as well as continuous follow-up as an out-patient. Thus, the experiences pertaining to these periods of treatment have been divided accordingly to afford greater discernment. From the quantity of contributions, more attention is clearly paid to out-patient experiences, which may reflect the fact that most surgery (necessitating in-patient admissions), was undertaken during the early pre-school years.

Experiences as an in-patient
> *I used to cry when my mum used to leave me, ... and after a while I just got used to it ... time after time.'*

> *... I just seem to have spent my entire life in and out of hospital.*

> *Can you imagine what that feels like ... as you go into the op. (operation), ... you know that you're going to come out looking different, ... I had this fear of coming out looking worse than what I went in, ... almost used to get ... paranoid about it, but ... I never did, it just became a way of life.*

Experiences as an out-patient When asked about the extent to which the interviewees felt involved in their treatment programmes, two aspects repeatedly emerged, namely, the congeniality of the Cleft Palate Team members, and the patients' own pre- and post-surgery photographs. Some ex-patients seized this opportunity to thank the hospital for their treatment, whilst others vented their dissatisfaction.

> *... I was almost sixteen ... sat in the chair, and he (surgeon) talked to my Dad, well, what we're going to do Mr. X, and I was saying excuse me ... Dad, I'm here ... tell him to talk to me, ... and I thought now I can understand how handicapped people feel in wheelchairs and when people say does he take sugar.*

> *... even a ten year old appreciates it when they say, right we've talked over the ... technical bits with your parents, would you like me to tell you now exactly what we're going to do to you, ... extra sensitive because you're walking into somewhere, where not only do you know you're different, they know you're different, and its because you're different that you're there, ... you almost get this inferiority complex.*

> *They should be asked if they want to see them (photographs), ... I didn't want to see any photos ... of when I was a baby ... not even when I was a teenager, ... They didn't actually show them to me ... I was sat on the chair and they got them out, and they was passing them ... to one person from another person to see, ... and that's really upsetting ... finished me off ... for the rest of the day.*

168

... I've spent so long from sort of like childhood up to ... mid twenties coming to hospital, and then all of a sudden that's it, there's no contact ... it would be a good idea ... even if it was only ... once every five years or something, ... would you like to come in and we'll just have a chat, see how you're getting on.

Plastic surgery

References made to plastic surgery relate to a variety of matters. Most predominant, however, is the interviewees' recollection that during childhood they had little idea of what their treatment entailed. The implication of this, is that as children they tended to accept and adjust to whatever happened to them more easily than when they were older.

I don't think its any good asking a seven year old if he wants an operation which is going to improve his facial features, ... at that age they're not going to have any real conception of what's going on.

I had my last operation when I was twelve, so I think I had the childhood acceptance of whatever was going on.

(Regarding scar on hip following bone graft surgery) ... I wish they'd have said to me we can't guarantee what sort of scar you'll get, ... but to actually promise me this little tiny scar.

I've often thought I'd like to have another operation.

Orthodontic treatment

It is notable that, despite the extent of teasing reported during the interviews, some of the participants referred to their teeth as incurring the greatest problems. The wearing of orthodontic appliances, such as braces sometimes provoked ridicule as might be expected.

... the biggest problem I ever had is my teeth, you know I'm held up by scaffolding really. I've had more pain from my teeth than anything else.

(Regarding orthodontic appliances) ... I used to put them in my pocket when I went to school, and put them back in my mouth before I went back in home. ... (they used) to call me 'staple-chops' and things like that, ... they (dental braces) used to be really big clumpy things, you couldn't get your lips around them.

The Cleft Lip and Palate Association (CLAPA)

During the interview, the value and role of a support group, such as the existent Cleft Lip and Plate Association was discussed. Whilst many of the participants were unaware of the Association's existence, one particular perspective warrants documentation.

> ... its very difficult to know what to say on that, because ... I had a period of mental illness ... not so long ago, ... I got involved with groups there ... and in some ways it wasn't good for me really, ... I needed to get away from that sort of environment ... and so in the same way, I wonder whether ... although it may help in certain ... circumstances, ... wonder whether you should associate yourself with a group of people ... with cleft palates or whatever ... you become so sort of insular, and worry about your own problems, rather than just getting on with living your life.

Section F - Experiences and perceptions related to the cleft

This section incorporates insights into the implications of being born with a cleft at different developmental stages. Particular emphasis is placed upon the impact of the cleft deformity upon personal and social relationships, since previous sections have focused on medical, educational, and occupational aspects. In doing so, the concerns of this section are intended to correspond directly with section six of the postal questionnaire (entitled 'Your Experience of Having A Cleft Lip and/or Palate').

The interview data in the subsequent subsections are arranged in such a way as to reflect the progress of psychosocial development, commencing with birth, and concluding with adulthood. Thus, the problem areas encountered at various stages can be more easily discerned. The range of individual differences in both life experiences and reactions to those experiences is a significant feature of the following contributions, not least in the manner in which the participants' parents initially responded to the diagnosis.

Interviewees' perceptions of their parents' reaction to their birth

> ... it must have been very difficult and very brave, ... because no doubt people come round and look at the new baby, and if they don't see some little angelic creature that must cause problems and demand explanation.

> My mum ... said that she wished she knew what was happening, ... she just had the baby at home, and was left with this baby that she didn't know what to do with.

> ... my parents were lucky that they did have something like the family ... even the neighbours, ... they never really sheltered me away even then.

170

... my father's a G.P.(General Practitioner) ... and my mum did a medical degree, ... and I suppose they could talk at a medical level to each other.

Childhood relationship with parents

... its a dreadful thing to say, but I can't actually remember my mum ever cuddling me, ... I had the best of everything physically, ... I don't think I can remember my mother ever telling me she loved me. I expect she did tell me but I can't remember.

My parents never offered me any advice, any comforts ... I was very fortunate I went to a private school, ... I was very much told that's it get on with it.

(Older sister also has a cleft) ... my dad, he was always the one behind us ... On Sunday afternoons in the summer, everyone put on their best dress,and we'd always go for walks, ... dad used to have one of us on each hand and mum had my brother on her hand, ... we literally walked around the whole of X ... we used to meet everybody. And my dad said he was so proud of us ... (aged) about five and six and seven, ... Now he says ... he's so proud of (his) children ... but you never hear my mum say it.

Parental explanation of the cleft and the need for hospital treatment

All the way along it was explained to me what was happening and why.

It would have been nice then for my mum to have said to me, you are a little bit different, but that makes you more special to me, or something along them lines ... just to give me that tiny little bit of grounding, but I waddled into junior school thinking I was exactly the same as everybody else.

Relationship with siblings

Whilst some interviewees alluded to the protection afforded them by their siblings during their school days (please see Section B concerning education), further insight into the diverse nature of sibling relationships is evidenced by the following comments.

(Regarding two older sisters) ... what my mum said was one of my sisters ... used to try to ... protect me from everybody, ... and the other one used to give me a really hard time, because she thought ... people out in the world are going to give him a hard time, so you'd better get used to it.

(Regarding older brother) ... before I had my nose done ... he used to call me 'boxing nose', ... I think maybe (this did affect me) because I was younger ...

I thought big brother's picking on me, ... He did occasionally call me 'bent lip' and things like that.

(Regarding older brother) ... I think in his mind he did sort of think well, she gets a lot of attention, and things like that, especially when I was in hospital and people were buying presents and giving me cards, ... got to him then.

Personal and social relationships with peers during teens

As suggested in the literature review (chapter two), the cleft-impaired may experience particular diffidence and anxiety about personal and social relationships. The unease surrounding socialization is borne out in the subsequent disclosures with only one exception.

I was in an all-boys school, ... until I was eighteen I had no previous connection with girls ... and onto university, ... I had one or two relationships, but I think I was very shy ... extremely nervous, ... very conscious of my appearance, ... I presume that was greater than most people would have, ... I tended to lead a fairly active life, so it didn't bother me to the extent that I was busy doing other things, ... but certainly ... relationships were very slow in coming, that was because of me and my self-consciousness.

... I think it affected me, ... I often felt ... will I be left on the shelf ... will anyone want to go out with me, and that's where I think counselling is needed, ... I can remember going on holiday with a friend and ... I'm sure my cleft palate affected it, ... about twelve, thirteen ... I remember going off with her but always feeling apart, not actually joining in ... because I was frightened they would tease me, ... and another time ... she set up a date with me ... I was about fifteen, ... the whole evening folded because of my speech ... I was definitely very, very worried until I actually had a boyfriend.

... I've never personally had an awful lot of problem with boys anyway.

Adult experiences and perceptions about living with a cleft

Personal The following comments allude to the participants' self-perceptions in relation to other people, particularly to their peers.

... a lot of the time now in spare moments ... I try and analyse what's gone by, ... I've often wondered if it was worth going to the doctor and seeking some psychiatric help, ... if I perhaps might need some counselling of some sort, but its something I've always put off because I've always been too embarrassed about asking about it, ... having spent all my life in hospitals it doesn't bother me at all, and that's why I was quite prepared to come today.

(Regarding coping) ... its a question of having to really, I mean really I've got no choice ... people take the mickey and that, I mean I could just stay in here and shut the door and not go out again, ... I'm not the type of person that would do that ... because I always go out, and no-one will ever stop me ... going out with my friends.

... I think as time goes on I see myself as a lonely old man, ... I can see it coming to that, and I often make a conscious effort to change, to actually ... go out, socialize more, make a start, and then I might do for a couple of weeks, and then I can always find something ... and then before I know where I am I'm back in the same old routine, ... I've got no real friends at all now.

I could talk to you for hours because I've never had the opportunity to talk, ... its really nice to open up, ... all one's life ... its been instilled in you ... that you're very different, ... so you tend to take a back seat anyway.

Social In contrast to the previous contributions, those incorporated under this subheading refer to the interviewees' perceptions of how they are perceived by others, especially their peers.

One thing that I find hard now is ... my son is actually teased because of me. So, although it affected me as a child it also affected him, ... still hurts me, ... before I went into nursing I was working at a boys' school, and I would get teased there as well by teenage children, ... that was only five years ago ... I still find teasing the most hurtful thing ... and mimicking.

... sometimes I feel very laid back and relaxed, and at other times I do get very nervous ... so it sort of differs with me, ... its people of the opposite sex actually ... the most nervous thing for me, ... its first impressions ... this is the trouble, ... People seem to think oh he looks out of the ordinary or strange, ... Its really younger people think this anyway.

... you realize you're different from a very early age, ... and other people know that you're different. I find sometimes that people .... are quite shy or awkward about talking to me, ... because I obviously give off ... that I feel awkward about talking, ... I feel that I ... have to loosen people up a bit really make them feel I'm alright, its a funny sort of feeling.

Current outlook upon life As the analysis and discussion of the postal questionnaire data suggest, despite the majority of respondents reporting adverse experiences when younger in conjunction with having a cleft, there appears to be a marked change in perception and attitude on reaching adulthood. The cause of this positive change is described by some individuals in terms of their improved circumstances, whilst others attribute it to increased life experience and maturity. However, as the ensuing remarks indicate such optimism is not universal.

> *... if there was one person that I could give just a little bit of confidence to, and say go out there, grab the world by the throat, shake it and take what you want, then that would make all the little bits of upset, the hurt, and the pain that I've had as a kid worth it.*

> *I think it makes you sort of more aware that there are people that are worse off than you, ... I'm walking around and I'm fine, ... it makes you want to care about people more ... because you know what its like to be teased, ... and people do need to know that they're wanted, ... I think it helped me a lot.*

> *I've got an attitude problem ... I've ... come to accept it.*

Impact of the cleft upon appearance and cleft-related problems Although in general, the interviewees exhibited a mature and resolved approach to their cleft deformity, references made to moments of insecurity and self-consciousness intimate that the cleft cannot ever be fully accepted.

> *You can't blame yourself, but ... sometimes you wish that ... you had a balanced face and that, just to see what it was like.*

> *... its only I suppose extremely recently that I've ... almost accepted my appearance, ... it sounds terrible at ... twenty-eight to say that, ... but I actually had a moustache for a long time ... I'm not quite sure why I shaved it off, anyway I did and I suddenly felt very, very exposed indeed ... I'd had it for five or six years, ... it was actually quite difficult to shave it off I was very surprised.*

> *... when I was younger in photographs I noticed I would try and stretch my smiles, ... but I'm much more ... confident than what I was in that respect, because I know its all finished, and its all been done for the best.*

Reaction to other people with a cleft Comments regarding the interviewees' reactions on meeting other people with clefts were entirely volunteered, and clearly diverse in nature.

> *I know a girl I was at school with she had a hare lip and cleft palate, and we tended to help each other, ... she was a lot younger than me ... I took her on as a friend, ... because I knew what it was like myself to be in that situation.*

> *... we had a BCG ... injection ... and the bloke had a cleft palate, ... and the first thing you do is like a mate ... its like a brotherhood syndrome, it becomes a brotherhood thing.*

I find it hard to sit in the same room with a person with a hare lip, certainly felt very conscious.

... there was a girl assistant ... in the shop, ... and she had a cleft palate ... looked straight at me and ... she looked down, and she really looked ashamed ... it upset me a little bit ... I don't think you should be ashamed.

Recurrence of the cleft in participants' own children and genetic counselling

The possible recurrence of the cleft deformity in the participants' own children was discussed during some of the interviews. In some instances, the outcome of these conversations could be seen to constitute projections of the interviewees' self-esteem and feelings of acceptance by others. That is, if the speaker possesses a sense of self-worth and acceptance by other people (particularly parents), he/she is more likely to display a positive attitude towards the notion of parenting a child with a cleft.

... when I was carrying X I said to my husband, what if I have one that's got the same as I've got? He said it won't matter, ... you will love it and after ... we sat down and talked, ... I felt better to think that he'd married me for how I was and not how I should be.

That has worried me actually ... I don't really know how I'd cope at the moment. I think I'd cope in the way knowing that something could be done, ... it is in the back of my mind wondering ... whether my children will have it, or whether it will skip my generation and go into their generation, ... it is a fear really in my mind, but I think I probably would cope because I've had to, and my parents had to. Knowing ... my parents coped ... I think it would probably be easier, because they would help me as well ... and they would ... know what I was doing wrong.

Absolutely devastated ... if I wait nine months for this lovely baby to come out, having just experienced it I know I was holding my breath, ... I was thinking is he going to come out with a cleft palate, ... it was quite a nerve-wracking few minutes.

Suggestions relating to the study

More media coverage of cleft lip and/or palate was suggested by one individual in commenting: *... there's nothing really on the telly.*

The involvement of parents in the study was recommended by another participant.

I would have thought your enquiries would have to include asking parents how they felt, the problems they had ... its the parents who actually deal

175

with the practicalities and the problems, so I would have thought that would be fairly essential.

One of those interviewed suggested that the participants' own children should be interviewed as part of the study, to gain their perspective on the parents' cleft impairment. This advice followed the disclosure that the participant's daughter had never asked nor discussed her mother's cleft with her.

Recommendations

Emerging from the data collected by postal questionnaire and personal interviews, are three specific areas of need. According to the participants these areas have been insufficiently addressed in clinical practice, and as such have been incorporated into proposed recommendations for improving the current management of cleft patients. Each recommendation will be now examined, in the light of pertinent anecdotal data, prior to further discussion in the following chapter.

It should be noted that the recommendations for the professional service providers, are generated entirely from the composite voice of the interviewees (or consumers). Thus, the proposals are conceived by those who have personal experience of being on the receiving end of cleft-related treatment, and who have been given the opportunity to share those experiences. Needless to say, the suggestions made reflect retrospective treatment provision, which has clearly advanced over time.

Recommendation I - Parent education/counselling

With the benefit of hindsight, many participants recognized the crucial need for parents of cleft-impaired babies, to receive more professional support in the first weeks of infancy. This support could incorporate increasing the parents' understanding of the longer term implications of clefts, counselling (where applicable), and introduction to other parents in a similar position. The way in which the initial news of the cleft diagnosis was delivered to parents was also deemed significant to the parents' subsequent adjustment to the deformity.

a) *Delivering the initial news of the diagnosis to parents*
    I think I would probably say to them ... its ... awful at the moment but it is a process, ... as the child gets older explain to them exactly what's happening to them, and what is going on so that they know ... that it does get better, and that its worth it all in the end.

176

*You have to be light about it, ... you have to say you've got a beautiful child
... its got a cleft, ... it has to be completely diffused from being serious ... Its
got to be made light of because it isn't everything, ... its only skin and flesh,
... people have got to be made aware of that ... and that its not an
imperfection of the parents.*

*I don't think there is a correct way ... because some people will react to it
differently to others.*

b)   *The nature of subsequent parent education / counselling*
     *... the main thing I would say ... the child who's got a hare lip and a cleft
     palate, there will be some minor speech defects but obviously you've got to
     help a child work at them, ... what you really need to do is to try and build
     the confidence up to tell the child ... that with surgery it can be vastly
     improved, then its not something they will have to live with for the rest of
     their life.*

     *... I suppose its a matter of someone going along and saying if you feel like
     this that's alright, because a lot of people feel like that ... and we know why
     you feel like that, and you shouldn't judge yourself too harshly for
     thinking that.*

     *... I think early on perhaps its the parents who need the support more than
     the actual child.*

     *... I think they should ... right from the word go ... have counselling for
     people.*

Recommendation II - Early teenage counselling

Whilst Recommendation I seeks to capitalize upon the present professional
advice given to parents of infants with clefts, Recommendation II addresses
a comparatively neglected area of provision. Since the onus of clinical
treatment in Great Britain tends to be placed upon the correction of
appearance and speech, insufficient attention may be given to the
psychosocial difficulties which arise, especially as the patient approaches
adolescence. The need for such help and advice at this particular stage is
clearly identified in the following excerpts, which highlight the diversity of
pressing concerns.

a)   *The need for teenage counselling*
     *... I suppose in the teenage years you don't need someone necessarily to tell
     you what to do, you just need to know that there's someone there if you
     don't know what to do, ... the analogy of families being a chair in the
     middle of a dark room, and you have to learn to get the courage to move
     away from the chair, but you have to know that the chair's there, ... To some*

177

extent you need a sort of substitute chair, because of ... psychological side of things ... important.

... there were a few times when I did get ... depressed or worried and just felt so unsure, ... if there was this sort of thing (counselling) when I was in my early teens, I would have gone in and said ... are there different ways that I can ... help myself feel strong mentally, so that I can cope with other things that are going to come ... especially schooling.

I think that would be very, very difficult unless you've actually had it yourself, ... I think because every person is different, and there again, you don't know how each child reacts or feels inside, ... and that is the difficult side.

b) *The form teenage counselling should take*
   ... if I lived in an area where they had a counselling, or ... call it something else I would definitely have gone ... and perhaps taken a friend, ... or another member of the family, ... I think it would have to be after school ... Probably have it more like a social thing, although the emphasis being on counselling, and talking and sharing.

   ... what I would have been happy doing is if you had a very informal, even sort of like a club, ... why not a youth club in a hospital? ... where you can at least be you, now you know you're not going to have an awful lot of problem with people staring at you, because you're all the same ... and chances are out of a whole crowd, you're bound to find somebody that you get an affinity with, and possibly who's to know ... providing you don't live too far away that could possibly become a real friendship, ... you have a really awful day, either at college or something, ... you meet up ... and at the end of an hour you're rolling around at the other one's expense, ... no harm because you know you're both in the same boat, but I think to go for an actual formal counselling is going to be dreadful, because what's happening is you've got your normal person saying, you're not normal but I know how we can overcome this, and I wouldn't go.

   ... a one-to-one conversation I think ... instils confidence, ... At the end of the day ... that's what its all about is instilling confidence, ... talking to ... somebody like you on a one-to-one basis.

c) *How and when to counsel cleft-impaired teenagers*
   Its got to be informal then they can be themselves, ... you'll get the confident ones ... and they'll walk in, ... and chances are they're going to pick on the shyest one in there, that thinks no-one's going to talk to them because they look funny, ... and they think ... this person's asking all these questions ... and they're exactly the same as me, now why can't I be like that, ... and then

178

your mind starts going if they can do it, what on earth's stopping me from doing it, and they all boost each other up, and you're off.

... if you can have a group of clefters that would be brilliant, ... I don't think I ever met anyone actually in eight years who had a cleft palate, ... that makes it worse, because you walk around going I'm the only one like this.

... self-confidence ... you could include this, ... definitely when they start secondary school to convince them, the kids that they're not any different from anybody else, it doesn't stand out regardless of what they think when they look in the mirror, ... get them to come to terms with it say look you know so and so, look at the size of their ears, look at the size of their nose don't you think they're worried about that?

Recommendation III - involvement of school staff

Similar to the previous Recommendation, the third proposal breaks new ground in exploring the potential for school involvement in the patient's cleft management. The school has been identified as an additional source of support to the patient, since as a child and an adolescent the individual spends a large proportion of his or her waking hours in the school environment. Moreover, it is within this environment that much of the traumatic teasing appears to take place, which has implications for possible intervention by the school staff. Views as to the value of such intervention, however, are mixed as the ensuing comments indicate.

... That sounds absolutely wonderful, but have you any idea how embarrassed I would have been, sat in the middle of the class while my teacher is telling everybody else to stop teasing me? ... I would have died ... you're not going to ever stop teasing. I think you'd be best off from my personal point of view, going for the teaching to cope with teasing, rather than ... going for the stop teasing, ... because if they don't do it (teasing) openly, they're going to do it on the way home.

... educating them at school, but without ... making it overtly ... this person is ... in need of your sympathy, ... we're not in need of sympathy we're just in need of ... tolerance.

a) *Infant school level*
    ... start at infants' school explain to the children, ... even if its only the ones in their class, then they can turn round and say oh look, oh he's alright this is what happened to him, ... obviously its down to the school staff.

    ... up until that age (four and a half to five years old) I didn't know that I had it (cleft), if children would have teased me, ... I don't think I would have cottoned on to what they were teasing me about, ... I think after the age of

about eight and nine then they do. But saying that ... things were different, ... now ... everything is coming forward isn't it, so saying that to children of ... five and six (years old), it could be an advantage to them.

b) *Primary school level*
... I think with teachers some of them are too frightened to say anything to the children about bullying and that sort of thing, but I think they should be ... involved more, ... not so much to the children that have been bullied, but to the children that are bullying, and make them understand its not right, ... I think maybe do it to the class in general, not actually specifically pinpoint the bully and the person that he's bullying, ... sort of how to deal with things if they see somebody being bullied.

... I think if it could be instituted in all schools, ... what could you call it, social awareness, ... If you could just give all the children half an hour or whatever discussion on it, ... these people have got this wrong with them ... they're no different from anybody else, its just that they're suffering for one reason or another, they're exactly the same and there's no reason to pick on them, ... its never going to change ... People are always going to find something wrong with somebody else, ... even people who've got nothing wrong with them get bullied.

... there's a risk there isn't there, ... it would have to be done very subtly, ... the danger is that ... if it appears that the teacher is sticking up for a particular individual who is getting bullying, rather than stop bullying ... probably going to make it worse.

c) *Secondary school level*
... they need to be ... talked to once a month if someone with a cleft palate is at a big secondary school, ... the teacher has to be incorporated and to just say how are you getting on, ... its got to be someone they can trust.

... I'm not so sure about that, because if you take a situation where in a school of ... five hundred children you've got one child with a hare lip, cleft palate whatever, then all of a sudden all the teachers are going to say right, here we've got Joe Bloggs, he's got this problem ... don't upset him, so immediately he's marked teacher's pet, ... by all means counsel the teachers separately, but don't have them getting up and saying ... don't upset the kid, because it marks him out straightaway.

This particular quotation serves to highlight a fundamental assumption encountered throughout the investigation, which emanates from the disability literature. That is, the assumption that the cleft and its potentially adverse connotations are largely the problems of the individuals concerned. In this way, society as a whole (including the school classroom) can renounce any responsibility for its stigmatizing and victimizing response to the cleft population. In that the school environment is a microcosm of society, the teachers' perceptions and hence treatment of the cleft-impaired, can wield significant influence. The way in which their influence can be used to actively expiate the plight of those with a cleft, will be addressed in proposing recommendations for change (chapter nine).

8 The implications of the findings

Experience is what you do with what happens to you.
(Aldous Huxley)

Introduction

The purpose of the present chapter is to examine the validity of the hypotheses delineated in the Introduction (chapter one) in view of the findings. On this occasion, the term 'hypothesis' is defined in its broadest sense of comprising a 'supposition made as a starting-point for further investigation from known facts' *(The Concise Oxford Dictionary)*. The suppositions being presented have evolved from BNH's research. This interpretation differs from that adopted by experimental methodologists, who seek to prove or disprove 'null' hypotheses. Within the developmental framework pursued throughout the study, the hypotheses will be discussed in a chronological rather than a hierarchical sequence.

Factors relating to the participants' psychosocial development and functioning during the developmental years (hypotheses i-vi)

Factors relating to the home environment

Hypothesis i The home environment of the cleft population implicated in the study, has distinguishable features which are attributable to the cleft defect.

The findings of the current study suggest that whilst the majority of participants had a propitious early home background, some of them were raised in circumstances which were less conducive to optimum psychosocial development. For example, evidence of an 'unfavourable' family environment, a 'detrimental' parental attitude, little or no explanation of non-attendance at hospital clinics for cleft-related treatment, and personal adjustment problems have all been documented in previous chapters. All of these early influences are related to the care which parents were able to offer their children, and as such reflect the environment in which a disadvantaged minority appear to have been reared.

In addition to the close relationship between a 'detrimental' parental attitude and an 'unfavourable' family environment ($p < 0.01$), strong associations were similarly found between these two dimensions, and sporadic or no explanation of non-attend at the requisite hospital appointments (non-significant and $p < 0.05$ respectively). Alongside these findings should also be placed the evident correspondence between an adverse parental attitude and/or a deleterious family environment, and personal adjustment difficulties ($p < 0.01$ and non-significant respectively).

Therefore, it appears that the home circumstances of a minority of participants were undoubtedly wanting. Having established this, one needs to ascertain to what extent the adversity could be conceivably attributed to the cleft defect. In doing so, attention is turned to the two primary deficits characterizing the condition, namely, impaired communication (including speech) and impaired appearance.

Regarding the implications of impaired communication, the literature provides some insight into the ways in which the nature of family dynamics may be affected by the presence of the cleft in one family member. Various sources infer the disruption of effective communication caused by cleft-related problems of feeding, speech and hearing (for example, Phillips and Stengelhofen, 1989; Albery and Russell, 1990). Other authorities refer to the adverse effects of developmental language delay upon family interaction, not least in the mother's altered behaviour towards the cleft-impaired child (for example, Wasserman et al., 1988).

Sibling rivalry may also effect family friction. For instance, literature focusing upon the implications of disability, documents tense relations between siblings and the impaired child, such as hostility (Podeanu-Czehofsky, 1975), jealousy, anxiety and aggression (Kew, 1975). One needs only to contemplate the 'extra' attention seemingly devoted to the child with a cleft, (such as frequent hospital visits), to appreciate how such rivalry can escalate.

The strain which impairment can place upon the family is also indicated by Strauss and Broder (1991, p.154), who speak in terms of the wider population.

> There is evidence that children with special needs elicit considerable family stress, possibly affecting parental marital status and family harmony (Scheper-Hughes, 1987b). Furthermore, research suggests that children with special needs are more likely to be neglected or abused than are other children (Gothard et al., 1985). Scheper-

Hughes (1990) has asked whether child maltreatment is merely the developed world's response to the impulse to control deviance.

In addressing the particular demands placed upon the family by a child with a disability, Philp and Duckworth (1982, p.33) refer to a model based on the work of Harrison (1977) and Bradshaw and Lawton (1978), which demonstrates how the disabled individual can produce stress in the parents (Figure 8.1).

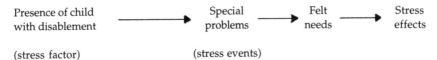

Presence of child   ⟶   Special   ⟶   Felt   ⟶   Stress
with disablement   problems   needs   effects

(stress factor)   (stress events)

Figure 8.1 Model of how a child with disablement produces stress in the parents

Philp and Duckworth (1982, p.33) explain that 'special problems' include emotional and physical stress, and transport difficulties (for hospital visits). 'Felt needs' are exemplified by financial pressures, and the seeking of relevant information and support, and the 'stress effect' reflects the emotional, physical and financial consequences of the disability.

Other literature suggests that the parents and family impose a certain role upon the impaired child within the home environment. Stengelhofen (1989, p.27) describes how this role evolves.

> Spriestersbach's (1973) findings show that cleft palate children tend not to be treated in the same way as their potentially normal communicating peers. For example, they are given less encouragement to babble; given less chances to talk as much as they want; take less part in family conversations ... This list of factors gives clear indication that they may become poor communicators, less because of their specific speech problems, but more because they are given a role as a poor communicator and deprived of usual encouragement and opportunities.

Therefore, since the communication problems experienced in the homes of some of the cleft population typify cleft-related difficulties, they can be directly attributed to the cleft per se. It must be stressed that it is the existence of the defect, rather than the presence of the impaired individual which is under scrutiny. Although these two concerns are inextricably linked, the former appears to be a fundamental influence regarding family dynamics.

The second area of impaired appearance is relevant only to instances of cleft lip and palate on this occasion. In the course of data analysis, the significance of the cleft's visibility has become increasingly apparent. For example, the majority of participants incorporated into the categories of 'detrimental' parental attitude and/or 'unfavourable' family environment, presented with a visible cleft. As postulated earlier, these results suggest that those with a visible cleft, may be subjected to particular adversity from birth.

Whilst it could be advocated that babies with cleft lip and palate, tend to be born to households where parental attitude towards the children and the family environment are not conducive to child rearing, the literature suggests the converse. That is, the visibility of the cleft may actually influence the quality and the quantity of family interaction taking place.

In addition, it transpires that most of the young patients assessed by BNH as displaying personal adjustment problems to the cleft presented with a visible defect ($p < 0.05$). In that the preponderance of those whose parents exhibited a 'detrimental' attitude towards them experienced adjustment difficulties, it appears that the visibility of the cleft can directly affect personal circumstances.

Supplementary evidence of the differing parental attitudes shown towards 249 children having a visible or non-visible cleft, emanates from the work of O'Riain and Hammond (1972, p.386).

> We found a tendency for parents of children with a post-alveolar cleft only to be less concerned than those of children with lip involvement also. The highest percentage of both 'encouraging' and 'detrimental' influences was found in those children having bilateral lip clefts and therefore presenting the more distressing visible deformities at birth.

The distinction between the visibility and the severity of the cleft diagnosis should be noted. Whilst the former refers to the conspicuousness of the cleft, and most notably to cleft lip, the latter denotes the extent of clefting. Needless to say, cleft lip can range from being a relatively minor defect (incomplete), to a more extensive one (complete). Furthermore, the severity of the cleft corresponds to its visibility in that the manifestation of a bilateral complete cleft may be more obvious than a unilateral incomplete cleft. The connotations of this distinction for the individuals concerned may be contrary to expectation, as discussed under hypothesis vii.

McWilliams (1982) suggests that the parents' acceptance of the infant's condition, may be determined by the severity of the cleft, which reinforces the earlier findings of Clifford (1969), Clifford and Crocker (1971) and Spriestersbach (1961a; 1973). Similarly, Tisza and Gumpertz (1962, p.87) found that the psychological trauma was greater for parents giving birth to a baby with cleft lip compared to one having cleft palate only. 'The baby with the cleft lip creates a much more immediate trauma for the parents than the baby who has only cleft palate.'

Natsume et al. (1987) likewise highlight the significance of cleft type upon the mother's reaction to the neonate. A higher proportion of mothers of cleft lip babies denied their child's existence as a human being and harboured suicidal thoughts, when compared with mothers of the cleft palate only group. The former mothers also tended to be more preoccupied with anxieties about the child's future socialization than the latter group.

Data elicited by personal interviews undertaken for the purposes of the present study, reinforce these findings. The reader is referred to interviewees' accounts of the reactions of their parents (especially their mothers) to their birth (chapter seven). Whilst some parents felt stigmatized, and wished to keep their impaired baby indoors for fear of being seen, others apparently received the necessary support from family and friends.

The particularly disadvantaged plight of individuals with a visible cleft is also evidenced by the feeding complications associated with cleft lip, which are additional to those of cleft palate (for example, Hathorn, 1986; Drillien et al., 1966). The implication of feeding difficulties in threatening parent-child bonding and interaction was mentioned in chapter two.

In reviewing the literature, Brantley and Clifford (1980) refer to the documented relationship between negative parental affect and visible defects in the child. In addition to the observations of the current investigation, this finding suggests the persistence of adverse parental attitudes towards those born with a visible cleft. One explanation for this tendency is that the child's detectable abnormality continues to insult the parents' perceptions of their ability to produce a 'normal' child. The feelings of inadequacy and disappointment experienced by some parents, which can lower their self-esteem and competence as parents, has been already implicated in the literature review (chapter two).

In summary, evidence suggests that the early home environment of the cleft population does contain distinguishable features, which may be attributed to the presence of the defect. Furthermore, the features identified in the writer's study accord with those documented in the literature, which indicate that the participants involved in the investigation are representative of the wider cleft population. Whilst the home environment is heralded as one of the most potent influences upon the individual's psychosocial development, the role played by the cleft impairment in determining the nature of that environment should not be underestimated.

Hypothesis ii A 'detrimental' parental attitude towards the cleft-impaired patient identified during the child's pre-school years, has an adverse effect upon his or her psychosocial development and later psychosocial functioning.

Having established how and why the cleft defect can influence the family environment (including parental attitude), the second hypothesis focuses on the consequent implications of doing so. Attention is paid to elucidating the nature of the influence exerted by a 'detrimental' parental attitude, upon the child's psychosocial development and later functioning.

In attempting to define the relationship between adverse causes and effects, it is necessary to conceive the way in which the disadvantage is internalized by the child. The emerging picture is that the deformity may effect or reinforce an adverse home environment, rather than the child being born into deleterious circumstances per se. Thus, a 'detrimental' parental attitude may constitute a response to the child, as opposed to being a predisposing factor of his/her environment. Schaffer's (1977, p.30) observation offers insight into the interdependence of parent-child interaction.

Both parents and child operate within a system of mutuality where the behaviour of one produces effects on the other that in turn modify the behaviour of the first. One has to consider the whole network of interacting influences; not, as the critical period model attempts to do, skip all but the first and last link.

In addressing this issue, the reader is reminded that a statistically significant correlation was found between a 'detrimental' parental attitude and negative perceptions of school ($p < 0.05$), and also between an untoward attitude and subjection to teasing ($p < 0.05$). Similarly, a close correspondence emerged between an 'unfavourable' family environment and pessimistic impressions of school ($p < 0.05$), and/or peer victimization. These results suggest that exposure to unrewarding parenting at home, can make the individuals concerned more susceptible to unrewarding experiences with their peers at school.

In addition, reference is made to the consistent association between an unfavourable family environment (including 'unfavourable' parenting), and the potential for psychosocial problems during the pre-school, childhood ($p < 0.05$), adolescent and adulthood stages of development (chapters five and six). One cannot dismiss the fact that at all ages, those having an unsupportive home background, appear to be more prone to psychosocial dysfunction.

Regarding the impact of a 'detrimental' parental attitude upon the individual's adult self-esteem, Broder et al. (1992, p.262) state: 'Since parents are thought to have an indelible impression on the child's sense of self, parent perceptions are believed paramount in the child's self-esteem (Schonfeld, 1969).' These sentiments clearly reiterate the earlier theorizing of Erikson (1950; 1959) and Coopersmith (1967) regarding the determinants of self-esteem.

Likewise, Brantley and Clifford (1980) intimate that parental attitudes may jeopardize the individual's psychosocial maturation, and threaten family functioning. However, this thinking is contradicted by a larger proportion of the self-report measures of self-esteem supplied by the participants as adults. As depicted in the comparison of data (chapter six), those responding in the direction of low self-esteem tended to be associated with parents who had displayed a 'satisfactory', rather than a 'detrimental' attitude towards their children.

Therefore, whilst a 'detrimental' parental attitude towards the cleft-impaired child may increase his or her potential for psychosocial dysfunction, the potential is not necessarily realized. Indeed, it could be argued that the older and more mature the cleft-impaired become, the more likely it is that the realization of this potential will be assuaged for the majority of individuals. Thus, the implications for long term adverse effects can be reversed in most cases.

In discussing the impact of earlier adversity on adult life, Schaffer (1977) proposes that the circumstances experienced need to be constantly reinforced. Thus, the child who is consistently exposed to unpropitious parenting, is more vulnerable to later psychosocial maladjustment, compared with the child who has only sporadic exposure to it. In this context, Schaffer (1977, p.27) refers to the theorizing of Campbell and Jaynes (1966).

> ... an early experience can be perpetuated and incorporated into the adult personality only if it is periodically reinstated; that is, if a small amount of partial practice, or repetition of the experience, occurs throughout childhood.

Schaffer (1977, p.27) capitalizes upon this notion and continues:

> This applies, presumably, to the case where one misfortune sets in train a whole sequence of further misfortunes, each confirming the child's expectation of what life has to offer him, and each giving him further reason to adopt whatever behaviour ... Under such circumstances one can predict the final outcome with rather more confidence, for a child in this situation is sustained and encouraged in the response he originally adopted.

In that parental overprotectiveness and indifference are both regarded as 'detrimental' (according to BNH), evidence of their possible long term impact can be found amongst the interview data. For example, with hindsight, parents (especially mothers) are blamed for individuals' distressing experiences at school and beyond, the consequences of which feature vividly in their long term memories. In particular, mention is made of the fact that as children, it was not explained why nor how they differed from their peers regarding the cleft. Therefore, when the individuals concerned encountered victimization, they were apparently ignorant of the probable cause. The obvious anger which such memories engendered in the interviewees, evidences the adverse influence which a 'detrimental' parental attitude can exert upon later life. The reader is referred to chapter seven for further details.

Having examined data pertaining to the second hypothesis, it appears that the relationship between the cleft-impaired child and his/her parents is characterized by a complex network of variables. Whilst there is evidence that a 'detrimental' parental attitude towards the child, may exert an adverse long term effect upon the individual, there is also documentation to suggest that such consequences are not inevitable.

In summary, it would seem that although 'unfavourable' parenting has the potential to hamper the individual's psychosocial development and functioning, other factors serve to reinforce or diminish its likelihood. In the context of the present study, a primary factor concerns the nature of the school environment. It is to the elucidation of this environment, that attention is now turned.

Factors relating to the school environment

Hypothesis iii The school environment of the cleft population implicated in the study, has distinguishable features which are attributable to the cleft defect.

It is important at the outset, to distinguish between data relating to the participants' home environment and personal circumstances, and those relating to their school environment and socialization with peers. Whereas the former largely originate from assessments made by BNH and her colleagues during the patients' developmental years, the latter have been gathered from the retrospective stance of the adult participants. Although this variation may invite controversy regarding the accuracy of the adults' school perceptions, the time 'lapse' enables study of the impact of adverse experiences upon later life.

In evaluating the extent to which the participants' school environment was influenced by the presence of the cleft, the reader is reminded of their responses relating to past school experiences. The most notable of these concern the vast proportion of individuals who had been subjected to teasing (n=174, 80.2% of respondents), and/or who harbour negative perceptions of school as adults (n=130, 60.0% of respondents). The close relationship which appears to exist between experience of teasing and negative school perceptions ($p < 0.01$), suggests that teasing largely determines the nature of the school perceptions. Indeed, this is borne out by the preoccupation with reporting teasing-related aspects of schooling, evidenced by both questionnaire respondents and interviewees, when asked about their school experiences.

Further evidence of the role played by the deformity in the participants' schooling, derives from the strong association between the perceived influence of the cleft upon education and subjection to teasing ($p < 0.01$), and/or negative impressions of school ($p < 0.01$). In each instance, where the defect was estimated as having exerted a 'high'/'very high' influence upon education, the majority of respondents had been teased and/or reported adverse perceptions of school (chapter five).

The notion that the cleft thwarted the individuals' learning and educational progress, is reinforced by data elicited by personal interview, at both primary and secondary school levels (chapter seven). This idea warrants some qualification, since various reasons are advanced by the participants. For example, treatment-related factors (such as out-patient appointments or hospitalization) are held responsible for instances of disrupted schooling. Far greater significance is attached, however, to problem-related factors notably impaired speech, appearance and/or hearing associated with having a cleft.

By implication, cleft impairment at school necessitates the withdrawal of the individual from his or her peers for treatment purposes. It may also compel the withdrawal of peers from the individual concerned, on the grounds that the defect has an alienating effect and the deformed person is thus perceived as being 'different'. In this way, the presence of the cleft per se can actively mitigate against the individual's 'safe' passage through school.

Published literature in this field highlights the vulnerability of the cleft population's socialization. However, little reference is made to how personal and social relationships may be impoverished by peer victimization. In this respect, the findings of the current study both support and extend the literature, by providing insight into aspects of socialization to which the majority of participants are especially susceptible.

The purpose of schooling is not only to provide the opportunity for intellectual learning, but to offer youngsters a forum for social learning. Since a large proportion of the developmental years is spent in school, it follows that the experiences gained there are likely to characterize the individuals' lives at this stage. Therefore, alongside experiences of classroom learning, experiences of interacting with peers can be expected to exert a major influence upon the individuals' psychosocial development and functioning. This is exemplified by the participants' particular concern with the nature of their personal and social relationships with peers at school.

The same emphasis is apparent in published research. For example, in summarizing the findings of various studies, Goodstein (1968) advocates that although there is little evidence of psychopathology, children born with a cleft palate may suffer from problems concerning social acceptance. Similarly, Stricker et al. (1979) identify the cleft population's difficulties in establishing and maintaining social relationships, as opposed to exhibiting deviant personality traits.

Other authorities note the anxieties expressed by cleft-impaired adolescents surrounding social interaction, which may be evidenced by social inhibition (for instance, Harper and Richman, 1978; Kapp, 1979). Clifford and Clifford (1986) surmise that the increased susceptibility of the cleft population to peer pressure and perceptions, may account for the common feelings of stigmatization and victimization by peers. Incidents of teasing are also reported by Noar (1991).

At the same time, self-consciousness about the defect can reinforce the individual's sense of being socially unacceptable. In this way, peer perception can directly influence the person's self-perception and self-esteem to his or her detriment. Broder et al. (1992) refer to the relevance of social learning theory in this context. According to this theory, children perceive themselves as others perceive them (Videbeck, 1960).

Moreover, personal and social relationships in addition to school performance can be threatened by compounding cleft-related problems, such as impaired communication skills, hearing loss and/or instances of nasal regurgitation (during eating and/or drinking), due to an unrepaired fistula. The reader's attention is drawn to the interview data (chapter seven) for examples of such occurrences. These factors can actively mitigate against the development of stable relationships, since they label the individual as 'different' which affects their desirability as a potential friend.

According to the literature, in addition to deleterious peer attitudes towards the cleft impaired, the perceptions and expectations of school teachers can also adversely affect their school experiences and educational performance. For instance, Clifford and Walster (1973) and Shaw and Humphreys (1982) document that the presence of the cleft defect may incite teachers to have low academic expectations of impaired pupils. This finding reflects the realization of a self-fulfilling prophecy, that disfigurement (speech and/or appearance) implicates inferior intellectual functioning. Needless to say, there is evidence that the cleft population responds to this expectation, by harbouring a poor perception of their own abilities with consequent underachievement (for example, Richman and Eliason, 1982).

Therefore, there is sufficient evidence to suggest that for the majority of participants in the study, their school days did not prove to be the proverbial 'happiest days' of their lives. Indeed, with hindsight the converse may be a more realistic evaluation. It could be advocated that in some instances the collective prejudices of school contemporaries and teachers, compel those born with a cleft to encounter negative experiences at school. Whilst the former may be responsible for engendering victimization in terms of teasing and social isolation, the latter may promote the expectation of low educational attainment.

In that these adversities reflect the responses of peers and school staff to the presence of the cleft, it is postulated that the defect can influence the school environment of the cleft-impaired to their detriment. The following two hypotheses are concerned with identifying the individuals most vulnerable to such stigmatization, and to examine the broader consequences for their psychosocial development and functioning.

Hypothesis iv The victims of teasing portray a particular personality 'type'.

The participants' preoccupation with the experience and implications of being teased, when asked about their school days has now been established. Moreover, the association between home background, and visibility of the cleft, and victimization have also been documented. The particular vulnerability of those encountering adversity at home for peer victimization, is further reinforced by the finding that individuals who exhibited personal adjustment problems to the defect, were the most susceptible to being teased.

Collectively, these findings suggest that deleterious personal circumstances predispose an individual to deleterious school experiences, in that peers seek out those they perceive as vulnerable as targets for their ridicule. Although this may be a viable interpretation, one needs to remember that teasing was not exclusive to those with unsatisfactory personal circumstances. Indeed, the vast majority of the participants were apparently victimized to some degree (chapter five). This suggests that the presence of the cleft itself appears to provoke some form of negative reaction in most instances.

In view of this, it is regrettable that information relating to personality measures (including self-esteem) was not recorded at the time of the teasing. Although the respondents' self-reports regarding personality traits and self-esteem are available (chapter five), they are essentially retrospective indications, and therefore, evidence the long term impact of being teased. In considering supplementary findings, the reader is referred to the interviewees' hindsight accounts of the factors surrounding instances of teasing (chapter seven).

With respect to the paucity of published research concerned with teasing, almost exclusive reference is made subsequently to literature published in conjunction with the national Anti-bullying Campaign. This event was launched in May 1992, to raise public awareness and to offer guidance on bullying. Attention has been given to various aspects of the problem, such as the circumstances surrounding bullying, including definition of the perpetrators and their victims. In the present study, the terms 'bullying' and 'teasing' (verbal bullying) are used interchangeably, as this reflects the practice adopted by the questionnaire respondents. In characterizing the injuring and injured parties involved in the act of bullying, Tattum and Herbert (1990, p.19) pose and then attempt to address two pertinent questions.

> Is there a typical bully? Bullies are usually bigger and stronger than average and older than their victims. They are characterised by impulsiveness and a strong need to dominate others. Bullies are associated with general anti-social, rule-breaking behaviour in school and the community. They are often aggressive towards parents, teachers and siblings.

Bullies are thought to learn their bullying tactics from their home environment. They may be the children of past school bullies, and become the parents of future bullies. The choice of victim, however, cannot always be anticipated as the authors suggest (p.21).

> Is there a typical victim of bullying? Contrary to popular belief, bullying victims don't always differ much from other children. Children who wear glasses, are overweight, have red hair, speak with a pronounced accent of stutter, do not automatically invite bullying attacks. Generally, the bullied are physically weaker and often younger than their persecutors. They are more anxious and insecure than pupils in general - often cautious, sensitive and quiet. Many are lonely children with few friends (which may be by choice) and have difficulty asserting themselves in the peer group. Compared with boys in general victimized boys have a closer contact and more positive relations with their parents, in particular their mothers.

Regarding the psychosocial implications of being subjected to teasing, Tattum and Herbert (1990, p.21), sound a pessimistic but realistic note when they caution:

> The long term effects of persistent bullying can make youngsters feel isolated and wonder what is wrong with them. They may begin to feel that they deserve the teasing and harassment, so that they become withdrawn and less willing to take social, intellectual or vocational risks.

These sentiments are clearly borne out by the findings of the current study, which suggest that low self-esteem and socially undesirable personality traits are commonly detected in the victims of teasing (chapter six). Moreover, the fact that these characteristics are more apparent in the visible, than in the non-visible cleft groups, suggests that the visibility of the defect (cleft lip) per se may provoke teasing. Having examined the evidence as to whether or not those subjected to teasing portray a particular personality 'type', attention is turned to the impact such tribulation may exert over the victims' psychosocial development and later functioning.

Hypothesis v Negative experiences of interaction with peers during childhood and/or adolescence, exert an adverse influence upon his or her psychosocial development and later functioning.

In addressing this hypothesis, one needs to contemplate the significance of personal and social relationships formed (or failing to form) at school, for psychosocial maturation. For example, if such relationships are transient, it may be of no fundamental consequence if they prove to be problematic and unrewarding. If, on the other hand, interaction with school peers forms the basis from which all other social relationships proceed, the nature of them is integral to the individuals' personal and social functioning thereafter, since man is essentially a 'social animal' (Demetrius the Cynic, 1st century A.D.).

Prior to consulting the findings of the present study, reference is made to literature which sheds light upon the predicament of the cleft-impaired, especially those with an additional visible defect (cleft lip and palate). Various authors have expounded the close relationship existing between self-perception and peer perception (such as Broder et al., 1992). In seeking to explain why many members of the cleft population suffer adverse social experiences, reference is made to the facial attractiveness literature, which highlights the discriminatory processes operating in the selection of potential friends by peers. For example, Lerner and Lerner (1977) suggest that adolescents tend to befriend contemporaries whom they consider attractive. By implication, peers who are perceived as unattractive are deemed unworthy of friendship.

In explaining the phenomenon of 'person perception theory' which this behaviour exemplifies, Tobiasen (1984) indicates that an individual's physical appearance is endowed with inferences concerning his/her personality and behaviour. Therefore, whilst physical attractiveness connotes socially desirable attributes, physical unattractiveness (including disfigurement) is associated with socially undesirable characteristics (Schneider et al., 1979; Patzer, 1984 amongst others). As Eliason et al. (1991, p.190) point out: 'Facial characteristics have been long used as a means of judging an individual's overall attractiveness, desirability as a friend or romantic partner, and as a means of judging personality (Patzer, 1985).'

Eliason et al. refer to MacGregor's (1974) observation that the greatest obstruction to the psychological adjustment of those with a facially deviant appearance, is society's attitude towards them as marginal or 'forgotten' people. Similar reports emanating from the literature, include that of Bull and Rumsey (1988), who advocate that individuals with an unattractive or an abnormal facial appearance, are generally perceived as less friendly, less intelligent and exhibiting less socially desirable personality traits. In view of this, the evidently strong relationship which exists between visibility of the cleft and adverse school experiences can be better understood.

Furthermore, as Tobiasen (1984) delineates, the implication is that attractive and unattractive children and adolescents are treated differently, and thus have different experiences of social interaction. Indeed, the former tend to receive preferential treatment, whilst the latter may be actively discriminated against. Consequently, the differential treatment by others can effect differential behaviour by the individuals concerned, such that those perceived as unattractive may exhibit a socially undesirable demeanour. In doing so, other people's perceptions and expectations of the unattractive or disfigured population are fulfilled, and both parties thereby promote a persisting cycle of disadvantage.

Strauss and Broder (1991, p.153) document that one of the most consistent findings to emerge from research studies, is the association between appearance, consequent social stereotyping and expectations (for example, Byrne, 1971; Berscheid, 1980; Langlois et al., 1987). The authors refer to Goffman's (1963) pioneering work on the theory of stigmatization and handicap, in attempting to unravel the essence of this association. Physical appearance which differs in some respect from the norm tends to engender negative evaluations by the onlooker.

From the literature, there can be little doubt that these evaluations contrive to alter the quality of interaction taking place between the affected individual and non-affected peers. Indeed, the interaction is not aided by the uncertainty with which the impaired individual approaches it, sensing potential stigmatization. As Strauss and Broder recommend: 'Studies of school performance, career attainment, dating, peer social relations, teasing, and discrimination may be done to determine how stigma experience results in altered interactions and self-concept' (p.153). The apparent distress and awkwardness which deformity causes has been found to be a cross-cultural phenomenon according to Shaw (1981).

In accordance with this theorizing and as anticipated, individuals with a visible cleft, whose facial appearance is thus disfigured, tend to be less acceptable to others than those with a non-disfigured appearance (for example, Tobiasen 1987). In Tobiasen's study, the cleft impaired were perceived as being less popular with peers, less sociable and less appealing as a potential friend, than their non-cleft contemporaries.

One consequence of these findings is that stigmatization directly affects the victim's self-perception. As Clifford and Clifford (1986) suggest, negative peer perceptions can adversely influence the relationship between self-esteem and self-concept. Thus, peers have a significant role to play in determining the psychosocial functioning of the cleft impaired.

Moreover, as the literature suggests, if peers perceive an individual to possess socially desirable attributes, that individual is likely to benefit as his or her friendship is an appealing acquisition (for example, Patzer, 1984; Tobiasen, 1989). If, however, the individual is visibly disfigured, the implications are less favourable since even first impressions can be stigmatising. Rather than enjoying rewarding friendships, this individual may internalize his or her disadvantaged status to such an extent as to believe that his/her friendship is not worth attaining (as a child, adolescent or adult). Unfortunately, such self-perceptions can convey subtle messages of rebuffal to all potential befrienders.

With respect to the data of the present study, the findings appear to support the literature. For example, the close association between visibility of the defect (deviant appearance) and subjection to teasing and negative perceptions of school, has been described in conjunction with the previous hypothesis.

The long term impact of stigmatization at school is suggested by the relationships between adult respondents' negative school perceptions and reports of being teased, and measures of their current self-esteem and personality traits. In almost all instances, the majority of those exhibiting low self-esteem in adulthood felt negatively about their school days, and/or had been subjected to peer victimization.

In similar vein, the majority of those (for most opposing pairs of adjectives) responding in the direction of socially undesirable personality traits, had experienced teasing and/or reported negative perceptions of school. At the same time, one must bear in mind that the majority of participants evidenced high self-esteem, and socially desirable personality characteristics, regardless of their experiences and memories of school (chapter five). It would seem, therefore, that whilst a minority subgroup are still conceivably suffering from their earlier adversity, the majority of participants are not hampered in the same way.

Further evidence that negative experiences of peer interaction at school, have a long term and deleterious impact upon only a minority of adult respondents, derives from data pertaining to changed perceptions on leaving the school environment. For example, most of those reporting unhappy impressions of school, report increased self-confidence since their school days ($p < 0.01$). A similar trend exists for almost all of those who were subjected to teasing. The suggestion that later life experience can undermine earlier tribulations, is reinforced by the finding that the majority of participants who expressed pessimism about their school years and/or had been victimized, were also able to proffer optimistic and positive advice to parents of a cleft-impaired baby (chapter five).

Regarding the relationship between peer and self-perceptions, it is noteworthy that many respondents volunteered that they had noticed a fundamental change in other people's attitudes towards them since leaving school. Similar sentiments were expressed in the course of conducting personal interviews (chapter seven). In view of this, whilst stigmatization of the facially disfigured may persist into adulthood, it appears most potent during the impressionable formative years, when friendships may be based on more superficial criteria than in adulthood.

In summary, it seems that inexpedient interaction with school peers, may be expected to exert a profound and a long term influence upon the psychosocial development and later functioning of those experiencing it. Having said this, further elucidation is preserved until discussion of hypothesis x, which addresses the reasons why in the face of adversity, some individuals metaphorically 'sink', whilst others apparently 'swim'.

Implications for clinical practice

Hypothesis vi Developmental trends amongst the participants in the study can be identified from information gleaned from independent data sets. Consequently, an 'at risk' group of individuals for psychosocial maldevelopment/malfunction can be detected during the developmental years, on the basis of their diagnosis, personal circumstances and/or social experiences.

The purpose of this supposition is to advocate that a group of participants were 'at risk' for psychosocial dysfunction during their developmental years. In doing so, a distinction must be made between at risk 'factors' and an at risk 'group', since it is the former which define the latter. For instance, whilst the cleft impairment itself is considered by some to put the cleft population 'at risk' in psychosocial terms, others specify particular factors which make the individuals especially vulnerable. Furthermore, not all those deemed to be 'at risk' on the basis of at risk factors (or warning signs), potentiate their status as such. The influences which contrive to keep the individual 'at risk' into adulthood, will be discussed under hypothesis viii.

Broder et al. (1992, p.262) highlight the vulnerability of the cleft population, by reviewing the evidence.

> Children with clefts are at risk for social rejection (Tobiasen, 1987), introversion (Richman, 1983), low self-esteem (Broder and Strauss, 1989), speech difficulties (Van Demark and Harden, 1990), negative body images, (Strauss et al., 1988), unrealistic perceptions about their facial appearance and behavior (Richman et al.,1985), and poor school achievement (Richman et al., 1988).

Similar sentiments are expressed by Kapp-Simon et al. (1992), in conjunction with congenital craniofacial anomalies. They endorse the notion that it is the existence of the impairment per se, which places affected children and adolescents 'at risk', rather than particular subgroups within the cleft population (for example, Wallander and Varni, 1989; Varni et al., 1989b). It is regrettable that the findings are not discussed in terms of visibility and non-visibility of the defects diagnosed.

Amidst the diverse aspects of development, there appears to be general consensus that it is the individual's psychosocial development which is most at risk. Some authorities indicate that the cleft impaired are susceptible to low self-esteem and socially undesirable personality traits (for example, Broder and Strauss, 1989). Other sources are more specific, and advocate that the visibility of the cleft renders the individual especially at risk for psychosocial dysfunction (such as Steinhausen, 1981). According to McWilliams and Musgrave (1972) and Fox et al. (1978), it is the severity of the cleft which is associated with the greatest risk for developmental problems, including language skills.

In contemplating how to allay individuals from being 'at risk' in the future, Clifford and Clifford (1986, p.118) state: 'We can only conclude that effective cleft palate treatment and psychological support early in life provides a basis for successful adaptation in adolescence.' In similar vein, Bickel (1970) points to the need for assistance to be offered as early as possible to the patient's family, especially the mother. In doing so, reference is made to the direct association between parental acceptance of the child and the child's personality.

Further recommendation of greater attention to the family is cited by Kapp-Simon et al. (1992, p.352), in conjunction with their study of chronically ill children, which includes youngsters with cleft lip and/or palate.

Varni and his associates have attempted to identify factors that are associated with better psychological functioning (Varni et al., 1988: 1989a; 1989b; Varni and Setoguchi, 1991). They suggested that variability in adjustment may be related to family functioning, childrens' self-perception, interpersonal skills, and the quality of social support available to the children.

On the basis of their investigation of the craniofacially disfigured, Pillemer and Cook (1989) state that this population is at risk for future psychological dysfunction. In particular, they attribute maladjustment to years of earlier adversity, as do Clifford and Clifford (1986) in their identification of a group of malfunctioning cleft-impaired adolescents.

In addressing the implications of an 'at risk' group, Kapp-Simon et al. (1992, p.356) emphasize the need for longitudinal research to identify factors which can predict adjustment over time.

Cross-sectional studies currently available suggest that there may be periods of time when children with CFA (craniofacial anomalies) are at greater psychological risk (e.g., when entering adolescence). Yet at each period of time there are children who appear to be functioning well based on the measures of adjustment available to us. Further identification of the factors that protect the child from psychological distress would enable professionals to screen families for those specific factors and establish intervention strategies geared to provide the support families need.

Consideration of the clinical implications in preventing the further demise of those most at risk, has been given by Strauss and Broder (1991). In heralding clinicians' attempts to highlight the need to evaluate psychological factors of the craniofacially-impaired, mention is made of the consequent increase in mental health workers and range of psychosocial services available (Broder and Richman, 1987). The enterprising developments include family support groups, relevant literature distributed to the affected families and schools concerning cleft conditions, and assessment of patients and family dynamics. The authors continue: 'We believe that these efforts reduce stress, increase awareness, decrease fear of the unknown, improve self-concept, and promote positive communication and family stability, yet no published data exist that verify these beliefs' (Strauss and Broder, 1991, p.152). The clinical implications of the findings are considered in chapter nine.

Therefore, there is evidence to suggest that information gathered from independent sources, identifies developmental trends which deem the cleft-impaired to be 'at risk' for psychosocial dysfunction. However, whether those at risk constitute the whole cleft population on the basis of the defect per se, or a particularly disadvantaged minority subgroup within that population is unclear from the published literature. At this stage, the findings of the current study implicate the emergence of a vulnerable subgroup, entrapped in a cycle of disadvantage. It is for this reason that the same hypothesis is presented for consideration in the subsequent section, since its relevance for the adult participants can be thereby addressed (hypothesis viii).

The adult participants' retrospective perceptions of being born with a cleft, and factors relating to their current psychosocial functioning (hypotheses vii-viii)

Factors relating to the type of cleft diagnosed

> It is only shallow people who do not judge by appearances.
> (Oscar Wilde)

Hypothesis vii Participants born with a cleft lip and palate experience greater and more persistent psychosocial trauma, than participants born with cleft palate only.

Previous discussion of the findings has focused upon the ature of the participants' personal circumstances and social experience during their developmental years. In doing so, the apparent significance of the visibility of the cleft defect has been highlighted. That is, regarding personal circumstances, the majority of those associated with an 'unfavourable' family environment and/or a 'detrimental' parental attitude, and/or personal maladjustment ($p < 0.05$) have a visible cleft. In similar vein, untoward experiences encountered at school, such as negative school perceptions and victimization by peers, seem to be more common in individuals having a visible than a non-visible defect ($p < 0.01$ and $p < 0.01$ respectively).

Whilst these results pertain to the participants' earlier years of life, it is notable that the same trend is evidenced by their self-report measures of self-esteem and personality as adults. Those responding in the direction of low self-esteem and/or socially undesirable personality traits, tended to have a visible as opposed to a non-visible cleft. Given that the pattern of responses is so consistent across variables, the psychosocial implications of having a visible cleft warrant further investigation.

In seeking deeper insight into the cleft population, some researchers have paid particular attention to the extent of the cleft defect as a significant variable, as Strauss and Broder (1991, p.152) comment.

> Recent work (Tobiasen, 1987) points to the need for standardized and broadly available measures of facial appearance for psychosocial research use. Extent of defect (disfigurement) may be an intervening variable that could affect self-perception, as well as observer perception (impression formation) (Tagiuri, 1969). Such data could impact on team treatment recommendations for patients and their families.

By way of clarifying the terminology prior to consulting further literature, a distinction can be drawn between two different descriptions of the cleft defect. The writer has referred already to the first of these, in discussing the 'visibility' versus the 'non-visibility' of the impairment. However, published research findings also allude to a 'mild' versus a 'severe' cleft. Since the terms represent different aspects of the condition, the relationship of one with the other can be broadly tabulated as follows. The diagnostic descriptions used in the table are in accordance with the classification delineated in chapter one (Hathorn, 1986). Table 8 denotes the extreme cleft types only, so, for example, an incomplete cleft lip and palate does not feature since it conceivably rests between the 'mild' and 'severe' forms of visible impairment.

With reference to Table 8.1 below, it will be noted that the participants involved in the investigation, are incorporated into three of the four cells. In that none of them has a cleft lip only, the 'visible/mild' combination is not applicable on this occasion.

Strauss and Broder (1991) promote the value of speaking in terms of the cleft's visibility (Broder, 1982; Broder and Strauss, 1989). However, in doing so they allude to the 'invisible' cleft to denote cleft palate only. On this matter, the writer prefers the use of the term 'non-visible', since although a cleft palate may not be visible to the layman, examination of the oral cavity renders it a non-visible, rather than an invisible defect.

Table 8.1
The association between visibility
and severity of the cleft

Visibility of the cleft	Severity of the cleft	
	'Mild'	'Severe'
Visible (cleft lip)	Incomplete/partial cleft lip (unilateral or bilateral)	Complete cleft lip (unilateral or bilateral with or without cleft palate)
Non-Visible (cleft palate)	Incomplete cleft palate only	Complete cleft palate (with or without cleft lip)

Other researchers focus on the severity of the cleft. Amongst them is Lansdown et al. (1991), who explore the challenging notion that severe facial disfigurement may be less psychologically traumatic for the individual than a milder disfigurement. They cite various authorities whose findings support this hypothesis. For instance, MacGregor (1970) states that a milder defect may be more difficult to cope with, in comparison with a severe defect. Similarly, Epsteen (1958) surmises that a relatively minor facial deformity can produce psychological distress which is disproportionate to the severity of the anomaly. This finding is later reinforced by Harper et al. (1980).

In interpreting these results, an especially notable explanation has been advanced by Reich (1969), which centres on the theme of predictability. That is, those with a severe facial defect can confidently predict that they will receive an adverse response from the majority of people they meet. However, because the mildly facially impaired cannot predict others' reactions to them with such accuracy, their anxiety levels are raised in anticipation which reinforces feelings of tension (MacGregor, 1990). As Lansdown et al. relate (1991, p.170):

> These results, contradicting the general public's assumptions, may speculatively be construed in terms of predictability. If children with a severe facial deformity know they will be stared at, called names, shunned or pitied, then they have to learn to cope with this consistent reality. However, children with a mild facial deformity may spend time and energy worrying whether or not their deformity has been noticed. An inability to predict other people's responses is well known as an underlying factor in anxiety (Kelly, 1955) and could explain previously anecdotal conclusions as well as those reported here.

In accordance with the concept that psychosocial distress may be caused by the unpredictability of other peoples' reactions, Strauss and Broder (1991, p.153) refer to the 'theme of uncertainty in interpersonal interaction.' Having said this, they do not denote the potentially greater trauma associated with milder deformity.

Whilst severity of the impairment may not be a valid predictor of psychological trauma, some authorities argue that visibility is of more significance. In their study of burns patients Williams and Griffiths (1991) discovered that visibility was a notable predictor of psychological welfare. Other findings show no correlation between visiblity and severity of the disfigurement (for example, White, 1982).

Needless to say, the revelation that a linear relationship does not appear to exist between the degree of facial disfigurement and the degree of psychological distress caused, has enormous implications for those treating the cleft population. The fact that the findings mitigate against general expectations infers that unless the Cleft Palate Team has access to such knowledge, the vulnerability of those with relatively mild anomalies may be grossly underestimated.

At this point, reference must be made to an observation proffered by a plastic surgeon involved in cleft management. On discussing the hypothesis under scrutiny with the writer, the surgeon stated that in his experience, those with an asymmetrical facial appearance (unilateral cleft lip), are perceived by others to have greater facial abnormality, than those with a symmetrical appearance (bilateral cleft lip). Thus, the relationship between perceived abnormality and severity of the cleft seems to be contrary to expectation.

With reference to the interview data of the present study, one person highlighted the particular predicament experienced by the mildly facially disfigured.

Perhaps they think well, if it wasn't just for that little nick everything would be perfect ... If you got a major one, then there's not much you can do.

Reference to the idea that the expectations of those with a mild defect may differ to those with more extensive clefting, is made by BNH's former colleague.

I think perhaps too with just a little cleft ... their expectations are higher, whereas with a severe cleft the result is so ... miraculous that ... they worry less about that.

Another former colleague who worked with BNH, remarked that the realization that the mildly impaired may be suffering a disproportionate amount to their disfigurement, spurred a change in operative techniques.

... if you look at the history of the development of the actual surgery, you'll see that ... partial lip surgery changed several times in order to get rid of the problem which we ... noticed.

On further questioning, it transpired that the objective of the changes was to obtain 'unnoticeable scarring', with the scars being incorporated into the natural contours of the upper lip.

I think a lot of that depended ... on a better knowledge of the anatomy of the obicularis oris muscle ... by altering the approach to the operation ... gradually, you know, it became obvious we were getting better results, and they were important because ... the owners of these partial clefts were unhappy.

Strauss and Broder (1991, p.153) discuss the role disfigurement may play in the individual's psychosocial functioning. They suggest that in striving for undetectable scarring, the surgeon may be relinquishing the patient's psychological 'crutch'.

The impact of having had a deformity may remain a psychosocial issue even if only a minor scar persists as a physical reminder. Perhaps surgical repair that is effective in reducing the deformity may leave the patient adrift without the emotional protection or hiding place the defect provided (Peter and Chinsky, 1974; Schneiderman and Auer, 1984; Schneiderman and Harding, 1984).

Similarly, Bradbury et al. (1992, p.99), studied the psychosocial outcome of children undergoing prominent ear correction. In reporting their findings they state: 'During the postoperative interview there was some suggestion of more distress than before, as they could no longer find a reason for their problems.' The authors conclude that levels of patient distress cannot be predicted from the degree of prominence.

Therefore, in addressing the hypothesis that individuals born with a cleft lip and palate, experience more psychosocial trauma than their less impaired counterparts, various considerations need to be borne in mind. Since cleft lip constitutes a visible facial disfigurement, those with additional cleft lip do appear to experience greater tribulation in their personal and social lives.   Having established this, with respect to the visible cleft population, it is advocated that those with milder facial disfigurement may encounter more psychosocial distress than those with more severe clefting. Although this notion may contradict expectation, there is convincing evidence that it is a feasible explanation in view of the research findings, and one which is also applicable to other forms of facial disfigurement.

Regarding the present investigation, the results increasingly point to the existence of a vulnerable minority subgroup amongst the participants. With respect to those seemingly entrapped in a cycle of disadvantage, their plight might be exacerbated by the mildness, rather than the severity of a visible cleft.

Implications for clinical practice

Hypothesis viii   An 'at risk' group of individuals for psychosocial maldevelopment/malfunction can be identified during the adult years, on the basis of their diagnosis, personal circumstances and/or social experiences.

In discussing hypothesis vi, the existence of an 'at risk' group of individuals during the developmental years was advocated. At the same time, however, uncertainty was expressed as to whether the vulnerable group applied to the cleft population per se on account of the defect, or to a particularly disadvantaged subgroup within that population. The purpose of the current hypothesis is to examine this issue with the benefit of hindsight, from the participants' adult perspective.

Regarding the data elicited by the adult participants, the majority of them responded in the direction of high self-esteem, and socially desirable personality characteristics, regardless of cleft type and earlier adversity (chapter five). Moreover, most of those who expressed negative school perceptions and/or had been subjected to teasing, reported increased self-confidence since leaving school ($p < 0.01$ and non-significant respectively). In addition, the preponderance of those facing tribulation at school were now able to proffer positive advice to the hypothetical parents of a baby with a cleft.

Further evidence of the apparent psychosocial health of the majority of the adult respondents, is found in their levels of current satisfaction with speech and appearance, and the perceived influence of the cleft upon various aspects of life. In these instances, the emerging trend is that regardless of the quality of the participants' lives during the developmental years, most of the participants are functioning well as adults.

The trend, however, does not incorporate the unfortunate minority who began life in disadvantaged personal circumstances, encountered further tribulation at school, and appear to continue to do so in adulthood. Indeed, one needs only to peruse the findings of the data mentioned above, to realize that on every occasion, there is a subgroup of participants who respond in the direction of disadvantage. For example, with respect to advice to parents, the vast majority of those who emphasized the negative aspects of having a cleft, harboured unhappy memories of school and/or had been victimized by peers (chapter five).

Thus, it is advocated that although the cleft defect itself may predispose the individual towards vulnerability, in terms of personal circumstances and social experiences, this susceptibility is not necessarily realized in adulthood. Having said this, for a minority of the cleft impaired, the realization of this potential is apparent during the developmental years, and continues to be apparent in adulthood.

In proposing the notion that 'time heals wounds', Bjornsson and Agustsdottir (1987, p.156) suggest that the impact of earlier trauma diminishes over time. That is, the painful memories of childhood, are pushed into the recesses of the subconscious mind (for example, Edwards and Watson, 1980; Heller et al., 1981). Needless to say, this is the authors' explanation for their subjects' relatively high levels of satisfaction with cleft-related treatment. Other authorities advocate that adjustment to disfigurement over time is a natural progression, involving various psychological processes (Patterson et al., 1993). In view of the minority subgroup mentioned above, however, time does not appear to heal all wounds universally.

One of the most notable insights into the psychosocial functioning of the adult cleft population is offered by Heller et al. (1981, p.464).

> ... the results for these patients are consistent with the picture of prolonged dependence on the family and of lower levels of social integration reported by others (Spriestersbach, 1973; Peter et al., 1975). These young adults with CLP (cleft lip and/or palate) also appear to be disadvantaged with respect to their peers. Half of this sample were less than completely satisfied with their social life, almost half had few leisure activities, and one quarter had few friends. Other studies document fewer friendships, decreased participation in social activities, and a later and lower marriage rate (McWilliams and Paradise, 1973; Peter and Chinsky, 1974). If we consider those rated as 'marginally adequate' along with those judged to display clearly inadequate psychosocial functioning, the figure for maladjustment is 33% - considerably higher than that reported for adult Montrealers (Roberts et al., 1970), but somewhat lower than the figures given for Midtown Manhattan (Langner and Michael, 1963).

Continued problems in the realm of social and personal functioning are also reported by Noar (1991). In his study of cleft-impaired young adults (aged 16-25 years), particular difficulties were expressed regarding the acquisition of a girl or a boy friend.

Therefore, whilst the majority of adults with a cleft manage to cope satisfactorily in psychosocial terms, there is evidence that a residual group of those perceived to be 'at risk' during their earlier lives remain 'at risk' in their adult lives. In this respect, Fox et al. (1978) claim that it is possible to predict the problems exhibited by older children and adults with cleft palate, during the first three years of life. If this is so, it heralds optimistic implications for those most 'at risk', since this finding can instigate improvements in clinical practice.

In summary, the purpose of considering the existence of an 'at risk' group during the developmental years (hypothesis vi), and in adulthood (hypothesis viii), has been to establish the feasibility of predicting problems in psychosocial development for later functioning. The fact that a disadvantaged minority in adulthood is associated with 'at risk' factors, such as having a visible cleft and experience of earlier victimization, deems the factors to have predictive qualities. It is precisely because the nature of these factors are themselves predictable, that predictions can be made early on in the child's development, with the expectation that further tribulation can be allayed.

Even if the nature of the disadvantageous personal circumstances and social experiences encountered by the cleft impaired cannot be improved directly, once those at risk have been identified, steps can be taken to equip them with the necessary psychosocial 'survival kit'. In this way, the prediction of long term adversity can, at least be thwarted. Further elucidation of this fundamental issue and its implications for clinical intervention, can be found in the following section.

Factors determining the impact of circumstances and experiences encountered during the developmental years, upon the participants' psychosocial functioning in adulthood (hypotheses ix-x)

On reaching this stage of the discussion, a consistent pattern of findings has been established, concerning the psychosocial functioning of the participants involved in the study. In its broadest sense, this pattern indicates that the majority of individuals appear to be functioning satisfactorily, regardless of their previous circumstances and experiences, whilst a minority still bear the scars of earlier disadvantage and adversity. In this way, a cycle of disadvantage that was set in motion during the developmental years, gathers momentum and impact by persisting into adulthood.

The opportunity now arises to tackle the fundamental question as to what determines whether an individual is incorporated into the well functioning majority, or the poorly functioning minority. By addressing this issue with the benefit of hindsight, observations can be made which will have direct relevance for clinical practice, in that early identification of the vulnerable subgroup may forestall later psychosocial dysfunction.

In doing so, the two areas to be studied are not so much 'hypotheses' as theoretical tenets, which emerge from the preceding discussion of data and pertinent literature. In posing intrinsically significant questions regarding cause and effect relationships in accounting for developmental trends, they underpin the theoretical infrastructure of the whole investigation.

Hypothesis ix Coping mechanisms are a function of innate and/or learned behavioural responses to environmental stimuli.

Examination of the data suggests that differences in long term outcome, may be attributable to intrinsic differences in the participants' psychological disposition. These variations are evidenced by the responses shown to adverse environmental stimuli, such as being teased by peers.

Regarding the range of responses to teasing in the data, the participants seem to fall into three distinct groups. Emphasis is placed upon the nature of the response made, since it reflects the way in which the individuals coped with their predicament. As will become apparent, whilst some individuals appear to possess naturally resilient personalities, others have had to learn resilience, or have been unable to learn it for some reason. Indeed, those implicated in the 'at risk' group discussed in conjunction with hypotheses vi and viii, may be precisely those who lack the necessary psychosocial means to break the cycle of disadvantage in which they are evidently trapped. The three groups are delineated below.

Group 1   Innate/'natural' resilience: e.g. humouring the bully.

Group 2   Learned resilience: e.g. learning to ignore the bully.

Group 3   'At risk': lacks innate or learned resilience to avert psychological injury.

Each of these groups will be discussed in accordance with pertinent data and literature. Needless to say, the discussion is largely speculative in view of the paucity of literature in this area.

Group 1 - Innate or 'natural' coping strategies

According to Clifford and Clifford (1986), the ability to cope effectively with the challenge of disfigurement, stems from early and satisfactory psychological adjustment to being born with a defect. With reference to the data, there is abundant and predictable evidence of the close correspondence between a 'favourable' home background, parents who display an 'encouraging' attitude towards the cleft-impaired child, and healthy personal adjustment. The hospital records indicate that most participants did not show signs of psychosocial maladjustment during the various developmental stages (chapter four). In the majority of instances, the individuals' early environment was conducive to psychosocial development, with supportive relationships being formed between the impaired child and other family members.

In contrast and by implication, the inability to cope effectively with the challenge of disfigurement, may stem from early and unsatisfactory adaptation to the defect. This probability has been discussed in conjunction with earlier hypotheses.

Regardless of the nature of home circumstances and family relationships, however, most participants encountered adversity outside the home environment. Therefore, the way in which these individuals responded to (and thus coped with) the untoward experiences encountered, may explain why some of them were able to deflect the potentially venomous intimidation by peers.

With respect to the interview data, various coping strategies were imputed in discussing the interviewees' response to being teased (chapter seven). It is advocated that individuals with a natural resilience were prepared to take a more active role than their less outgoing counterparts, by humouring the bullies or offering reciprocal retorts. In that an active response requires a degree of assertiveness, this behaviour is most likely to be displayed by individuals with a natural ebullience, who are not easily intimidated.

Having conducted the interviews, it is clear that those who reported using these particular coping mechanisms during their youth, were the most extravert and self-confident of the interviewees. Indeed, one member of this 'naturally resilient' group volunteered that he relied upon his sense of humour and personality more than anything else. He, like others with his disposition, had obviously naturally acquired his psychological 'survival kit' long before it was needed.

During the course of other interviews, constant reference was made to the role self-confidence played in coping with adverse situations. It is notable that this retrospective observation tended to derive from those who had fared less well during their developmental years. For instance, with the benefit of hindsight, self-confidence was perceived as the key to coping effectively: '... confidence ... that's what its all about' (chapter seven). For those fortunate enough to possess this coveted attribute, life seemed more benevolent and altogether less traumatic.

Having said this, although self-confidence may be inextricably linked to self-esteem, where applicable, an 'unfavourable' home background did not appear to dampen the individuals' resilience. Indeed, if anything, earlier disadvantage may have enhanced their determination to assert themselves. It would seem that some people have the innate capacity or predisposition to survive in psychosocial terms, by possessing natural coping strategies which ensure their survival whatever their situation.

Perhaps the underlying 'secret' of this competent group, is that the teasing is not sufficiently internalized as to play havoc with their sensibilities. That is, the significance of being the target for victimization by peers is undermined and considered of little consequence to them. In characterizing the other two subgroups, the extent to which the ridicule is internalized by those subjected to teasing, may prove to be the distinguishing factor.

Group 2 - Learned coping strategies

Whilst some individuals appear to be 'blessed' with innate/natural coping mechanisms for dealing with adversity, others may need to learn effective coping strategies in the process of encountering such experiences.

Examples of learned coping strategies are exemplified in the interview data. Responses to teasing include ignoring the comments made, avoidance behaviour, offering some explanation for the defect, and 'counting one's blessings' (such as others are worse off). In all these instances, the responses reflect reactions which have been advised or taught to the individuals concerned, by members of the Cleft Palate Team, school teachers, parents and so forth. Most interviewees felt that their strategies had effectively diminished the impact of victimization, and the extent to which they had internalized the insults.

In encouraging the learning of specific skills to cope with challenging experiences, the development of training programmes for the facially disfigured has been promoted. The instigation of such a scheme, in itself, gives credence to the notion that coping skills can be learned, and reflects the lack of innate coping strategies amongst some members of the cleft population. There is evidence to suggest that social skills are associated with psychological adjustment to disfigurement (Moore et al., 1993). This finding reinforces the work of Kapp-Simon et al. (1992, p.355) on children and adolescents with craniofacial anomalies (CFA), including cleft lip and/or palate.

> Increasing the social skills of children with CFA could potentially have a positive effect on overall adjustment. The child with CFA does not have much control over the reactions of others to his or her physical differences, but s/he can learn to behave in a more effective manner through specific social skills training (McGuire, 1990). Consistent with the experimental results of Rumsey et al. (1986), these findings lend additional support to the belief that improving the social skills of children with facial disfigurement could result in improved psychological adjustment and decreased social inhibition. Thus, a next step in understanding the relationships among these variables is to teach specific social skills to affected children, assess the effects of this training, and then measure the impact of skill acquisition on adjustment and social inhibition.

As mentioned earlier, self-confidence appears to be one of the prime components of effective coping. Needless to say, this particular attribute is inferred in the advice given to youngsters, and which is encouraged in social skills training. It is notable that a high proportion of the postal questionnaire respondents identified increased self-confidence when asked if and how their perceptions about school had changed since leaving school. When these data were cross-tabulated with those relating to negative perceptions of school and instances of teasing, on both occasions the vast majority of those reporting increased self-confidence since leaving school, expressed negative perceptions of school ($p < 0.01$), and/or had been subjected to teasing (as discussed in chapter five).

These findings clearly reinforce the notion that the learning of coping strategies in the face of adversity, can enhance psychosocial functioning. The fact that this attribute appears to develop on leaving school, suggests that some individuals are not naturally resilient, and need to learn to cope with threatening situations. Moreover, it is precisely by learning to cope and coping satisfactorily, that self-confidence is given the opportunity to flourish.

Although most of the adult participants in the study, are functioning satisfactorily in psychosocial terms, the residual subgroup continue to be enmeshed in a labyrinth of disadvantaged psychosocial functioning. Whilst the majority exemplify the use of innate and/or learned coping mechanisms delineated above, the lack of effective coping strategies is all too apparent in the vulnerable minority.

Evidence of the comparatively passive and subjugated existence of this minority, is found in the interview data. For example, references are made to responses to teasing which invited further victimization, by their inherent submission to the bullies. One individual divulged how he burst into tears and was *'hounded even more for crying'*. Another interviewee reported that he was *'very vulnerable psychologically'* at school, and harboured a defeatist attitude towards those who bullied him (chapter seven).

Allusion is again made to the significance of self-confidence in handling victimization effectively. In this context, one interviewee attributed his particular predicament to a lack of this esteemed facility:

> *... its something I've always lacked really ... a lot of confidence ... and that's ... held me back from ... certain situations.* (Results IV)

On examining the data, it is these individuals who continue to experience psychosocial problems as adults. For instance, one individual perceived that he has a long term 'psychological problem', and has contemplated seeing a psychiatrist or receiving counselling. By his own admission his social life is non-existent, and that he has got no 'real' friends to speak of. Another individual thought that she was always *'going to have a rough deal'*, since she felt that other peoples' attitudes cannot be changed.

Therefore, there is sufficient evidence to suggest that a minority of participants are 'at risk' in psychosocial terms, and that they will continue to be 'at risk' unless some form of intervention is offered to them. Perhaps the most significant factor which distinguishes between the optimistic or pessimistic outcomes experienced by the participants, is the degree to which the victimization is internalized. Whilst the previous two groups appear to be able to avert the impact of their negative experiences, those at most psychological risk are vulnerable because of their tendency to personalize and internalize the verbal abuse slung at them.

Although these individuals have now reached adulthood, their predicament may be reversible with appropriate intervention. Indeed, the 'successful' outcome of a recent programme aimed at addressing the problems of facially disfigured adults, has proved the efficacy of such a programme (*Changing Faces: Workshops and Advice for the Facially Disfigured*, conducted by James Partridge, 1992). Preliminary evaluation of the training programme suggests that it can enable the participants to become more self-confident, and less anxious in socializing with other people (Partridge et al., 1994).

In addition to providing a forum for discussing individual problems, the programme can effect fundamental and desirable changes if targeted at the appropriate individuals, at the appropriate time. However, in assisting in running the workshop, the writer discovered that potential candidates were not always willing, nor ready to be helped. In offering any form of help, the professional must always respect the participant's decision as to whether or not he or wishes to participate.

Social skills training is also proposed by Kapp-Simon et al. (1992), who found that psychological adjustment was most accurately predicted by the degree of social skills exhibited by adolescents with craniofacial anomalies (CFA) including cleft lip and/or palate. That is, maladjusted individuals were more likely than their well-adjusted contemporaries to display inadequate social skills.

> These findings suggest that adjustment and ultimately the level of inhibition displayed by children with CFA is related to their social skills and social behaviors rather than their feelings about their appearance, their perception of school performance, or even their own sense of self-worth. Additionally, children rated by their parents as possessing better social skills were more likely to feel socially accepted. (Kapp-Simon et al., 1992, p.355)

In view of the findings and the available literature, it is feasible to advocate the existence of three discrete subgroups within the cleft population. Whilst two of these enclaves incorporate individuals who 'survive' in psychosocial terms, by deploying innate and/or learned coping mechanisms, the third subgroup appears to lack the necessary survival 'equipment'.

Although efforts have been made to identify the nature of the 'survival kit', it appears that an ability to deflect the potentially injurious teasing comments is especially significant. Kobasa (1979) has advanced the useful concept of 'hardiness', to describe the resilience with which some individuals are able to cope with adverse situations. This notion implicates a sense of psychological 'detachment' (Roger, 1992) from the incident during the incident, and as such is identified as an integral component of adaptive 'coping style'.

Further insight is gained by consulting the locus of control theory (Rotter, 1966), which distinguishes between internal and external sources of control. That is, people who feel in control of their own lives and destiny (internal), contrast with those perceiving their lives to be controlled by external forces (external). This theory has direct implications for characterizing those who apparently cope, or fail to cope with challenging situations. For example, individuals with an internal locus of control, are more likely than their externally controlled counterparts to be in charge of their responses to events. Therefore, by undermining the implications of being teased by peers, their sense of self is controlled and maintained by their own behaviour, rather than being deranged and determined by the bullies' behaviour. The close association between taking responsibility for one's actions, and a positive self-perception and high self-esteem cannot be underestimated.

The evident benefits of possessing an internal locus of control are discussed by Hopson and Scally (1981, p.75), who describe the attempts of school teachers to encourage more youngsters to adopt this perspective.

A number of studies (de Charms, 1972) have demonstrated how teachers can be taught to teach children to increase their self-perceptions of internal self-control. They are taught to set realistic goals and to take personal responsibility for their actions. They discuss things that have happened in their lives and learn to ask questions like, 'Did I allow that to happen to me?, 'What could I have done about it?'. These programmes have been found to result in increased motivation for learning and in improved academic achievement.

In defining factors predisposing an individual towards internality, the authors identify characteristics associated with the early family environment, namely, nurturance, warmth and protection, in addition to consistent parental reinforcement. 'Absence of these or too much nurturance and protection can lead to a belief in external control' (Hopson and Scally, 1981, p.75). By implication, in the context of the present study, a 'detrimental' parental attitude epitomized by indifferent or overprotective parenting, could have conceivably encouraged externality in the children concerned.

The theme of taking responsibility for one's self is now pursued, in discussing the way in which professionals and patients perceive each other in the course of cleft-related treatment.

Hypothesis x The cleft impaired are perceived as a 'normal' rather than a pathological population, by professionals involved in cleft-related treatment.

The issue to be addressed on this occasion concerns the way in which the professionals on the Cleft Palate Team perceive the cleft population. On examining this area, it will be seen that the professionals can actually shape the patient's (and his or her parents) own perception of the defect. The implications of this are of fundamental significance to the parents' attitude towards the impaired individual and cleft-related treatment, which is in turn, integral to the patient's emerging self-perception and self-esteem.

The discussion will be extended subsequently, to consider the way in which the patient and his or her parents perceive the Cleft Palate Team, since this can also exert a profound effect upon the patient's psychosocial development.

By way of clarifying the terminology, the term 'pathological' attributes physical or mental disorder as the cause of an anomaly. On the other hand, 'normal' alludes to that which conforms to a standard type, and is regarded to be 'free from mental or emotional disorder' *(The Concise Oxford Dictionary)*. It is notable that this definition makes no reference to physical disorder. The fundamental difference between them becomes obvious in considering their implications not only for the cleft population, but also those with other forms of disfigurement.

To take the two extremes, the defect can be regarded as a birth defect which can be largely normalized by surgery and other appropriate interventions, or as a gross and lifelong deformity. The sometimes lengthy course of hospital treatment may be seen as reinforcing the pathological implications associated with a cleft. It is no coincidence that in illustrating the opposing perspectives, reference is made to the deformity, rather than to the person with the deformity. The emphasis upon symptoms as opposed to the their implications for the individual, infers that the individual may be perceived in terms of the defect. Thus the 'correctability' of the predicament may determine whether the person born with a cleft, is seen as a 'pathological' case or one who is inherently 'normal'. Such perceptions may carry implicit value judgements.

At face value, the dichotomy may seem straightforward and based upon personal opinion. On closer examination the matter of professional perception is not only a complex issue, but one which warrants some justification in view of its potential impact upon the patient. Although sporadic, the literature reflects this complexity and the divided opinion as to whether the cleft population should be placed into the 'normal', or the 'pathological' camp.

By way of highlighting the different implications of the two perspectives, Table 8.2 below compares their relative strengths and weaknesses. As will become apparent, the two perceptions convey intrinsically different messages to the patient and to his or her parents.

Table 8.2
Different perceptions of the cleft population held by members of the Cleft Palate Team

Cleft population perceived as 'normal'	Cleft population perceived as 'pathological'
Professionals anticipate the hospital intervention offered to 'normalize' the patient with a cleft, thereby enabling him/her to lead a 'normal' life.	Professionals anticipate that the patient with a cleft may require their expertise for many years, due to the multiplicity of potential cleft-related problems.
Since psychological problems are not anticipated, emphasis is placed upon correcting the visible and/or audible defects associated with a cleft	If the patient has adequate support from family/friends, psychosocial problems which do emerge may be minimized. However, there exists a hospital-based support network available if necessary
Therefore, the potential for psychosocial problems which cleft-related is underestimated. Insufficient attention may be given to the cleft-impaired patient when psychosocial problems do arise.	Therefore, potential cleft-related problems are anticipated and it is conceivable that too much emphasis may be placed upon detecting possible signs of psychopathology.
Consequently, complications may arise from problems being inadequately addressed.	Consequently, complications may arise from problems being overly addressed.

Depending upon the Cleft Palate Team's perception of the cleft defect, patients and the patients' parents are unwittingly relegated to either the 'normal' or the 'pathological' groups (Table 8.2). As suggested earlier, this consignment does not depend so much upon the individual's psychosocial functioning, as upon notions of the cleft condition per se. Thus emphasis is placed upon the indications for medical or paramedical intervention, rather than the implications of the defect for the patients' integration into the 'outside' world.

Some members of the Cleft Palate Team may conceive that a pathological view of the cleft population would create further problems, by encouraging the patient (and his or her parents) to indulge in their predicament. At the same time, however, other professionals feel that treating the patient as one who essentially conforms to the standard of 'normality', may undermine potential problem areas to the detriment of the patient and his or her parents.

Needless to say, where the different perceptions are held by members of the same Cleft Palate Team, the cohesion of treatment objectives may be confounded. Attention is turned first to discussing the implications for perceiving the cleft population in terms of its 'normality' with subsequent consideration given to its possible 'pathological' status.

One of the prime advocates for highlighting the normality of the cleft population, is Clifford (1983) who poses the challenging question 'Why are they so normal?'. Based on research findings that the cleft impaired do not show signs of psychopathology (for example, Goodstein, 1968; Strauss and Broder, 1991), and are able to function satisfactorily in psychosocial terms, Clifford suggests that their cleft-related problems have been overestimated by those treating them. 'It is possible that by their very availability cleft palate teams influence adaptation to the circumstances of cleft lip and palate' (p.83).

Thus, by promoting notions of goal-orientated treatment, applauding improvements in the patient's speech and/or appearance, and emphasizing the importance of monitoring these concerns, professional interest in the cleft condition may enhance attention to potential problems areas. Other evidence that the cleft population exhibit normal psychosocial functioning, has been documented by Clifford and Clifford (1986) and Stricker et al. (1979) amongst others.

One of BNH's former colleagues reinforces how the professionals may distinguish the cleft population from other in-patients:

> ... the children weren't sick children, which does make a great deal of difference.

This view in itself demonstrates the emphasis placed upon the redemptive powers of corrective surgery.

If the cleft is regarded as a remediable defect in an otherwise 'normal' person by the professionals involved, the individual may experience a contradictory viewpoint when socializing with peers. As the literature expounds, impeded speech and/or appearance can provoke victimization and social isolation, which suggests that the social encounters of the cleft impaired may not experience 'normal' interaction. Where the professionals encourage the patient and his or her patient's parents to think in terms of the child's normality, the individual may have a rude awakening on entering school. As the personal account of Brown (1983, p.85) poignantly illustrates.

They (parents) tried so hard to show me that I was alright. 'You're OK. You are not different. We do not see you as being different'. I start to believe that I am alright because I believe my parents. Then I go back to school and the teasing would start; I'd get on the subway, people would stare.

Another paradox to emerge is that whilst professionals may encourage normalization of the cleft population, this message is discredited by the sometimes prolonged treatment programme, and insistence that regular review clinics should be attended. The 'hidden' agenda of these implications clearly convey to the individuals concerned, that they are still very much regarded as 'patients', requiring the expertise of the Cleft Palate Team until they are officially discharged.

In contrast, however, other authorities suggest that the cleft population should be incorporated into discussion of youngsters with chronic illnesses. A particularly notable contribution by Kapp-Simon et al. (1992), includes children and adolescents with cleft lip and/or palate in the study of craniofacially anomalies (CFA).

... children with CFA share many of the potential stressors that have been associated with having a chronic physical illness. These include such factors as repeated clinic evaluations throughout childhood, multiple hospitalizations, and differences in physical appearance (Wallander et al., 1989, Varni and Setoguchi, 1991). These similarities suggest that children with CFA should rightly be considered children with chronic illness and that theories about their psychological functioning should draw on the broader literature available on children with chronic illness. (p.352)

In attempting to assuage value judgements at this point, one needs to define more precisely, what constitutes a pathological existence, as opposed to a pathological symptom. Within the broader context of disability, Philp and Duckworth (1982, p.2) refer to the dichotomy which exists between the terms 'primary' and 'secondary' handicap. They explain that allied to the obvious manifestation(s) of a (primary) handicap, 'secondary' handicap is seen as incorporating:

... an important facet of disadvantage, ie adverse professional and public reaction to the presence of primary handicap by way of labelling and stigma.

Thus, by implication, an individual's handicap should be seen in terms of its wider personal and social implications, in addition to its physical symptoms.

In view of the misrepresentation of what 'handicap' may imply, the World Health Organisation (WHO, 1980b) has addressed the problems of definition in its trial scheme of terminology, based on Wood's (1975) preparatory work in Britain. The scheme presents a conceptual framework for a trial *'International Classification of Impairments, Disabilities, and Handicaps' (ICIDH)*.

In the scheme, the idea of handicap as equivalent to disadvantage consequent on disease, defect or disability is given a much more precise definition by means of a terminology of 'disablement' (Wood and Badley, 1978). Disablement is regarded as consisting of three consecutive but distinguishable 'planes' of experience - that of impairment, that of disability and that of handicap. (Philp and Duckworth, 1982, p.2)

The way in which these planes relate to each other is outlined below (Philp and Duckworth, 1982, p.3).

Disablement (experience summarized)

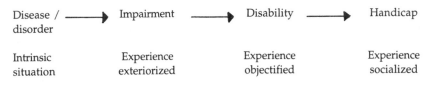

Figure 8.2   The concepts in the World Health Organisation trial scheme

The three planes of experience are described in terms of the physical, functional and social implications for the individuals concerned. In this scheme, 'handicaps' no longer refer to a subgroup of disabilities, but represent the disadvantages which result from disabilities.

- *Impairments (experience exteriorized)* describe the individuals' physical anomalies and abnormal appearance.

- *Disabilities (experience objectified)* describe the way in which the individuals' everyday functions and their execution are hampered.

- *Handicaps (experience socialized)* describe the disadvantages which prevent the individuals from carrying out roles which are characteristic of normal life (determined by sex, age, social and cultural factors).

The paradigm proposed above deliberately moves away from the classification of intrinsic and extrinsic handicap. In reporting upon the working party's instigation, Philp and Duckworth (1982) state that whilst the significance of the intrinsic/extrinsic distinction was diminishing, it continued to reflect the primary interests of 'medical' and 'social' workers.

215

That is, the former tend to treat intrinsic handicap, and the latter extrinsic handicap. In this regard, the reader is reminded of the writer's reference to the comparable terms 'overt' and 'covert' problems (chapter one). Whilst this categorization is useful, and served the purpose of delineating the primary concerns of the present study, it is now superseded by the more refined scheme compiled by the World Health Organisation working party.

The dichotomy between 'normal' and 'pathological' perceptions of the cleft population, therefore, raises complex issues as to how impaired, disabled and/or handicapped this population is in reality. Much appears to depend upon each individual's personal experience of living with a cleft, information to which the professionals may have little access, other than patients' (and their parents') word of mouth reports. Indeed, it could be advocated that members of the Cleft Palate Team are only aware of the finer details of this information, when they encounter instances of psychosocial dysfunction. That is, such insight is only gained when problems arise. In view of this, it is feasible to suggest that intervention for psychosocial difficulties, is generally provided on a curative, rather than a preventative basis.

Regarding the implications of the WHO model for the participants in the current study, whilst all of them can be legitimately regarded as exhibiting 'impairments' and 'disabilities', the vulnerable minority are most susceptible to experiencing 'handicaps' as well. As Philp and Duckworth (1982, p.5) explain:

> ... under the new WHO scheme, 'handicap' is not a label that should be automatically and permanently applied to any child with impairments, however severe. Rather it should be used as a precise description of last-resort disadvantage and unmet needs.

This conceptualization gives insight into how the cycle of disadvantage can persist into adulthood, as the following extract endorses.

> Handicap is characterized by a discordance between the individual's performance or status and the expectations of the particular groups of which he is a member. Disadvantage accrues as a result of being unable to conform to the norms of his universe. Handicap is thus a social phenomenon, representing the social and environmental consequences for the individual stemming from the presence of impairments and disabilities. The essence of an adverse valuation by society is discrimination by other people, but the concept is, nevertheless, essentially neutral as regards its origins. Thus the individual's own intention is of no immediate concern; disadvantage can arise when the individual deviates in spite of his own wishes, but it can also develop when the deviation is inadvertent or as the product of his own choice. (Philp and Duckworth, 1982, p.6).

In profiling the cleft population, it is notable that Tobiasen (1991) also recommends adoption of the WHO nomenclature, especially in widening the horizons of psychological research in this field.

Since the perceptions of the Cleft Palate Team can influence the perceptions of cleft-impaired patients, the former are responsible for promoting a realistic perspective. Whilst the perception of the cleft population as 'normal' or 'pathological', may be a matter of professional judgement and experience, a compromise position may be the most conducive for the patient. In accordance with the research findings, the message conveyed by the professionals to the patients, could implicate the increasing likelihood of living a 'normal' life with maturation, whilst acknowledging that this may be more challenging for some individuals than others.

Allied to the question concerning the most apposite way for the Cleft Palate Team to perceive the cleft population, is the issue concerning how the patients and their parents perceive the professionals responsible for providing cleft-related treatment. More precisely, this issue hinges on what roles are adopted by the patients (and their parents) and the professionals during the course of hospital intervention.

In examining the various options, Stengelhofen (1989) describes three distinct models of interaction which derive from the work of Cunningham and Davis (1985). Although these are proposed as models of parent-professional relationships, it is anticipated that with time the patient will be responsible for pursuing his or her own treatment. The paradigms described refer to the 'expert', the 'transplant' and the 'partnership' models of parent-professional interaction.

The expert model, incorporates the traditional medical model in assuming that the professionals are the experts, responsible for controlling the course of treatment. In contrast, the patient/patients' parents are expected to adopt a passive stance, accepting whatever received wisdom the experts feel appropriate to divulge. To the detriment of the patient, his or her passivity becomes inextricably linked with increasing dependence upon the professionals, who may unwittingly encourage the dependency by controlling the situation. This model of interaction is evidenced by many Cleft Palate Teams operating in the United Kingdom today.

A viable alternative to the traditional relationship, concerns the transplant model in which the professional adopts the role of teacher. Although the necessary treatment is still determined by the experts, the patient and/or his or her parents are involved in its execution. It is more apparent amongst health and educational personnel today, but its popularity is gradually gaining momentum in some aspects of cleft-related treatment. Perhaps the best example of this is seen in the context of speech therapy. Whilst the speech and language therapist conducts the appropriate assessments and plans treatment, the patient's and his or her parents' assistance in undertaking the advised activities at home, is considered essential if treatment objectives are to be fulfilled. In detailing this model, however, Stengelhofen cautions that lack of negotiation can result in resentment and power struggles between the parties concerned, particularly if parental interest and/or ability is questionable.

With respect to the multi-disciplinary nature of the Cleft Palate Team, and the sometimes extensive cleft-related treatment, the third type of parent-professional relationship appears to be the most conducive to the cleft population. The partnership model of interaction, is so-called because of its emphasis upon the adoption of active roles by all concerned in the individual's hospital intervention, including the parents.

Moreover, the parents are encouraged to express their opinions as to what they regard appropriate treatment, since they are most familiar with the child and thereby possess parental 'expertise'. According to this paradigm, the professional's role is one of a 'catalyst', which enables and supports the wishes of the parents (Pugh, 1985). As Stengelhofen (1989) points out, some parents may not wish to accept their role as partners. In such instances, the professionals should try to ascertain their reasons.

It is conceivable that parents may be reluctant to become active participants in the treatment process, because they prefer the implications of the expert model. Indeed, it could be speculated that those who offered only partial, or no explanation for non-attendance at hospital clinics (chapter five), wished to be non-committal regarding their role in the proceedings.

Having said this, since the data reflect trends which took place some twenty to forty years ago, it is likely that the treatment adhered to the traditional, expert model, where the patient and his/her parents were expected to adopt a passive role of compliance. Although in hypothetical terms the partnership model of interaction may be the most conducive to cleft-related treatment, the fulfilment of its objectives relies upon the mutual interest and commitment of both parties to the treatment process.

As Russell (1989, p.37) indicates in conjunction with speech and language therapy, in view of the sometimes lengthy treatment programme:

> There is the need to establish the foundations of a long term relationship with the parents and to provide them with accurate and comprehensible information.

However, this can only be established and maintained with the parents' assistance, as Oldfield and Tate (1964, p.8) remark:

> Speech results and prognosis after operation are rather unpredictable. They depend almost as much upon the intelligence and keenness of the mother as upon the anatomical result in the child's palate.

Therefore, with respect to the opening question as to whether patients and their parents regard the professionals as professionals or as partners, it seems that the reply lies with the patients and their parents. That is, if they are sufficiently interested in the treatment, they may perceive the professionals as partners, jointly investing their efforts for the ultimate benefit of the patient. If, however, they are indifferent towards the patient's hospital intervention, and dependent upon the professionals to do whatever is necessary, they will probably view the professionals as professionals. In this way, the stereotypical roles of the active professional and the passive patient are maintained. One implication of this, is that following hospital discharge the individual may feel vulnerable and a sense of loss in that he or she no longer has contact with the Cleft Palate Team. This perception may be especially strong where, due to the lengthy treatment programme, the hospital has been seen in terms of a 'very old family' (chapter seven).

In summary, in addressing a variety of hypotheses, this chapter has sought to enhance understanding of the participants' past and present psychosocial functioning. On speculating what determines present perceptions in view of past influences and experiences, it appears that it is not just a matter of luck whether an individual copes, or fails to cope with the challenge of disfigurement. Rather, the more optimistic probability infers that the individual can learn to cope, and can learn to cope effectively. Furthermore, this learning can take place at various stages of life with the appropriate guidance.

As the writer's own experience proves, having identified those most at risk, whether during the developmental or adult years, coping strategies and counselling can offer the individual the means by which to arrest the cycle of disadvantage. However, perhaps the greatest test is whether or not the individual wishes to be helped.

It is suggested that whilst the majority of participants were learning how to cope with adversity in their youth, the vulnerable minority were learning helplessness (Seligman, 1975). To use the terms adopted by Hopson and Scally (1981), those who can learn 'self-empowerment', whilst those who cannot are 'depowered'. As Lencione (1980) indicates, where psychological and social dysfunction does occur, it may be more handicapping for the individual than the cleft itself. The extent to which the depowered members of the cleft population may be helped to become self-empowered is the focus of the final chapter.

9 Conclusion and recommendations: what now?

If I tell you, you will forget,
If I show you, you will remember,
If I involve you, you will understand.
(Police Sergeant, Henley Training Centre)

Introduction

In culminating the study, this final part of the study has two objectives. Firstly, it seeks to conclude all that has gone before it in preceding chapters. Secondly, it proposes recommendations as a beacon for the future. In action research, conclusions are inextricably linked with heralding pertinent changes for the future.

Thus, in addition to formulating a conclusion, recommendations will be proposed for improving current clinical practice. In accordance with the data, the priorities for clinical intervention concern the early identification of those most 'at risk' in psychosocial terms (based on predictive factors), and where necessary reversing the cycle of disadvantage evidenced by older individuals. The recommendations to be discussed are delineated below.

- Parent counselling/education
- School involvement

- Support during adolescence
- The importance of continuity
- Indications for future research

In considering how the proposed recommendations can be potentiated, the reader's attention is drawn to the compilation of a hypothetical 'job description', for a hypothetical 'Specialist Liaison Professional' presented in Appendix 4. As implicated by the job description, it may be more expedient for one member (preferably a psychologist, or a speech and language therapist with a psychology background) of the Cleft Palate Team to assume responsibility for ensuring that the recommendations are implemented. In this way, proper attention can be given to the psychosocial aspects of patients' lives, as opposed to being disparately contemplated by all members of the team, as and when, the caseload permits.

The role designated to the 'Specialist Liaison Professional', is essentially borne out of the findings of the follow-up study. That is, whilst greater attention may be paid to the psychosocial implications of the cleft population in other countries, notably the United States of America, the current recommendations do not seek to directly emanate any one model of patient care. Indeed, the fundamental distinction between State provided and privately financed treatment provision serves to differentiate the treatment approaches adopted in the United Kingdom and the United States of America respectively. Thus, at this stage, it would appear to be expedient to recommend improvements which are tailor-made to the British National Health Service. Once the psychosocial needs of the cleft population have been more fully acknowledged, the constitution of the Cleft Palate Team in the United Kingdom might begin to resemble those found in the United States of America.

Parent counselling/education

> There are only two lasting things we can give our children -
> one is wings, the other roots.' (Richard Whitfield, 1988)

The objectives of recommending more attention to educating and/or counselling the parents of a cleft-impaired child from birth are as follows.

•   To provide a supportive and affirming role to the parents, and where necessary to encourage and enable the parents to adopt a positive attitude towards their child.

•   To offer help in addressing problems of a psychosocial nature if and when they arise. For example, this may include addressing the psychological aspects of poor parent-child, unsatisfactory feeding and/or impoverished communication and interaction.

•   To foster realistic expectations of the hospital treatment available, and to establish the need for sustained parental interest and

222

commitment to the patient's cleft-related treatment programme, which may span many years.

- To increase the parents' knowledge of the nature and implications of the cleft condition.

- To provide an advisory role for queries and anxieties which may arise. This includes making the parents aware of the existence and aims of the self-support groups run by the Cleft Lip and Palate Association (CLAPA), and the literature produced by the Association. Access to other information should also be made available to parents.

The underlying assumption in presenting these recommendations, is the perceived need to improve both the quantity and quality of the help proffered to the cleft-impaired child's parents. Whilst some guidance is given to the parents as part of the responsibilities of the Cleft Palate Team, the national picture of such provision continues to be very diverse and idiosyncratic across the country. The notion that a psychologist should be automatically included in every Cleft Palate Team, continues to be viewed with some scepticism by other more established members of the team. This uncertainty may stem from a general misunderstanding and underestimation of both the need for, and the role of such an essential presence on the team.

Alongside these recommendations must be acknowledged the invaluable part played by health care professionals working with the pre-school population, notably, speech and language therapists, social workers and health visitors. It is envisaged that rather than being perceived as a 'rival' by these disciplines, the creation of a 'Specialist Liaison Professional' (for whom the recommendations are largely proposed), would be welcomed as a means of supplementing and alleviating their already pressurized timetables.

By providing the parents with the necessary support and advice for coping with psychosocial difficulties from the child's birth, future problems may be assuaged if not prevented altogether. In addition, by equipping parents with adequate knowledge of the cleft condition, their expectations regarding the professionals' ability to perform 'miracles' can become more realistic. In this way, the parents can be enabled to feel more in control of their situation, and have a better understanding of the treatment implications.

This 'ideal' scenario is more likely to take place where the parents perceive that their part in the treatment process is valued by the professionals. In this way, a partnership model of hospital care may gradually evolve, with the potential for a joint 'contract' to be negotiated on the understanding that adherence to the child's treatment programme will be a mutual investment. That is, a contract in which both parties are required to invest their available resources and expertise for a common purpose. Therefore, as the development of a partnership becomes more feasible, less credence is attributed to the passive patient/active professional paradigm epitomized by the traditional medical model.

By conceptualizing treatment as a mutual investment, the cleft is treated by combining the efforts of the various experts. Whilst the professionals apply the skills of their particular profession, the patient and his/her parents have first hand experience of the implications of being born with a cleft, and the ensuing cleft-related problems encountered in everyday life.

Accordingly, each 'partner' can support the other in persevering through the sometimes lengthy treatment programme. The professionals can do this by affording the patient the best and most appropriate cleft-related treatment throughout. The patient and his or her parents on the other hand, can support treatment objectives by attending the specified hospital appointments, and by carrying out the advice offered, such as practising speech therapy activities at home. It should be noted, that there are diverse reasons other than parental indifference as to why opportunities for treatment (at follow-up clinics) may be missed, such as fear of the professionals, a chaotic life style, emotional instability, or inconvenience (amongst others). These reasons require a pro-active, rather than a reactive caring attitude from the professionals concerned if the partnership is to flourish.

Furthermore, parents' commitment to treatment during the patient's formative years, may be rewarded by the patient's own emerging commitment to it. This will become particularly apparent at the time of hospital discharge (usually during late adolescence or early adulthood), when the patient will be in a position to take responsibility for him/herself. Instead of experiencing the withdrawal symptoms of a dependant on discharge, the person will have gained the independence and confidence to cope effectively with the cleft defect. Perhaps the greatest benefit of the partnership approach to cleft-related treatment, is that the patient on discharge has learned how to be his or her own therapist.

In view of these implications, the need for greater attention to be given to the parents of the cleft-impaired child from the earliest possible stage cannot be disputed. Indeed, the consequences for the patient of committed and interested parents may contrast dramatically with the converse. The subsequent perpetuation of the cycle of disadvantage, may be only too apparent in the patient whose parents have not shown interest, nor been able to achieve commitment to the cleft-related treatment. Beginning with negative feelings towards the child with a cleft, perhaps from birth, the parents may pursue a parenting style which reflects and communicates their indifference to the youngster. Although this communication may be unspoken and relatively subtle in its expression, the young patient is usually sensitive to the message being conveyed.

If these vulnerable parents are not given sufficient support and affirmation in the early stages of the baby's life, the negative emotions and attitudes may be harboured and proliferate unchallenged. Early parent counselling has an invaluable role in identifying those most 'at risk' in psychosocial terms, and in addressing the emerging problems.

In presenting these recommendations, the consistent message of the literature in the arena of child psychology and psychiatry is heeded. That is, the attitudes, perceptions and behaviour of parents exert a significant influence upon the attitudes, perceptions and behaviour of their offspring, and evidence of this influence can be detected from infancy.

School involvement

The face is the image of the soul. (Cicero)

The focus of the second set of recommendations is upon the school environment, since it is here that the patient with a cleft spends a large proportion of the childhood and adolescent years. The recommendations to be made in conjunction with the school environment in general, are succeeded by those relating to the different levels of schooling. Underlying all of them is the aspiration to involve school staff in evaluating and advancing the progress of all cleft-impaired pupils.

The school environment in general

• To involve the school staff in adopting a holistic approach to treating the patient, since school plays a significant role in the patient's psychosocial development.

• To encourage the school staff to act as 'watch dogs' in detecting those at most risk for psychosocial maldevelopment and future malfunction, alerting the relevant professionals when and where necessary. In this way, the staff can be inspired to take a more active role in monitoring the progress of those, whose untoward personal circumstances and social experiences predict a persisting cycle of disadvantage.

The pre-school stage

At the pre-school stage, the young child may attend a playgroup or a nursery school, amongst the most common options. Within this early school environment, attention could be given to the following areas of development:

• Discussion of the child's speech and language skills, and the extent to which interaction with others is disrupted by impoverished communication skills and impaired hearing (where applicable). Suggestions could be proposed for optimizing opportunities for communication and social integration if necessary. In this way, the Cleft Palate Team has access to an additional source of information concerning the impact of the cleft defect upon the child's social and educational activities, and can thereby monitor the young patient's progress from the earliest stages of socialization.

• Discussion regarding the extent to which nursery or playgroup staff perceive the pre-school child with a cleft to be 'at risk', based upon their observations of the child's behaviour, such as withdrawal from social situations.

- Discussion regarding the benefit of talking about body image, and the implications of being different and disfigured, including instances of bullying.

- Encourage the use of stories which incorporate stigma and disfigurement of various kinds in positive presentations. There are various young childrens' books available which focus upon particular difficulties associated with sounding and looking different to others. For example, Althea's titles include *I Can't Talk Like You* and *I Use A Wheelchair*. Others consider the expression of feelings, such as Anita Harper's book entitled *What Feels Best*.

Initiatives are also being developed to raise the self-esteem of pre-school children, by exploring the value of self awareness group work known an 'Circletime' (White, 1989). A further resource is material addressing the problem of bullying, which incorporates Toni Goffe's *Bully for You ...*, and Angela Grunsell's *Let's Talk About Bullying* amongst others.

The primary and secondary school stages

At the primary and secondary school stages, liaison could be undertaken with schools attended by those with a cleft. The predominant areas of interest are those which reflect the individual's psychosocial development and functioning, as outlined below.

- Discussion of the impact of impaired articulation and/or nasal speech upon the child's communication and interaction with peers. Advice could be given as to how the school environment could be improved, where applicable, to maximize opportunities for communication and socialization.

- Discussion of emerging language problems which may be related to the cleft, and how they impact upon the individual's school life.

- Discussion of the child's hearing acuity in class, which may be impeded by the cleft condition. Factors such as whether the child sits in an optimum place in the classroom for hearing the teacher, and how the hearing loss affects classroom and peer interaction could be addressed.

- Discussion of the pupil's personal and social relationships within the school context, such as susceptibility to peer victimization and social isolation.

- Discussion of the school's policy for dealing with teasing and other forms of stigmatization. This could be centred on the literature produced in conjunction with the national Anti-bullying Campaign in May 1992 (for example, that supplied by Kidscape and Tattum and Herbert, 1990), which offers practical guidelines on how the bullied, the bullies and school staff can address the problem of victimization in schools. Other recent literature includes that produced by the National Society for the Protection of Children (NSPCC), which gives advice on how to alleviate the stress caused by bullying (such as, *Tips To Beat Stress*, 1992). Pertinent suggestions are also extended to the parents of the victims, which suggest the possibility for concerted efforts to be made in tackling this distressing area.

• Discussion as to the extent to which teachers and peers are cognizant of the individual's need for hospital treatment, such as hospitalization, and missed schooling due to attendance at hospital clinics. The school staff (including the Education Welfare Officer where applicable) can play an invaluable role in minimizing the potentially adverse impact of these events upon the child's school performance, by supporting the youngster awaiting hospital admission, and discussing the implications of being hospitalized. Relevant material in the form of stories about preparing for hospitalization is available (for example, Juliet Bawden's book *When I Went To Hospital*, 1989). Having said this, in undertaking these recommendations, school staff must beware of increasing the chances of classmates further labelling cleft-impaired pupils by affording the latter 'special' attention.

Since school teachers may have daily contact with the patient, they are in a unique position not only to alleviate problems faced by the patient/pupil, but also to discern signs of psychosocial distress and disadvantage. For these reasons, their co-operation needs to be sought throughout the patient's schooling. In doing so, they may be considered to represent the educational component of the Cleft Palate Team.

Support during adolescence

I can imagine nothing we could do that would be more relevant to human welfare, and nothing that could pose a greater challenge to the next generation of psychologists, than to discover how best to give psychology away. (Miller, 1969)

In addressing the diverse factors associated with adolescence, attention is first turned to how the Cleft Palate Team can assist the cleft-impaired teenager in general terms, before focusing upon its role in specific areas.

The Cleft Palate Team's role in assisting the adolescent cleft population

• To provide a supportive and affirming role to patients, and where necessary to encourage and enable patients to adopt a positive attitude towards themselves.

• To offer help in addressing problems of a psychosocial nature if and when they arise.

227

- To increase the patients' knowledge of the nature and implications of the cleft condition.

- To encourage realistic expectations of the hospital treatment available, and to establish the need for patients' consistent commitment to cleft-related treatment, which may span many years.

- To provide an advisory role for queries and anxieties which arise.

In perusing the above objectives, it is no co-incidence that they resemble those outlined for the first set of recommendations (parent counselling / education). However, the fundamental distinction between them is the shift of attention from the patient's parents to the patient him/herself. This shift reflects the development of the individual from one who is wholly dependent upon his/her parents, to that of an increasingly independent person. Therefore, in addition to the patient, the recommendations address care of the parents during the patient's formative years, and care of the patient when considering the years of adolescence and beyond.

The Cleft Palate Team's role in addressing specific cleft-related problems encountered by the adolescent cleft population

It has been established that psychosocial dysfunction during adolescence can be predicted from the accumulation of identifiable 'at risk' factors. The Cleft Palate Team, therefore, has a particular responsibility in detecting evidence of those factors in cleft-impaired patients. Such detection could incorporate attention to the following areas.

- The patient's personal adjustment to the cleft defect, and his/her response to the requisite cleft-related treatment.

- The patient's self-perception as measured by assessment of self-esteem and other personality traits at specific ages.

- The circumstances characterizing the patient's home environment.

- The experiences characterizing the patient's school environment and social life.

- The patient's intellectual development and school performance, which may be adversely affected by the presence of the cleft.

Having identified those whose psychosocial development is considered to be 'at risk', the individuals concerned can be offered help in addressing the problems encountered. It is anticipated that the most common problem areas will relate to the development of personal relationships and social interaction with peers. In response, the help available could incorporate training in specific aspects of socialization, which have proven value in enhancing the personal and social lives of the cleft-impaired. The primary components of the proposed training, which encompass the development of coping strategies for dealing with adverse situations are outlined below.

- Social skills training, which focuses upon the following:

  - Improved communication skills.

  - Discussion regarding the patient's personal and social relationships, with emphasis placed upon notions of self-esteem, self-confidence, self-perception and self-concept, which often challenge the cleft-impaired during adolescence.

  - Discussion regarding peer perception of the cleft-impaired individual, and how this need not determine self-perception.

  - Discussion regarding the nature of awkward situations in general, and how the adolescent's response to such situations may be altered for their ultimate gain.

- Assertiveness training, such as learning to challenge or deflate the protagonists of peer victimization.

Underlying these recommendations, is the assumption that by providing the patient with the necessary 'psychological equipment' and self-knowledge, the person is empowered to begin to take responsibility for him or herself. Whilst this approach to reversing the cycle of psychosocial disadvantage is still in its infancy, invaluable material is currently being developed by the charity 'Changing Faces', which offers rehabilitation for those with a facial disfigurement of all ages. As the charity's director, James Partridge (1992) explains in the literature, 'skills workshops' are being set up throughout the country, to enhance the self-confidence and social composure of the facially disfigured. In addition, the workshops provide the opportunity for the participants to meet others experiencing similar problems, and for supportive friendships to be cultivated.

The workshops seek to address the psychosocial difficulties associated with both acquired trauma (such as facial tumours and burns), and congenital anomalies (such as cleft lip and/or palate and birth marks). As evidenced by the participants, whilst the actual cause of the impairment may differ, the problems encountered can be very similar in essence.

In supporting the cleft-impaired during adolescence priority is given to identifying those at most risk for psychosocial dysfunction now and in the future. By countering present difficulties, such as peer victimization, with the assurance of learned coping skills and a more positive self-perception, it is anticipated that the cycle of disadvantage may be reversed.

Therefore, as with parents in the child's early years, by developing further insight into the cleft condition and its implications, the patient may experience greater control over his or her particular situation. Concepts of investing in treatment and adopting a partnership role with the Cleft Palate Team discussed in relation to the earlier recommendations have direct relevance here.

A variety of recommendations has been presented. Between them, they offer proposals for development which relate to the patient, the patient's parents, and the professionals. Suggestions targeted at the school, implicate that this relatively untapped source has a potentially significant part to play in addressing the patient's psychosocial needs.

The importance of continuity

The patient born with a cleft may require hospital treatment from infancy into adulthood, depending upon individual circumstances. In view of this, the recommendations previously outlined should not be regarded as a checklist of tasks, which can be 'ticked off' once they have been attempted. Rather, the objective of the specifications is to provide a profile of the ongoing responsibilities, pertaining to the Cleft Palate Team's psychosocial management of the cleft population. Therefore, although the recommendations address different ages of development (and hence different stages of management), the responsibilities should be seen as long term, in addition to short term aims and objectives.

Indications for future research

In identifying and addressing the predominant implications of the findings for improved clinical practice, the limitations of the present study become especially apparent. Therefore, in concluding the study, the limitations must be incorporated into projections for future research.

In claiming to be a retrospective follow-up study, one of the most obvious weaknesses of the current research is its heavy reliance upon essentially subjective data. One needs only to consider the nature of the first two data sets pertaining to the assessments and clinical observations (as recorded in the hospital notes) of BNH and her colleagues, to appreciate the lack of objective assessment materials. Although the information reflects the personal perceptions of the Cleft Palate Team, it also represents the professional expertise of the assessors, albeit from medical and paramedical disciplines (rather than from psychology).

Therefore, ideally, in conducting a retrospective follow-up study of this nature, rigorous attempts should be made to deploy objective measures, which are both valid and reliable for the purposes of monitoring patient progress over time. Although not existent at the time of BNH's research, such instruments are now readily available. For example, speech and language therapists today have access to sensitive and sophisticated assessments for recording impaired articulation (and phonology) and nasality. The relative paucity of research 'tools' available to BNH compared with those on offer today, serve to highlight the time lapse and the advances made in research methodology since then. Needless to say, research continues into the refinement of assessment materials.

The data base which has accumulated in the course of the current study could be extended in various ways, thereby increasing its potential for understanding the psychosocial implications of being born with a cleft. For example, exhaustive attempts could be made to trace the remaining participants in BNH's original survey involving over 501 patients, commencing with consultation of the Central Register. Given the available time and financial resources, the writer's methodology could be replicated, to enable comparisons to be made with the wider cleft population. In addition, the similarities and/or differences emerging between the cleft population and other disfigured groups (such as people with congenital birth marks) could be investigated.

Furthermore, additional personal interviews could be conducted to supplement those undertaken for the present research. On the basis of the findings, more attention could be paid to elucidating the circumstances surrounding incidents of teasing, as this aspect may have application to all those with some form of craniofacial disfigurement.

Indeed, given the nature and the wide range of the information elicited for the purposes of this investigation, the focus of the writer's attention has been upon obtaining an overview in attempting to identify developmental trends. The objective of future research, however, could be to pursue a case study approach within the longitudinal research paradigm, by selecting a smaller number of participants for detailed study, on the basis of specific criteria.

A further possibility in extending research into the psychosocial aspects of cleft lip and/or palate, might be to conduct a cross-sectional study of the cleft population, by concentrating on those falling within a particular age band and/or cleft type. In doing so, the feasibility of including a control group could be considered, a feature which has not been plausible in the writer's study since it was instigated by an earlier researcher.

Amongst the recommendations made in this chapter, is the suggestion that greater attention should be paid to the psychosocial welfare of the patient's parents from birth. Future research could include seeting up trials which seek to put the recommendations into practice. For example, a hospital-based parent support group could be instigated by a member of the Cleft Palate Team (such as the 'Specialist Liaison Professional'), with the aim of offering parents a forum for discussing cleft-related problems and supplying relevant information. Such provision could conceivably enhance parental low self-esteem and raise self-confidence.

The identity of such a group would be fundamentally different to the more socially orientated function of the self-support groups run by CLAPA (Cleft Lip and Palate Association). Whilst the ethics of establishing a control group need to be addressed, providing the hospital parent group adheres to specific and measurable objectives, its benefits to both parents and patients could form the focus of an invaluable research project, deploying some form of assessment to evaluate progress.

Having identified those who are at most risk for psychosocial dysfunction, future research could study the efficacy of offering social skills training to adolescents and to the disadvantaged minority amongst the adult cleft population. As mentioned earlier, the writer has already taken part in such an exercise with promising results. To be undertaken on a trial basis, consideration would have to be given to valid and reliable methods of measuring changes in the participants' perceptions and behaviour (amongst other aspects). This approach to countering psychosocial difficulties is still in its infancy, but it has enormous potential for development, especially in offering help and support to those with clefts, and to the wider craniofacially-disfigured population.

In conjunction with the suggested research, the reader will recall that various interviewees taking part in the present study, volunteered to help in setting up an informal group for cleft-impaired adolescents. The primary objective of this notion was to offer the facility to meet others in a similar situation, in order to share experiences and difficulties with those who expressed an interest in doing so.

Whilst it would be inappropriate to 'use' such a group for a demanding research study, the short and long term value of establishing a hospital-based meeting place for the participants could be evaluated in an unobtrusive way. One means of doing this would be to invite the adolescents involved to express their feelings about having a member of the Cleft Palate Team (such as a speech and language therapist or hospital-based social worker in the absence of a psychologist), playing a participatory role in the group. The ethical issues relating to the organizational concept of 'user groups' may be of relevance in this context. In providing a resource for disseminating information and discussing issues relating to everyday life, the group's function should not be exploited nor deflected for extraneous purposes, such as research.

In view of the apparent significance of the visibility of the cleft defect to psychosocial development and functioning, this area warrants further examination. In particular, future research could refine the variables studied, by distinguishing more rigorously the degrees of visibility. One possible focus for research in this field would be to investigate a hypothesis which emerges from the findings of the present study. That is, it is conceivable that cleft-impaired and unimpaired individuals respond to different aspects of the defect. Thus, the individual born with a cleft seems to be more preoccupied with how visible the cleft appears to be to others, with comparatively more anxiety being displayed over a 'mild' than a 'severe' deformity.

Therefore, providing the descriptive terms, such as 'mild' and 'severe' clefting were defined according to objective and universally agreed criteria, the proposed research could make a positive contribution to enhanced understanding of the cleft population, and those with other forms of craniofacial disfigurement.

On examining the indications for future research, it transpires that their realization depends on one fundamental condition, which is the same for all of the proposals mentioned. This condition concerns acknowledging the fact that the psychologist has a valuable contribution to make in enhancing understanding of the cleft population.

Although the professional worlds of the hospital and academia may exist independent of the other, in the case of research into cleft lip and/or palate, access to this population is usually through the hospital door. Accordingly, studies concerned with psychosocial aspects of the defect have been undertaken in a piecemeal fashion, by interested professionals involved in cleft-related treatment, notably speech and language therapists and orthodontists. Until such time as the psychologist is guaranteed a place on the Cleft Palate Team, routine research into the psychosocial implications of being born with a cleft, must await further attention with research proposals being relegated to the 'pending' tray.

Having said this, with reference to the introduction to this chapter, there is a promising 'beacon' for the future. This takes the form of an investigation of treatment provision for the cleft population, instigated in July 1991 by a Steering Committee of the Royal College of Surgeons. In undertaking the project for audit purposes, consideration is being given to the psychosocial aspects of cleft impairment, and a longitudinal study of patients with a cleft is now underway. A report on the findings and recommendations is expected to be produced in the near future. In the meantime, attempts are being made to further identify the psychosocial needs of the cleft population, using both quantitative and qualitative methods to do so.

Appendix 1

Survey of 249 children with a cleft conducted by Hammond and O'Riain (1968-1972) - basis of data set 1

Introduction

The material presented in Appendix 1 supplements the description of BNH's research given in chapter one (introduction), and provides background information on the present study. In doing so, the terminology used by BNH and her colleague O'Riain has been preserved as far as possible.

Selection of sample

O'Riain and Hammond's (1972, p.380) criteria for selection is below.

- Both the primary closure of the soft palate and the initial speech assessment, had been undertaken prior to 30 months old at Odstock Hospital.

- The child's progress had been continuously reviewed, until the time of assessment by the surgeon and the speech therapist at the age of 5 years.

- The child had not been diagnosed with any severe impairments, unrelated to cleft palate, which might affect speech, such as special learning difficulties ('mental handicap') or deafness.

The 249 children who fulfilled these conditions (out of a possible 352 children), were seen jointly by the surgeon and speech therapist during the period of 2-5 years old, on a minimum of four occasions. Those who did not make satisfactory progress were seen as often as necessary, whilst the others received at least a yearly review. Each child in the sample was allocated to one of the three groups identified by the researchers, depending upon the extent of clefting (Table 1 below).

Table 1
The composition of the sample according to extent of cleft

Type of Cleft	n	%
Complete Clefts (Unilateral or Bilateral)	126	50.6
Post-Alveolar Clefts	93	37.4
Post-Alveolar Clefts with Lip Involvement	30	12.0
Total	249	100.0

Assessment

Various assessments were made by the surgeon and the speech therapist, regarding each child's speech, linguistic and general development. The attitude, speech and behaviour of the patient's parents were also noted.

Assessment of speech

The method employed for speech assessment was devised by Hammond, and reported in O'Riain and Hammond (1972, p.380). Each child's speech was described in terms of one of the following four categories.

- *Perfect*   As agreed by the surgeon, the speech therapist and the parent on the same occasion.

- *Acceptable* Imperfect but not conspicuously so. Minor articulation defect or minimal nasality, or both of these.

- *Unacceptable* Intelligible but obviously imperfect. Appreciable articulatory defects or appreciable nasality, or a combination of both articulatory defects and nasality of varying proportions.

- *Grossly defective* Unintelligible. Multiple articulatory defects with or without nasality.

Assessment of linguistic and general development

These areas were assessed when the child was 2 years of age, and subsequently, when aged 5 years old. Linguistic and general development were classified as indicated below.

- *Satisfactory*

- *Specific language retardation*

- *Overall retardation*

Assessment of parental attitude towards cleft-impaired child

During the assessment made when the child was aged 2 years old, the attitude, speech and behaviour of the mother, and whenever possible of both parents, was observed and recorded. Further notes were made over the following three years. In explaining the nature of their asssessments in this domain, O'Riain and Hammond (1972, p.381) state:

> We endeavoured to assess not good or bad parents in general but emotional and environmental factors which are known to have an effect on any child's speech development and progress. This we called parental influence.

Parental influence was assessed according to the classification defined below (draft and publication of O'Riain and Hammond, 1972, p.381).

• *Encouraging* The parents appeared to have made an adequate adjustment to their inevitable sense of guilt and disappointment, following the birth of their imperfect baby. The child was being given sufficient language stimulation, and a feeling of security. The parents were generally co-operative, encouraging the child at home in appropriate ways, and attending regular clinic appointments.

• *Indifferent* Parental influence was considered to be negligible. The parents were not concerned about their child's speech progress, and they offered the child very little help at home. This group of parents were irregular clinic attenders.

• *Detrimental* Many of these parents had not been able to adjust to their personal feelings, and responded by grossly overprotecting their child. In contrast, in a few instances, the child was simply ignored by his/her parents. Notably more time and affection was paid to other members of the family. Other factors associated with this category, were cases of broken homes, unacceptable cleft palate speech, and illiteracy of the parents. Some mothers had poor physical or mental health which required hospitalisation, this meant leaving the child with relatives or in care at a vulnerable age.

Data collection

O'Riain and Hammond (1972, p.381) examined all the patient records retrospectively, coded the data, and then transferred them to a pro forma sheet for each child. In the process of data collection, 137 variables were taken into account, which were incorporated under specific headings, such as the patient's age, type of cleft and the operative procedure undertaken during palatal surgery (please refer to Tables 4.1-4.6 in chapter four).

Appendix 2

Additional data elicited on interviewing two of BNH's former colleagues

It was noted in chapter one (introduction) that the writer had the chance to interview two of BNH's former colleagues, who were also involved in cleft lip and palate management at Odstock Hospital, Salisbury, at the time of BNH's research. The data reported in Appendix 2 supplement those cited in chapter one, and offer further insight into the implications of cleft management. The writer would like to take this opportunity to acknowledge the value and privilege of discussing the research with the former members of the Cleft Palate Team. In preparing the transcriptions of the interviews, the same procedure was followed as that described in chapter seven, for example, the interview data were edited to exclude instances of redundant filler speech (such as 'you know').

On mentioning the fact that when interviewed one ex-patient spoke of Odstock Hospital as her 'family', one of BNH's colleagues commented:

That's nice ... we always tried to sort of create that atmosphere ... because it meant so much. After all's said and done, ... from a surgical point of view ... you can't make ... somebody speak perfectly, you can't, they've got to do that haven't they? ... So really, we based it all on the family environment.

The subsequent remarks relate to the involvement of patients and their parents in the cleft-related treatment.

... basically you were never talking to, or were seldom talking to the child by itself, you were talking to the child plus a parent or parents, and so we used to try and explain the whole situation to them ... I think ... its tremendously

important to get them to understand what the situation is, and what you're trying to do for them.

I think ... the earlier in life I could see a child after birth, and see the parents, it was so much easier to ... manage the whole period of treatment, because if you could talk to them when they were a fortnight old, ... this was a tremendous advantage. But somebody ... produced at three, four, six months ... the family had grown up with it, and they'd got all sorts of ideas about it. But when you got the kids young, very young, a matter of weeks ... you could sketch out the whole programme, put them in the picture.

When conversing about experiences on the plastic surgery children's ward, the subject was raised concerning the parents' reaction following the child's initial repair surgery for cleft lip (where applicable).

... one of the things that always used to interest me ... when you have a baby with a cleft lip, when they smile you have this lovely grin ... After the babies' lips have been repaired, ... I used to say to the mums ... oh super! ... they used to say yes, its lovely. I used to wonder at first at this slight flatness of tone you used to get. It took quite a long time before it dawned on me the thing they missed was this big wide grin ... They had got used to it, and immediately post-operatively, of course, the baby's face is very stiff, so they don't have this lovely grin.

Reference was made later on to the children's hospital admission for further cleft-related treatment.

Basically, the thing that surprised me most of all, ... going back to the fact that they're not sick children, was the way that they came back into hospital. I'm not going to say they wanted to come and were delighted to be there, but in actual fact they accepted it so easily.

The importance of self-confidence in living with a cleft was discussed.

I'm sure that's the key to the whole situation really isn't it ... I'm sure it is. For instance, the development of speech ... when the family were with you ... in trying to get things ... normal ... I think the development of speech was much, much better than it was when the parents couldn't care less. ... that cropped up so many times, and this was something ... that (BNH) used to talk about.

The potential impact of the cleft deformity upon the parents and family was also highlighted.

I think it was very much a question of either it brought the family a great deal closer together, or it drove them violently apart ... and also too its very

*difficult for the other members of the family ... Mum was always going off
with that baby and leaving the other children behind, she was going to
clinic, she was going to the speech therapist, she was going to the ENT
clinic ... and so this child was getting considerably more 'mum support'
than any of the others were, and I suppose occasionally they must have
resented it quite strongly ... And so this is why feeding was so important, to
get ... the baby on a feeding regime that wasn't too complicated, because
otherwise mother was spending hours and hours and hours feeding the
baby.*

The following observations are included in view of the fact that BNH
regarded overprotective parenting as 'detrimental' in her research.

*... (overprotection) is worse for the child in the long run, because at least if
they have a degree of rejection they learn to stand on their own two feet at a
very early stage, ... therefore, possibly to cope with things in the end better,
whereas if they are overprotected, oh boy! ... it is terribly difficult, because ...
there's no way that you can blame poor mum ... I'm quite sure that I would
feel exactly the same, myself, but it doesn't help the children in the long run
... You spend a lot of your time saying please try and treat them exactly the
same way as all the other children in the family, because its easier for them
if you do ... Overprotection can really be as much of a problem as not
having enough protection. But you do wonder what happened to them.*

Insight was also offered into the way in which the cleft might impinge
upon the cleft-impaired child's education.

*... perhaps ... another field in which we are not getting through is to the
schools ... the child doesn't ask questions because he can't speak properly,
the teacher doesn't ask him questions because she can't understand him
properly, and perhaps there's a slight hearing defect there.*

On the subject of teasing, the individual's personality was considered to be
of fundamental importance.

*... I used to come up against it (teasing) with the bat ears ... and children
who have sticking out ears do get teased, and sometimes very badly. But
thinking about children themselves as a whole, over a large number of years
... it wasn't quite so much the ears it was the child, because this is part of it,
it isn't just what is wrong, its the child who responds to the teasing ... if it
wasn't for the fact they'd got sticking out ears, then because their mother
had red hair, or their trousers were too long ... or something, because its the
child who responds to teasing, ... not just the fact that there is something
wrong, but if it wasn't that it would be something else.*

241

Appendix 3a

Data collection form: hospital records-data set 2

Plastic Surgery Unit Ref. No. [ ]   BNH Ref. No. [ ]   Case No. [ ]

Section A - Background details

1.   Source of information ——————————————— [ ]

2.   Sex ———————————————————————— [ ]

3.   Date of birth ————————————————————— [ ]

4.   Home area ——————————————————————— [ ]

5.   Extent of cleft ————————————————————— [ ]

6.   Maternal complications (patient's mother)————————— [ ]

7.   Medical complications (patient)————————————— [ ]

8.   a) Birth order of patient in family ———————————— [ ]

       b) Sex of siblings————————————————————— [ ]

       c) Younger siblings———————————————————— [ ]

Section B - N.H.S. hospital treatment

9. Number of hospital admissions ⬚

10. Correspondence relating to non-attendance at hospital follow-up clinics or Speech Therapy appointments ⬚

11. Other agencies involved ⬚

Section C - Psycho-social development

12. Reference to family environment ⬚

13. Reference to pre-school years ⬚

14. Reference to pre-teenage years ⬚

15. Reference to teenage years ⬚

16. Reference to adulthood ⬚

Section D - Details of hospital discharge

17. a) Age at discharge from Speech Therapy ⬚

    b) Age at discharge from Plastic Surgery ⬚

18. Situation at discharge ⬚

Appendix 3b

The postal questionnaire - data set 3

When completing the following questions, please tick the answers that are most appropriate to you, unless otherwise indicated. Thank you.

A. Personal details

1. Are you   a) MALE   b) FEMALE

2. Your date of birth _____

3. Are you

     a) SINGLE   b) MARRIED   c) WIDOWED   d) DIVORCED

     e) OTHER

4. Do you have children?   a) YES   b) NO

5. Who has a cleft lip and/or palate in your family?

     a) YOURSELF

     b) OTHERS (please explain who)_____

B. Education

1. At what age did you leave full-time education? _____ years old

2. What did you do after leaving school? (ie at the age of 15/16 years old)

_____

_____

3. How did you feel about having a cleft lip and/or palate when you were at school?

_____

_____

4. Have your feelings changed?   a) YES   b) NO   c) DON'T KNOW

If YES, could you try to explain how your feelings have changed since your school days?

_____

_____

C. Employment

1. Are you in paid employment now?

a) YESb) NO c) OTHER (please explain)_____

   If YES, what type of work are you doing?

_____

2. Please rate your satisfaction with the type of employment, if any, that you have at the moment.

a) VERY SATISFIED	d) DISSATISFIED
b) SATISFIED	e) VERY DISSATISFIED
c) SOMEWHAT SATISFIED	f) NOT APPLICABLE

3. If you were able to choose, what job would you like to be doing in 10 years time?

_____

Can you try to explain why you would like to be doing this?

_____

_____

D. Speech and appearance

1. Have you ever received speech therapy?

    a) YES   b) NO   c) DON'T KNOW

If YES, please rate your satisfaction with the speech therapy that you have received/are receiving now.

    a) VERY SATISFIED   d) DISSATISFIED

    b) SATISFIED   e) VERY DISSATISFIED

    c) SOMEWHAT SATISFIED   f) NOT APPLICABLE

2. What mattered most to you as a teenager?

    a) THE WAY YOU SPOKE

    b) THE WAY YOU LOOKED

    c) OTHER (please explain) _____

Has this changed since then? a) YES   b) NO   c) DON'T KNOW

If YES, please try to explain in what ways this has changed.

_____

_____

3. Please rate your satisfaction with the way you speak now.

    a) VERY SATISFIED   d) DISSATISFIED

    b) SATISFIED   e) VERY DISSATISFIED

    c) SOMEWHAT SATISFIED   f) NOT APPLICABLE

4. Please rate your satisfaction with your appearance now.

    a) VERY SATISFIED   d) DISSATISFIED

    b) SATISFIED   e) VERY DISSATISFIED

    c) SOMEWHAT SATISFIED   f) NOT APPLICABLE

E. N.H.S. treatment for your cleft lip and/or palate

1. How do you feel about the follow-up clinics that you have been or are being asked to attend for your cleft lip and/or palate?

_____

2. Please rate your satisfaction with the surgery that you have received for your cleft lip and/or palate.

    a) VERY SATISFIED   d) DISSATISFIED

    b) SATISFIED   e) VERY DISSATISFIED

    c) SOMEWHAT SATISFIED   f) NOT APPLICABLE

3. Please rate your satisfaction with the orthodontic treatment that you have received for your cleft lip and/or palate.

    a) VERY SATISFIED   d) DISSATISFIED

    b) SATISFIED   e) VERY DISSATISFIED

    c) SOMEWHAT SATISFIED   f) NOT APPLICABLE

F. How you see yourself now

1. Below there is a list of words in opposites. Please circle the number which best describes how you see yourself now.

eg:	If you are very CALM	circle 1
	If you are CALM	circle 2
	If you are mixed	circle 3
	If you are WORRYING	circle 4
	If you are very WORRYING	circle 5

a) CALM	1	2	3	4	5	WORRYING
b) RETIRING	1	2	3	4	5	SOCIABLE
c) CONVENTIONAL	1	2	3	4	5	ORIGINAL
d) SUSPICIOUS	1	2	3	4	5	TRUSTING
e) LAZY	1	2	3	4	5	HARDWORKING
f) EVEN-TEMPERED	1	2	3	4	5	TEMPERAMENTAL
g) SOBER	1	2	3	4	5	FUN LOVING
h) DOWN TO EARTH	1	2	3	4	5	IMAGINATIVE
i) STUBBORN	1	2	3	4	5	FLEXIBLE
j) AIMLESS	1	2	3	4	5	AMBITIOUS
k) SECURE	1	2	3	4	5	INSECURE
l) RESERVED	1	2	3	4	5	AFFECTIONATE
m)NARROW INTERESTS	1	2	3	4	5	BROAD INTERESTS
n) SERIOUS	1	2	3	4	5	CHEERFUL
o) UNSTABLE	1	2	3	4	5	EMOTIONALLY STABLE
p) COMFORTABLE	1	2	3	4	5	SELF-CONSCIOUS
q) QUIET	1	2	3	4	5	TALKATIVE

r) UNADVENTUROUS	1	2	3	4	5		DARING
s) PROUD	1	2	3	4	5		HUMBLE
t) UNENERGETIC	1	2	3	4	5		ENERGETIC

2. Please indicate how far you agree with the following statements, by circling the appropriate number.

ie: 1 = STRONGLY AGREE
2 = AGREE
3 = DISAGREE
4 = STRONGLY DISAGREE

a) I feel that I'm a person of worth, at least on an equal plane with others.	1	2	3	4
b) I feel that I have a number of good qualities.	1	2	3	4
c) All in all, I am inclined to feel that I am a failure.	1	2	3	4
d) I am able to do things as well as most other people.	1	2	3	4
e) I feel I do not have much to be proud of.	1	2	3	4
f) I take a positive attitude toward myself.	1	2	3	4
g) On the whole, I am satisfied with myself.	1	2	3	4
h) I wish I could have more respect for myself.	1	2	3	4
i) I certainly feel useless at times.	1	2	3	4
j) At times I think I am no good at all.	1	2	3	4

G. Your experience of having a cleft lip and/or palate

1. What involvement, if any, have you had with the Cleft Lip and Palate Association (CLAPA)?

_____

2. How could the services provided by Odstock Hospital, Salisbury for the treatment of your cleft, have been improved for you?

_____

_____

3. Have you ever been teased about your speech or appearance?

_____

4. How much do you think having a cleft lip and/or palate has influenced or affected your life? For each of the following areas, please circle the number which indicates how much your cleft has influenced it.

	Very High	High	Mixed	Low	Very Low
a) EDUCATION	1	2	3	4	5
b) DATING WITH OPPOSITE SEX	1	2	3	4	5
c) TEASING	1	2	3	4	5
d) OCCUPATION	1	2	3	4	5
e) APPEARANCE	1	2	3	4	5

5. Do you have any particular advice to offer parents who have just learned that their baby has a cleft lip and/or palate?

_____

_____

6. Your experiences are very valuable to us in our attempts to improve the service and advice we give to our cleft lip and/or palate patients. If you would like to add any further comments about your experience of having a cleft, they would be welcomed.

_____

_____

_____

THANK YOU AGAIN FOR YOUR TIME AND CO-OPERATION

IN ANSWERING THESE QUESTIONS.

Appendix 3c

The interview schedule - data set 4

As delineated in chapter three (design of the study), the interviewer used a pocket size photograph album in conducting the semi-structured interviews. This method facilitated an informal and partnership approach to data collection, in that the questions to be asked were selected from those presented in the album, which was placed open on a table in front of both the interviewer and the interviewee.

The following details show the main headings under which the questions were incorporated, and the questions comprising each section (or 'theme'). It should be stressed that a slection of the questions were asked during each interview. The interviewer assured the participant at the outset, that there was no compulsion to complete the whole schedule. Alongside each section (or right hand 'page'), the relevant data in percentages was placed on the corresponding left hand side for the interviewee's perusal.

Contents of the interview schedule

1. *Introduction: views on receiving the postal questionnaire*

a)   'How did you feel when you received the questionnaire?'

b)   'Do you have any further comments about receiving it?'

The interviewer then explained that she would like to focus on certain aspects regarding the questionnaire, and to ask the interviewee his/her opinion on them.

2. *NHS treatment for your cleft*

a) 'With hindsight, can you outline the 'ideal' service provision for the treatment of your cleft?'

b) 'How does this compare with the treatment you received?'

3. *Parents / home environment / siblings*

a) 'What are your earliest memories of your home life as:
    i) a child?'
    ii) a teenager?'

b) 'Do you have any brothers or sisters?'

c) 'How well did you get on with them as a child/teenager?' (if applicable)

d) 'Did you talk to your parents about your cleft?'

e) 'How did your parents feel about the hospital treatment you received?'

4. *Consideration of hypothetical situations*

a) 'Imagine that you had to deliver news of the cleft to the parents of a newborn baby. What words would you choose to tell them about the cleft?'

b) 'How do you think you would react if you were such a parent?'

5. *Perceived influence of the cleft upon aspects of life*

'In the questionnaire we asked you about the impact of the cleft on aspects of your life. Would you like to say anything further about the areas?' (i.e., teasing / dating / appearance / education / occupation)

6. *Experiences related to having a cleft at school*

a) 'Could you elaborate upon your most vivid memories of primary school?'

b) 'What about secondary school?'

c) 'With hindsight, how could your school days have been improved for you?'

7. *Perceived change(s) since leaving school*

'Could you tell me more about why you think your feelings changed / have not changed (as applicable) since leaving school?'

8. *Experience of being teased (if applicable)*

a) 'A large number of people in the questionnaire said that they had been teased. Could you expand a little, and say something about the circumstances in which it happened to you?' (if applicable)

b) 'How did you tend to react to being teased?'

c) 'What effect do you think the teasing had upon you if any?'

9. *Perceived change(s) since the teenage years*

a) 'Can you elaborate further about what mattered most to you during your teens?' (i.e., speech and/or appearance / other)

b) 'What are the possible reasons for a change / lack of change in those concerns since your teens.?'

10. *Perceived change(s) in personality (including self-esteem)*

a) 'Do you think that your personality has changed much since your teens?'

b) 'What about your self-confidence, has that changed at all?'

254

c) 'Are you generally satisfied with your life at the moment?'

11. *Employment*

a) 'Do you feel you have been discriminated against in employment due to having a cleft?' (i.e., speech and/or appearance affected)

b) 'Do you think that your cleft has affected your future aspirations / career in any way?'

12. *Advice based on your experience of being born with a cleft*

a) 'How would you put your advice to the parents of a newborn baby with a cleft into practice?' (e.g., as part of early parent education)

b) 'Can you identify the most important aspects to incorporate in offering help to new parents?'

13. *Maturation and the development of coping skills*

a) 'How have you learned to cope with difficult situations, such as being teased?'

b) 'How important are coping skills for dealing with these sort of experiences?'

c) 'Do you think that you need to learn to cope, or does it just come naturally?'

14. *What of the future?*

a) 'How do you think we could improve our hospital service to patients with a cleft?'

b) 'What are the main priorities for treatment?'

15. *Recommendations based on the questionnaire responses*

'Having received a large number of questionnaires, there appear to be three different areas where suggestions have been made for improvement. I would like to discuss these with you, and to hear your reaction to them.'

a)   'The first of these relates to the need to give parents advice and help very early on.' (i.e., early parent education/counselling)

b)   'Another area is helping patients in their early teens.' (i.e., early teenage counselling)

c)   'A further area concerns involving schools more, for example, in addressing problems of teasing.' (i.e., school involvement - staff and peers).

The participant was then thanked very much for his or her help and time.

Appendix 4

Quality and standards of job description for Specialist Liaison Professional

As a member of the Cleft Palate Team the Specialist Liaison Professional is responsible for ensuring that the following recommendations are put into practice. That is, recommendations for the establishment and development of the management of all cleft-impaired patients treated by the Cleft Palate Team. The Specialist Liaison Professional will have a special interest in the treatment and psychosocial welfare of cleft-impaired patients.

Code of practice : implementation of the recommendations

Recommendation I - Parent counselling / education

1. Every newborn baby with a cleft to be reported to Specialist Liaison Professional based at the plastic surgery unit run on a regional basis, within 24 hours of birth. This advocation is based on the premise that the earlier the Cleft Palate Team become involved, the greater the mutual benefit for patient/patient's parents and the optimal use of National Health Service resources.

2. The Specialist Liaison Professional will visit every newborn with a cleft within the region (i.e., including all peripheral hospitals served by the plastic surgery unit), as soon as feasible within the first week of birth.

3. The Specialist Liaison Professional will allocate 1-2 hours (excluding travel) for every initial visit to the parents and newborn with a cleft.

4. The objectives of the initial visit mentioned above are:

a) To counsel and support parents in their adjustment to the cleft.

b) To notify the parents of the available local support group(s).

c) To explain the nature of cleft lip and/or palate as appropriate.

d) To introduce and outline the Cleft Palate Team's responsibilities.

e) To describe the likely hospital management of the cleft.

f) To provide appropriate information relating to the cleft defect.

g) To establish a contract regarding parental commitment in carrying out the proposed hospital treatment for the cleft.

h) To give the parents a date and time for the first appointment with the Cleft Palate Team, (following liaison with the speech and language therapy/plastic surgery unit secretary), and the Specialist Liaison Professional's name and address for queries arising from the initial visit, or to arrange a follow-up visit if requested.

i) To begin to help the parents adopt a positive attitude towards the child, so that the self-esteem of both parents and child is not adversely affected by the presence of the cleft defect. e.g., to focus upon the child's normality, rather than his/her impairment.

5. The Specialist Liaison Professional will be responsible for making her/himself familiar, with the advice being given to parents of babies with a cleft at each of the peripheral hospitals. The object of this task is to enable the Specialist Liaison Professional to reinforce the advice if appropriate, and/or to educate the staff of the peripheral hospitals in adopting a universal approach within the region to cleft-related problems. For example, advice given in conjunction with the delivering of initial news of the diagnosis (by midwives, medical staff and so forth), feeding problems, speech and language development, and the likely course of hospital treatment, amongst other aspects.

Thus, team-building with the plastic surgery unit run on a regional basis can be enhanced, by offering guidance to the staff of peripheral hospitals, who may be less familiar with the intricacies of all aspects of cleft management. A booklet, such as that being compiled by the Audit Committee for cleft lip and palate, in conjunction with the Royal College of Surgeons could become the accepted handbook, given to all parents by the Specialist Liaison Professional during the initial visit. This measure should encourage maximum parent, and later patient co-operation regarding the fufilling of treatment aims.

6.   In developing point 5. above, the Specialist Liaison Professional will be responsible for offering and providing specialist training for all speech and language therapists within the region, who are treating children (especially pre-schoolers) with a cleft. Such training may take the form of workshops or regular meetings in the speech and language therapy department at the hospital. A specific interest group (SIG) for those working within the region could be instigated, with its members being encouraged to join, for example, the South East SIG, which meets regularly in London, and to attend the annual conference of the Craniofacial Society of Great Britain, as one means of keeping up-to-date with advances in clinical practice.

The available training will not only improve the expertise of each of the therapists involved, but also enhance the universal treatment approach adopted at the plastic surgery unit. The proposed training will seek to demonstrate that children with a cleft palate who are referred for local speech and language therapy by the Cleft Palate Team, require immediate attention. Given the nature of cleft palate, delay in therapeutic intervention may have a deleterious effect upon the child's development, and should, therefore, be given priority where possible.

7.   The Specialist Liaison Professional will be responsible for ensuring that he or she can offer up-to-date information on the following areas of cleft management, based on close liaison with the relevant professionals:

a)   Feeding.

b)   Hearing.

c)   Speech and language development, including pre-verbal stage.

d)   Surgical programme, including the dates of appointments and the nature of follow-up clinics.

e)   Orthodontic programme.

f)   Possible implications of treatment for education e.g., missed schooling.

g)   Parent/patient support groups and sources of information, e.g., Cleft Lip and Palate Association, Changing Faces, Let's Face It.

h)   Contact name and address and details of genetic counsellor.

i)   Social worker/Social Services involvement if necessary.

j)   Clinical psychologist/psychiatrist involvement if needed.

The Specialist Liaison Professional will be directly involved in, or be aware of other services involved in any particular patient's management, and therefore, be in a key position to act as chief liaison/co-ordinator where necessary, such as in holding case conferences.

Recommendation II - School involvement

1.   The Specialist Liaison Professional will be responsible for liaising with, and involving the school staff in evaluating and advancing the progress of pupils born with a cleft.

2.   At the **pre-school** stage, liaison will be undertaken with the relevant nursery schools or playgroups, and will entail attention to the following areas of development:

a)   Discussion of the patient's speech and language skills, and the extent to which interaction with others is affected by impaired communication.   In this way, the Cleft Palate Team has access to an additional resource and rich source of information about the impact of the cleft defect upon the child's social and educational activities, and can thereby monitor the young patient's progress from the earliest stages of socialization/interaction with peers (a potentially threatening aspect of their lives).

b)   Discussion regarding the extent to which nursery/playgroup staff perceive the child with a cleft to be 'at risk' i.e., based upon observations/factors emerging, such as withdrawal from situations.

c)   Discussion regarding the benefit of talking about body image/ teasing and bullying/implications of being different and disfigured.

d)   Encourage the use of stories which incorporate disfigurement of various kinds in positive presentations.

3.   At the **primary school** and **secondary school** stages, liaison will be undertaken with the relevant schools, and will entail attention to the following areas of development:

a)   Discussion of the impact of impaired articulation and/or nasal speech upon the child's communication/interaction with peers.   The Specialist Liaison Professional will be able to offer advice as to how the school environment can be improved, if necessary to enable optimum communication opportunities/experiences.

b)   Discussion of emerging language problems which may be related to the cleft defect.

c)   Discussion of the child's hearing acuity in class.

d)   Discussion of the child's personal and social relationships within the school context e.g., teasing problems, withdrawal.

e)   Discussion of the school's current policy for dealing with teasing/bullying.

f)   Discussion as to extent to which teacher and peers aware/up-to-date with child's hospital treatment programme e.g., regarding hospital admission, missed schooling for attendance at follow-up clinics, the impact of these events upon the child's school performance (e.g., fear of forthcoming hospital visit). Discussion of the merits of helping to prepare the child for hospital admission.

Recommendation III - Support during adolescence

1.   The Specialist Liaison Professional will be responsible for collecting evidence (from other Cleft Palate Team members) and identifying, patients (from pre- school years) whose future psychosocial development is deemed to be 'at risk'. Such identification will be based upon the Specialist Liaison Professional's own observations, and information regarding the patients' development, experiences, reaction to treatment and so forth, and will be largely based upon the following factors:

a)   Knowledge and experience of the patient during years of Cleft Palate Team management.

b)   Personality and self-esteem of patient (according to assessment).

c)   Parental and social background.

d)   Social and psychological development.

e)   Intellectual development and school performance.

f)   Response/adjustment to cleft defect and treatment.

2.   Having identified those whose psychosocial development is considered to be 'at risk', the Specialist Liaison Professional will receive training in the following areas, in order to be in a position to train others and offer these aspects as a means of psychosocial support:

a)   Social skills training.

b)   Communication skills training.

c)   Assertiveness training.

d)   Discussion regarding awkward situations and self-consciousness.

e)   Discussion based on perception of self by others, especially peers.

f)   Discussion regarding personal and social relationships, emphasis upon notions of self-esteem, self-concept, self-perception and self-image, which often challenge the individual during adolescence.

3.   The Specialist Liaison Professional will be instrumental in devising methods for assessing and evaluating the progress of those taking part in the training programmes outlined in point 2. above.

Recommendation IV - The importance of continuity

The patient born with a cleft may require hospital treatment from infancy into adulthood, depending upon individual circumstances. In view of this possibility, the recommendations previously outlined should not be regarded as a checklist of tasks, which can be 'ticked off' once they have been attempted. Rather, the objective of the specifications is to provide a profile of the ongoing responsibilities concerning the Specialist Liaison Professional's management of patients with a cleft. Therefore, although the recommendations address different ages of development (and hence different stages of management), the responsibilities should be seen as long term, in addition to short term aims and objectives.

Recommendation V - Research

1.   The Specialist Liaison Professional will be required to undertake, and to participate in research, in conjunction with the particular research interests of the multidisciplinary Cleft Palate Team.

2.   The Specialist Liaison Professional will be given the opportunity to develop and maintain a data base of detailed information, pertaining to patients with a cleft lip and/or palate being treated in the particular region concerned.   The primary purpose of the data collection is to enable continuity of treatment records, and to monitor patients' progress over time.

3.   In-service training will be provided to enable the Specialist Liaison Professional to gain competence in the relevant research methodology and computer skills. Close supervision by colleagues will also be available.

4. The Specialist Liaison Professional will be encouraged by the Cleft Palate Team, to submit articles for publication in the appropriate journals, in accordance with the research being undertaken. He or she will also be recommended to attend the pertinent conferences, such as the annual conference of the Craniofacial Society of Great Britain, in order to keep up-to-date with advances in the management of cleft lip and/or cleft palate.

Bibliography

Abramowitz, R.H., Petersen, A.C. and Schulenberg, J.E. (1984), 'Changes In Self-Image During Early Adolescence' in Lamb, H.R. (ed.), *New Directions for Mental Health Services*, Jossey- Bass, San Francisco.

Adams, G.R. (1977), 'Physical Attractiveness Research: Toward A Developmental Social Psychology of Beauty', *Human Devel.*, 20, 217-323.

Adams, G.R. and Huston, T.L. (1975), 'Social Perceptions of Middle-Aged Persons Varying In Physical Attractiveness'.*Developmental Psychol.*, 1 1 , 657-658.

Albery, E.H. (1986), 'Type and Assessment of Speech Problems' in Albery, E.H., Hathorn, I.S. and Pigott, R.W. (eds), *Cleft Lip and Palate: A Team Approach*, Wright, Bristol, 52-57.

Albery, E.H. (1986), 'The Management of Cleft Palate Speech' in Albery, E.H., Hathorn, I.S. and Pigott, R.W. (eds), *Cleft Lip and Palate: A Team Approach*, Wright, Bristol, 58-62.

Albery, E. and Russell, J. (1990), 'Cleft Palate and Orofacial Abnormalities' in Grunwell, P. (ed.), *Developmental Speech Disorders*, Churchill Livingstone.

Albery, E.H., Hathorn, I.S. and Pigott, R.W. (eds), (1986), *Cleft Lip and Palate: A Team Approach,* Wright, Bristol.

Allgood-Merten, B.A. and Lewinson, P.M. (1990), 'Sex Differences and Adolescent Depression', *J. Abnorm. Psychol.*, 99, 55-63.

Althea. (1982), *I Can't Talk Like You,* Dinosaur Publications Ltd.

Althea. (1991), *I Use A Wheelchair*, Dinosaur Publications Ltd., (Revised

Edition).

Anderson, E.M. and Spain, B. (1977), *The Child With Spina Bifida*, Methuen, London.

Asterita, M.F. (1985), *The Physiology of Stress*, Human Sciences Press, New York.

Baker, L. and Cantwell, D.P. (1985), 'Psychiatric and Learning Disorders In Children With Speech and Language Disorders: A Critical Review', in Gadow, K.D. (ed.), *Advances in Learning and Behavioral Disabilities*, vol. 4, Jai Press, Greenwich, CT.

Bamford, J. and Saunders, E. (1985), *Hearing Impairment, Auditory Perception and Language Disability*, Edward Arnold, London.

Bardach, J., Morris, H. and Olin, W. (1984), 'Late Results of Primary Veloplasty: The Marbug Project'. *Plast. Reconstr. Surg.*, 73, 207-222.

Barker, R.G., Wright, B.A., Meyerson, L. and Gonick, M.R. (1953) *Adjustment To Physical Handicap and Illness. A Survey of The Social Psychology of Physique and Disability*, Social Science Research Council, New York, Revised Edition.

Baron, R. and Byrne, D. (1991), *Social Psychology: Understanding Human Interaction*, Allyn and Bacon, 6th Edition.

Bates, E., Camaioni, L. and Volterra, V. (1975), 'The Acquisition of Performatives Prior To Speech'. *Merrill-Palmer Quarterly*, 21, 205-226.

Bates, E. (1976), *Language and Context, The Acquisition of Pragmatics*, Academic Press, New York.

Battle, R.J.V. (1954), 'Past, Present and Future In Surgery of Clef Palate'. *Brit. Jour. Plastic Surgery*, 7, 217-228.

Baumgartner, R.M. and Heberlein, T.A. (1984), 'Recent Research On Mailed Questionnaire Response Rates' in Lockhart, D.C. (ed.), *Making Effective Use of Mailed Questionnaires*, New Directions For Program Evaluation, no. 21, Jossey-Bass, San Francisco.

Bawden, J. (1989), *When I Went To Hospital*, Little Mammoth Publications.

Bell, J. (1987), *Doing Your Research Project: A Guide For First-Time Researchers in Education and Social Science*, Open University Press, Milton Keynes.

Bell, R., Kiyak, H.A., Joondeph, D.R., McNeil, R.W. and Wallen, T.R. (1985), 'Perceptions of Facial Profile and Their Influence On The Decision To Undergo Orthognathic Surgery'. *Am. Jour. Orthod.*, 88, 323-332.

Berkovitz, B.K.B. ((1986), 'Embryology' in Albery, E.H., Hathorn, I.S. and Pigott, R.W. (eds),*Cleft Lip and Palate: A Team Approach*, Wright, Bristol, 1-9.

Berscheid, E. (1980), 'Overview of The Psychological Effects of Physical Attractiveness' in Lucker, G.W., Ribbens, K.A. and McNamara, J.A. (eds),*Psychological Aspects of Facial Form*, Craniofacial Growth

Series Monograph no.11, Ann Arbor: Centre for Human Growth and Development, 1-23.

Berscheid, E. and Walster, E. (1974), 'Physical Attractiveness', *Advances in Experimental Social Psychology*, 7, 157-215.

Berscheid, E., Walster, E. and Bohrnstedt, G. (1973), 'The Happy American Body: A Survey Report'. *Psych. Today*, 7, 119-131.

Bhatia, S.N. (1972), 'Genetics of Cleft Lip and Palate', *Br. Dent. Jour.*, 32, 95-103.

Bickel, J. ((1970), 'First Results In Early Speech Readiness Program In Cleft Palate Children', *Cleft Palate Jour.*, 7, 156-159.

Biglund, S. (1990), 'An Investigation Into The Source, Timing and Adequacy of Information Given To The Mothers of Children Born With A Cleft Lip and Palate'. *Unpublished BSc. (Hons), Dissertation*, Birmingham Polytechnic.

Birch, J. (1952 'Personality Characteristics of Individuals With Cleft Palate: Research Needs',*Cleft Palate Bull.*, 2, 2, 7.

Bjornsson, A. and Agustsdottir, S. (1987), 'A Psychosocial Study of Icelandic Individuals With Cleft Lip or Cleft Lip and Palate', *Cleft Palate Jour.*, vol. 24, no. 2, April, 152-157.

Blakeney, P., Portman, S. and Rutan, R. (1990), 'Familial Values As Factors Influencing Long-Term Psychological Adjustment of Children After Svere Burn injury', *Jour. Burn Care and Rehabilitation*, 11, 472-475.

Blattner, R.J. (1964), 'Congenital Defects: Impact On The Patient, Family, and Society', in Fishbein, M. (ed.),*Second International Conference On Congenital Malformations*, International Medical Congress, New York.

Blenkinsop, S. ((1989), 'Alligators Add Bite To Cleft-Palate Research', *The Sunday Times*, 17th December, P.D11

Bloom, L. (1973), *One Word At A Time: The Use of Single Words Before Syntax*, Mouton, The Hague.

Bowlby, J. (1973), *Attachment and Loss, Volume II. Separation: Anxiety and Anger*, Penguin, Middlesex.

Bradbury, E., Hewison, J. and Timmons, M. (1992), 'Psychological and Social Outcome of Prominent Ear Correction In Children', *Brit. Jour. Plastic Surgery*, 45, 97-100.

Bradley, D. (1977), 'Speech and Language Aspects: State of The Art', *Cleft Palate Jour.*, 14, 321-328.

Bradshaw, J. and Lawton, D. (1978), *Tracing The Causes of Stress In Families With Handicapped Children*, Social Policy Research Unit, University of York.

Brainerd, C.J. (1978), *Piaget's Theory of Intelligence*, Prentice-Hall, Englewood Cliffs, N.J..

Braithwaite, F. (1964), 'Cleft Palate and Lip' in Rob, C. and Smith, R. (eds), *Clinical Surgery*, Butterworths, London.

Brantley, H.T. and Clifford, E. (1979a) 'Cognitive, Self-Concept, and Body Image Measures of Normal, Cleft Palate, and Obese Adolescents', *Cleft Palate Jour.*, vol. 16, no. 2, 177-182.

Brantley, H.T. and Clifford, E. (1979), 'Maternal and Child Locus of Control and Field-Dependence In Cleft Palate Children', *Cleft Palate Jour.*, vol. 16, no.2, 183-187.

Brantley, H.T. and Clifford, E. (1980), 'When My Child Was Born: Maternal Reactions To The Birth of A Child', *Jour. Personality Assessment*, 44, 6, 620-623.

Breakwell, G.M. (1990), *Interviewing.* BPS Books, British Psychological Society and Routledge Ltd.

Brennan, D. and Cullinan, W. (1974), 'Object Identification and Naming In Cleft Palate Children',*Cleft Palate Jour.*, 11, 188-195.

Bretherton, I. (1985), 'Attachment Theory: Retrospect and Prospect' in Bretherton, I. and Waters , E. (eds), *Growing Points of Attachment Theory and Research*, Mono SRCD 50 (1-2, Serial No. 209).

Broder, H. (1982), 'Body Image of Individuals With Visible or Invisible Oral-Facial Disfigurement', *Paper presented at the Americal Meeting of The Psychological Association*, Washington DC.

Broder, H. and Strauss, R.P. (1989), 'Self-Concept of Early Primary School Age Children With Visible Or Invisible Defects',*Cleft Palate Jour.*, vol. 26, no. 2, April, 114-118.

Broder, H., Smith, F. and Strauss, R. (1992), 'Habilitation of Patients With Clefts: Parent and Child Ratings of Satisfaction With Appearance and Speech', *Cleft Palate-Craniofacial Jour.*, vol. 29, no. 3, May, 262-267.

Bronsted, K., Liisberg, W.B., Orsted, A. et al., (1984), 'Surgical and Speech Results Following Palatopharyngoplasty Operations In Denmark 1959-1977', *Cleft Palate Jour.*, 21, 170-179.

Brooks, A. and Shelton, R. (1963), 'Incidence of Voice Disorders Other Than Nasality In Cleft Palate Children',*Cleft Palate Bull.*, 13, 63-64.

Brown, H., (1983), 'Different? I'm Not Different. Am I?', *Cleft Palate Jour.*, vol. 20, no. 1, January, 85-86.

Bull, R. (1974), 'The Importance of Being Beautiful', *New Society*, 30, 412-414.

Bull, R. and Rumsey, N., (1988), *The Social Psychology of Facial Appearance*, Springer-Verlag, New York Inc..

Burton, L. (1975), *The Family Life of Sick Children*, Routledge and Kegan Paul, London.

Butler, N., Gill, R., Pomeroy, D. and Fewtrell, J. (1978), *Handicapped Children-Their Homes and Life Styles*, Department of Child Health, University of Bristol.

Byrne, D. (1971), *The Attraction Paradigm*, Academic Press, New York.

Bzoch, K.R. (1956), 'An Investigation of The Speech of Pre-School Cleft Palate Children', *Ph.D Dissertation*, Northwestern University.

Bzoch, K.R. (1959), 'A Study of The Speech of A Group of Pre-School Cleft Palate Children', *Cleft Palate Bull.*, 9, 2-3.

Bzoch, K.R. (1965), 'Articulation Proficiency and Error Patterns of Preschool Cleft Palate and Normal Children', *Cleft Palate Jour.*, 2, 340-349.

Bzoch, K.R. (1971), 'Categorical Aspects of Cleft Palate Speech' in Grabb, W. Rosenstein, S. and Bzoch, K.R. (eds), *Cleft Lip and Palate*, Little, Brown and Company, Boston.

Bzoch, K.R. (1979), 'Etiological Factors Related To Cleft Palate Speech' in Bzoch, K.R. (ed.), *Communicative Disorders Related To Cleft Lip and Palate*, Little, Brown and Company, Boston.

Bzoch, K., Kemker, J. and Wood, V. (1984), 'The Prevention of Communicative Disorders In Cleft Palate Infants' in Lass , N. (ed.), *Speech and Language Advances in Basic Research and Practice, vol. 10*, Academic Press, New York, pp.59-110.

Campbell, B.A. and Jaynes, J. (1966), 'Reinstatement', *Psychological Review*, 73, 478-480.

Campbell, M.L. and Watson, A.C.H. (1980), 'Management of The Neonate' in Edwards, M. and A.C.H. Watson, A.C.H. (eds), *Advances In The Management of Cleft Palate*, Churchill Livingstone, Edinburgh.

Cavior, N. (1970), 'Physical Attractiveness, Perceived Attitude Similarity, and Interpersonal Attraction Among Fifth and Eleventh Grade Boys and Girls', *Doctoral Dissertation,,* Houston.

Chang, C.C. and Herzog, B. (1974), 'Burn Morbidity: A Follow Up Study of Physical and Psychological Disability', *Ann. Surg.*, 83, 34.

Classification of Occupations (1980), *A Publication of The Government Statistical Service*, Office of Population Censuses and Surveys, HMSO.

Cleft Lip and Palate Association (CLAPA, Literature (not dated), 'One Out of Every 700 Infants Is Born With A Cleft Lip or A Cleft Palate. Help!', *CLAPA Literature*.

Clifford, E. (1967), 'Connotative Meaning of Concepts Related To Cleft Lip and Palate', *Cleft Palate Jour.*, 4, 165-173.

Clifford, E. (1969), 'The Impact of A Symptom: A Preliminary Comparison of Cleft Lip Palate and Asthmatic Children', *Cleft Palate Jour.*, 6, 221-227.

Clifford, M. (1975), 'Physical Attractiveness and Academic Performance', *Child Study Jour.*, 5, 201-209.

Clifford, E. (1979), 'Psychological Aspects of Cleft Lip and Palate' in Bzoch, K.R. (ed.), *Communicative Disorders Related To Cleft Lip and Palate*, Boston, Little, Brown and Company, Boston, p.37.

Clifford, E. (1983), 'Why Are They So Normal?' State of The Art - An Opinion, *Cleft Palate Jour.*, vol. 20, no. 1, 83-84.

Clifford, E. (1991), Editorial Commentary On Noar, J.H., (1991), (see Noar, 1991 below),

Clifford, E. and Brantley, H.T. (1977), 'When I Was Born: Perceived Parental Reactions of Adolescents' *Jour. Personality Assessment*, 41, 604.

Clifford, E. and Crocker, E. (1971), 'Maternal Responses: The Birth of A Normal Child As Compared To The Birth of A Child With A Cleft', *Cleft Palate Jour.*, 8, 298-306.

Clifford, E. and Walster, T. (1973), 'The Effect of Physical Attractiveness On Teacher Expectation', *Sociology of Education*, 46, 248-253.

Clifford, E. and Clifford, M. (1986), 'Social and Psychological Problems Associated With Clefts: Motivations For Cleft Palate Treatment', *International Dental Jour.*, vol. 36, no. 3, 115-119.

Clifford, E., Crocker, E.C. and Pope, B.A. (1972), 'Psychological Findings In The Adulthood of 98 Cleft Lip-Palate Children', *Plast. Reconstr. Surgery*, vol. 50, no. 3, 234-237.

Coggins, T., Henry, C. and Carpenter, R. (1978), 'A System For Coding Pragmatic Behaviors In Preverbal Children', *Paper presented at the American Speech and Hearing Convention*, San Francisco, California.

Conant, S. and Budoff, M. (1983), 'Patterns of Awareness In Children's Understanding of Disabilities', *Mental Retard.*, 21, 119-125.

Coopersmith, S. (1967), *The Antecedents of Self-Esteem*, W.H. Freeman, San Francisco.

Costa, P.T. and McCrae, R.R (1985b), *The Neo Personality Inventory Manual*, Psychological Assessment Resources, Odessa, F.L..

Costa, P.T. and McCrae, R.R. (1988), 'Personality In Adulthood: A Six-Year Longitudinal Study of Self-Reports and Spouse Ratings On The Neo Personality Inventory', *Jour. Personality and Social Psychol.*, vol. 54, no. 5, 853-863.

Cramer, B. (1976), 'A Mother's Reactions To The Birth of A Premature Baby' in Klaus, M.H. and Kennell, J.H., *Maternal-Infant Bonding*, The C.V. Mosby Company.

Crocker, E.C., Clifford, E. and Pope, B. (1973), 'The Cleft Palate Child Grows Up: An Analysis of The Adulthood of Former Patients' in Clifford, E. (ed.), *Psychosocial Aspects of Orofacial Anomalies: Speculations in Search of Data*, ASHA Reports no.8, American Speech and Hearing Association, Washington D.C..

Crystal, D. (1981), *Clinical Linguistics*, Springer Verlag, Wien.

Cunningham, C. and Davis, H. (1985), *Working With Parents. Framework For Collaboration*, Open University Press, Milton Keynes.

Davis, J.S. and Ritchie, H.P. ((1922), 'Classification of Congenital Clefts of Lip and Palate', *Jour. Am. Med. Assoc.*, 79, 1323-1328.

De Charms, R. (1972), 'Personal Causation Training In The Schools', *Jour. Applied Social Psychol.*, 2, 95-113.

DePaola, L.G. (1975), 'Cleft Palate Formation In The Human: A Critical Evaluation', *J. Baltimore Coll. Dent. Surg.*, 30, 82-89.

Dillman, D.A., Dillman, J.J. and Makela, C.J. (1984), 'The Importance of

Adhering To Details of The Total Design Method (TDM), For Mail Surveys' in Lockhart, D.C. (ed.), *Making Effective Use of Mailed Questionnaires*, New Directions For Program Evaluation, no. 21, Jossey-Bass, San Fancisco.

Dion, K.K. (1972), 'Physical Attractiveness and Evaluations of Children's Transgressions', *Jour. Pers. Soc. Psychol.*, 24, 207-213.

Dion, K.K. (1974), 'Young Children's Stereotyping of Facial Attractiveness', *Developmental Psychol.*, 10, 772-778.

Dion, K.K. and Berscheid, E. (1974), 'Physical Attractiveness and Peer Perception Among Children', *Sociometry*, 37, 1-12.

Dorf, D.S. and Curtin, J.W. (1982), 'Early Cleft Palate Repair and Outcome', *Plastic and Reconstr. Surgery*, 70, 74.

Dorner, S. (1975), 'The Relationship of Physical Handicap To Stress In Families With An Adolescent With Spina Bifida', *Dev. Med. Child Neurol.*, 17, 765.

Drillien, C.M., Ingram , T.T.S., and Wilkinson, E.M. (1966), *The Causes and Natural History of Cleft Lip and Palate*, Livingstone, Edinburgh.

Easson, W. (1966), 'Psychopathological Environment Reaction To Congenital Defect', *Jour. Neurol. Ment. Dis.*, 142, 453.

Edwards, M. (1980), 'Speech and Language Disability' in Edwards, M. and Watson, A.C.H. (eds), *Advances in The Management of Cleft Palate*, Churchill Livingstone, Edinburgh.

Edwards, M. and Watson, A.C.H. (eds), (1980), *Advances In The Management of Cleft Palate*, Churchill Livingstone, Edinburgh.

Eliason, M., Hardin, M. and Olin, W. (1991), 'Factors That Influence Ratings of Facial Appearance For Children With Cleft Lip and Palate', *Cleft Palate-Craniofacial Jour.*, vol.28, no.2, April, 190-194.

Elliott (not dated), *Kidscape Literature* (see Kidscape below).

Epsteen, C. (1958), 'Psychological Impact of Facial Deformities', *American Jour. of Surgery*, 96, 745-748.

Ericson, A., Kallen, B. and Westerholm, P. (1979), 'Cigarette Smoking As An Etiologic Factor In Cleft Lip and Palate', *Am. J. Obstet. Gynecol.*, 135, 348-351.

Erikson, E.H. (1950), *Childhood and Society*, Norton, New York.

Erikson, E.H. (1959), 'Identity and The Life Cycle',*Psychol. Issues*, 1, no.1.

Estes, R.E. and Morris, H.L. (1970), 'Relationships Among Intelligence, Speech Proficiency, and Hearing Sensitivity In Children With Cleft Palates', *Cleft Palate Jour.*, 7, 763-773.

Ferguson, M.W.J. (1988), 'Palate Development', *Development 103 Supplement*, 41-60.

Festinger, L. and Katz, D. (eds), (1953), *Research Methods In The Behavioral Sciences*, Dryden Press, New York.

Fishman, C.A. and Fishman, D.B. (1971), 'Maternal Correlates of Self-Esteem and Overall Adjustment In Children With Birth Defects', *Child Psychiatry Hum. Dev.*, 1, 4, 255-265.

271

Floyd, J. and Paynter, E. (1973), 'Linguistic Abilities of Children With Surgically Repaired Palatal Clefts', *Paper presented at the Annual Meeting of The American Cleft Palate Association*, Oklahoma City.

Fogh-Anderson, P. (1942), *Inheritance of Harelip and Cleft Palate*, Nordisk Forlag. Arnold Busck., Copenhagen, Nyt.

Fogh-Anderson, P. (1961), 'Incidence of Cleft Lip and Palate: Constant or Increasing?', *Acta Chir Scand.*, 122, 106-111.

Foster, T.D. (1980), 'The Role of Orthodontic Treatment' in Edwards, M. and Watson, A.C.H. (eds), *Advances in The Management of Cleft Palate*, Churchill Livingstone, Edinburgh.

Fox, D.A., Lynch, J. and Brookshire, B. (1978), 'Selected Developmental Factors of Cleft Palate Children Between Two and Thirty-Three Months of Age', *Cleft Palate Jour.*, vol. 15, no. 3, July, 239-245.

Fraser, F.C. (1970), 'The Genetics of Cleft Lip and Palate', *Am. Jour. Hum. Genet.*, 22, 336-352.

Fria, T.J., Paradise, M.D., Sabo, M.S. and Elster, B.A. (1987), 'Conductive Hearing Loss In Infants and Young Children With Cleft Palate', *Jour. of Pediatrics*, vol. 111, no. 1, July, 84-87.

Gamba, A., Romano, M., Grosso, I., Tamburini, M., Cantu, G., Molinari, R. and Ventafridda, V. (1992), 'Psychosocial Adjustment of Patients Surgically Treated for Head and Neck Cancer', *Head and Neck*, 14, 218-223.

Gilligan, C., Lyons, N.P. and Hanmer, T.J. (1989), *Making Connections: The Relational Worlds of Adolescent Girls At Emma Willard School*, Troy, New York.

Glaser, B. and Strauss, A. (1968), *The Discovery of Grounded Theory: Strategies For Qualitative Research*, Weidenfeld and Nicolson, London.

Glass, L., Starr, C.D., Stewart, R.E. and Hodge, S.E. (1981), 'Identi-Kit Model II - A Potential Tool For Judging Cosmetic Appearance', *Cleft Palate Jour.*, 18, 147-151.

Glastonbury, B. and Mackean, J. (1991), 'Survey Methods' in Allan, G. and Skinner, C. (eds), *Handbook For Research Students in The Social Sciences*, Allen and Unwin, London, Chapter 19, pp.225-247.

Gluck, M. (1977), 'Psychological Intervention With Preschool Age Plastic Surgery Patients and Their Families', *Jour. Pediatr. Psychol.*, 2, 23.

Gluck, H., Wylie, H. Mcwilliams, G. and Conkwright, E. (1965), 'Comparison of Clinical Characteristics of Children With Cleft Palates and Children In A Child Guidance Clinic', *Perceptual and Motor Skills*, 21, 806-810.

Goffe, T. (1991), *Bully For You...*, Child's Play Publications.

Goffman, E. (1963), *Stigma: Notes On The Management of Spoiled Identity*, Penguin, London.

Goodman, R.M. and Gorlin, R.J. (1983), *The Malformed Infant and Child. An Illustrated Guide*, Oxford University Press.

Goodstein, L.D. (1961), 'Intellectual Impairment In Children With Cleft Palates', *Jour. Speech Hear. Res.*, 4, 287-294.

Goodstein, L.D. (1968), 'Psychosocial Aspects of Cleft Palate' in Spriestersbach, D.C. and Sherman, D. (eds), *Cleft Palate and Communication*, Academic Press, New York.

Gothard, T.W., Runyan, D.K., and Hadler, J.L. (1985), 'The Diagnosis and Evaluation of Child Maltreatment', *Jour. Emerg. Med.*, 3, 181.

Grunsell, A. (1989) *Let's Talk About Bullying*, F. Watts Publications

Grunwell, P. and Russell, J. (1987a), 'Vocalisations Before and After Cleft Palate Surgery: A Pilot Study', *Brit. Jour. Disorders Communic.*, 22, 1.

Grunwell, P. and Russell, J. (1988), 'Phonological Development In Children With Cleft Lip and Palate', *Clinical Linguistics and Phonetics*, 2, 75.

Hakim, C. (1987), *Research Design, Strategies and Choices in The Design of Social Research*, Allen and Unwin, London.

Hammond, B.N. (BNH), (1970), 'Speech Results In Cleft Palate Surgery', *Paper presented at the meeting of The British Association of Plastic Surgeons*, Aviemore, June.

Hammond, B.N. (BNH), (1976), 'An Investigation Into The Causes and Management of Nasality In Non Cleft Palate Children', *Paper presentedby J. Harvey Kemble at the meeting of The British Association of Plastic Surgeons*, Windsor, June.

Hammond, B.N. (BNH), (1977), 'Hypernasality Among 561 Children With Cleft Palate-The Speech Therapist's View'. *Paper presented at the International Conference of Plastic Surgeons*, Toronto.

Harper, A. (1988), *What Feels Best*, Piccadilly Press.

Harper, D.C. and Richman, L.C. (1978), 'Personality Profiles of Physically Impaired Adolescents', *Jour. Clin. Psych.*, 34, 636-642.

Harper, D.C., Richman, L.C. and Snider, W. (1977), 'School Adjustment and Degrees of Physical Impairment', *unpublished manuscript* (available from D.C. Harper, N119 Hospital School, University of Iowa, Iowa City, IA 52242).

Harper, D.C., Richman, L.C. and Snider, B. (1980), 'School Adjustment and Degree of Physical Impairment', *Jour. Ped. Psych.*, 5, 377.

Harris, D. (1982), 'The Symptomatology of Abnormal Appearance: An Anecdotal Survey', *British Jour. Plastic Surgery*, 35, 312-323.

Harrison, S.P. (1977), *Families in Stress*, Royal College of Nursing, London.

Harter, S. (1983), 'Developmental Perspectives On The Self-System' in E.M. Heatherington, E.M. (ed.),*Handbook of Child Psychology: vol. 4. Socialization, Personality, and Social Development*, Wiley, 275, New York.

Harvey, D. and Greenway, P. (1982), 'How Parent Attitudes and Emotional Reactions Affect Their Handicapped Child's Self-Concept', *Psychol. Med.*, 12, 357-370.

Hathorn, I.S. (1986), 'Classification' in Albery, E.H., Hathorn, I.S. and Pigott, R.W. (eds), *Cleft Lip and Palate: A Team Approach*, Wright, Bristol, 17-19.

Hay, S. ((1967), 'Incidence of Clefts and Parental Age', *Cleft Palate Jour.*, 4, 205-213.

Heineman-De Boer, J.A. (1985), *Cleft Palate Children and Intelligence*, Lisse, Swets and Zeitlinger.

Heller, J.C. (1979), 'Hearing Loss In Patients With Cleft Palate' in Bzoch, K.R. (ed.), *Communicative Disorders Related To Cleft Lip and Palate*, Little, Brown and Company, Boston.

Heller, A., Tidmarsh, W. and Pless, I.B. (1981), 'The Psychosocial Functioning of Young Adults Born With Cleft Lip or Palate',*Clinical Pediatrics*, vol. 20, no. 7, July, 459-465.

Hewett, S. (with Newson, J. and Newson, E.), (1970), *The Family and The Handicapped Child*, George Allen and Unwin, London.

Hill-Beuf, A. and Porter, J. (1984), 'Children Coping With Impaired Appearance: Social and Psychologic Influences', Gen. Hosp. Psychiatry, 6, 294-301.

Holdsworth, W.G. (1970), *Cleft Lip and Palate*, 4th Edition, Heinemann, London.

Hopson, B. and Scally, M. (1981), *Lifeskills Teaching*, McGraw-Hill, London.

Horn, L. (1972), 'Language Development of The Cleft Palate Child', *Jour. South African Speech and Hear. Assoc.*, 19, 17-29.

Isaacson, R.J. (1962), 'Cortisone-Induced Cleft Palates In Inbred Mice', *Am. J. Orthod.*, 48, 626.

Jaehnig, W.B. (1974), 'Mentally Handicapped Children and Their Families: Problems For Social Policy',*Ph.D Thesis*, University of Essex.

Jenny, J., Cons, N.C., Kohout, F.J. and Frazier, R.J. (1980), 'Test of A Method To Determine Socially Acceptable Occlusal Conditions', *Community Dent. Oral Epidemiology*, 9, 424-433.

Kagan, K., Tyler, N. and Turner, P. (1974), 'The Process of Interpersonal Adaption Between Mothers and Their Cerebral Palsy Children', *Devel. Med. Child Neurol.*, 16, 518.

Kapp, K. (1979), 'Self Concept of The Cleft Lip and/or Palate Child', *Cleft Palate Journal*, vol. 16, no. 2, April, 171-176.

Kapp-Simon, K. (1980), 'Psychological Adaptations of Patients With Craniofacial Malformations' in Lucker, G.W. Ribbens, K.A. and McNamara, J. (eds), *Psychological Aspects of Facial Form*, Centre For Human Growth and Development, Ann Arbor, Michigan.

Kapp-Simon, K. (1986), 'Self-Concept of Primary-School-Age Children With Cleft Lip, Cleft Palate, Or Both',*Cleft Palate Jour.*, vol. 23, no. 1, January, 24-27.

Kapp-Simon, K., Simon, D. and Kristovich, S. (1992), 'Self-Perception, Social Skills, Adjustment, and Inhibition In Young Adolescents With

Craniofacial Anomalies', *Cleft Palate-Craniofacial Jour.*, July, vol.29, no.4, 352-356.

Kasner, K. and Tindall, D. (1984), *Bailliere's Nurses' Dictionary*, (20th Edition), Bailliere Tindall, London.

Katz, I. (1981), *Stigma: A Social Psychological Analysis.*, Lawrence Erlbaum, Hillsdale, N.J..

Kelly, G. (1955), *The Psychology of Personal Constructs*, Norton, New York.

Kernahan, D.A. and Stark, R.B. (1958), 'A New Classification For Cleft Lip and Palate', *Plast. Reconstr. Surg.*, 22, 435-441.

Kew, S. (1975), *Handicap and Family Crisis*, Pitman., London.

Kidscape (not dated), 'Stop Bullying!', *Anti-Bullying Campaign Literature*, Kidscape, London.

Kiyak, H.A., Hohl, T., West, R. and Mcneil, R.W. (1984), 'Psychological Changes In Orthognathic Surgery Patients: A 24 Month Follow-Up', *Jour. Oral Maxillofac. Surg.*, 42, 506-512.

Kleinke, C.L. (1975), *First Impressions: The Psychology of Encountering Others*, Prentice-Hall, New Jersey.

Kobasa, S.C. (1979), 'Stressful Life Events, Personality, and Health: An Inquiry Into Hardiness', *Jour. Personality and Social Psychol.*, January, vol.37, no.1, 1-11.

Knox, G. and Braithwaite, F. (1962), 'Cleft Lips and Palates In Northumberland and Durham', *Arch. Dis. Child*, 38, 66-70.

Kommers, M. and Sullivan, M. (1979), 'Written Language Skills of Children With Cleft Palate', *Cleft Palate Jour.*, 16, 81-85.

Lahti, A., Rintala, A. and Soivio, A. (1974), 'Educational Level of Patients With Cleft Lip and Palate', *Cleft Palate Jour.*, 11, 36-40.

Lamb, M.M., Wilson, F.B. and Leeper, H.A. (1973), 'A Comparison of Selected Cleft Palate Children and Their Siblings On The Variables of Intelligence, Hearing Loss, and Visual-Perceptual-Motor Skills', *Cleft Palate Jour.*, 9, 218-228.

Lamb, M.M., Wilson, F.B. and Leeper, H.A. (1973), 'The Intellectual Function of Cleft Palate Children Compared On The Basis of Cleft Type and Sex', *Cleft Palate Jour.*, 10, 367-377.

Langlois, J.H. and Stephan, C. (1981), 'Beauty and The Beast' in Brehm, S., Kassin, S. and Gibbons, F. (eds), *Developmental Social Psychology: Theory and Research*, Oxford University Press, New York.

Langlois, J.H., Roggman, L.A., Casey, R.J., Ritter, J.M., Rieser-Danner, L.A. and Jenkins, V.Y. (1987), 'Infant Preferences For Attractive Faces: Rudiments of A Stereotype?', *Devel. Psychol.*, 23, 3, 363-369.

Langner, T.S. and Michael, S.T. (1963), *Life Stress and Mental Health*, Thomas A.C. Rennie Series In Social Psychiatry. II The Midtown Manhattan Study, Collier-Macmillan Canada Ltd, Toronto.

Lanigan, S. and Cotterill, J. (1989), 'Psychological Disabilities Amongst Patients With Port Wine Stains', *British Jour. Dermatology*, 121, 209-

215.

Lansdown, R. (1981), 'Cleft Lip and Palate: A Prediction of Psychological Disfigurement?', *British Journal of Orthodontics*, vol. 8, April, 83-88.

Lansdown, R. and Polak, L. (1975), 'A Study of The Psychological Effects of Facial Deformity In Children', *Child: Care, Health and Development*, 1, 85-91.

Lansdown, R., Lloyd, J. and Hunter, J. (1991), 'Facial Deformity In Childhood: Severity and Psychological Adjustment', *Child: Care,Health and Development*, 17, 165-171.

Leahy, R.L. and Shirk, S.R. (1985), 'Social Cognition and The Development of The Self' in Leahy, R.L. (ed.),*The Development of The Self, A* cademic Press.

Leck, I. ((1969), 'Ethnic Differences In The Incidence of Malformations Following Migration',*Brit. J. Prev. Soc. Med.*, 23, 166-173.

Leder, S.B. and Lerman, J.W., (1985), 'Some Acoustic Evidence For Vocal Abuse In Adult Speakers With Repaired Cleft Palate', *Laryngoscope*, 95, July, 837-840.

Lefebvre, A. and Munro, I. (1978), 'The Role of Psychiatry In A Craniofacial Team', *Plast. Reconstr. Surg.*, 61, 546.

Leonard, B.J., Brust, J.D., Abrahams, G. and Sielaff, B. (1991), 'Self-Concept of Children and Adolescents With Cleft Lip and/orPalate', *Cleft Palate Jour.*, vol. 28, no. 4, October, 347-353.

Lencione, R.M., (1980), 'Psychosocial Aspects of Cleft Lip and Palate' in M. Edwards, M. and Watson, A.C.H. (eds), *Advances in The Management of Cleft Palate*, Churchill Livingstone, Edinburgh.

Lerner, R.M. and Lerner, J. (1977), 'Effects of Age, Sex, and Physical Attractiveness On Child-Peer Relations, Academic Performance, and Elementary School Adjustment', *Dev. Psychol.*, 13, 585-590.

Lewis, R. (1961), 'Survey of The Intelligence of Cleft-Lip and Cleft-Palate Children In Ontario', *Brit. Journal Disorders Communic.*, 6, 17-25.

Lin, N. (1976), *Foundations of Social Research*, McGraw-Hill.

Lindsay, W.K., Le Mesurier, A.B., and Farmer, A.W. (1962), 'A Study of The Speech Results of A Large Series of Cleft Palate Patients', *Plastic and Reconstructive Surgery*, vol. 29, no. 3, 273- 288.

Lissitz, R.W. and Green, S.B. (1975), 'Effect of The Number of Scale Points On Reliability: A Monte Carlo Approach', *J. Appl. Psychol.*, 60, 10-13.

Lockhart, D.C. (1984), 'The Stages of Mailed Questionnaire Returning Behavior' in Lockhart, D.C. (ed.), *Making Effective Use of Mailed Questionnaires*, New Directions For Program Evaluation, No. 21. Jossey-Bass, San Francisco.

Long, N.V. and Dalston, R.M. (1982), 'Gestural Communication In Twelve-Month-Old Cleft Lip and Palate Children', *Cleft Palate Journal*, vol. 19, no. 1, January, 57-61.

Lovius, B., Jones, R., Pospisil, O., Reid, D., Slade, P. and Wynne, T.

(1990), 'The Specific Psychosocial Effects of Orthognathic Surgery', *Jour. Cranio-Maxillo-Facial Surgery*, 18, 339-342.

Lowe, G.R. (1972), *The Growth of Personality: From Infancy To Old Age*, Penguin Books, London.

Lynch, J.I., Fox, D.R. and Brookshire, B.L. (1983), 'Phonological Proficiency of Two Cleft Palate Toddlers With School-Age Follow-Up', *Jour. Speech and Hearing Disorders*, 18, 274.

McCrae, R.R. and Costa, P.T. Jr. ((1987), 'Validation of The Five-Factor Model of Personality Across Instruments and Observers', *Jour. Personality and Soc. Psychol.*, vol.52, no.1, 81-90.

McDaniel, J.W. (1969), *Physical Disability and Human Behavior*, Pergamon Press, New York.

McDonald, E. and Baker, H.K. (1951), 'Cleft Palate Speech: An Integration of Research and Clinical Observation', *Jour. Speech Hear. Disord.*, 16, 9-20.

MacGregor, F.C., Abel, T.M. and Brynt, A. (1953), *Facial Deformities and Plastic Surgery: A Psychosocial Study*, Charles C. Thomas, Springfield, Illinois.

MacGregor, F.C. (1970), 'Social and Psychological Implications of Dentofacial Disfigurement', *Angle Orthodontist*, 40, 231-233.

MacGregor, F.C. (1974), *Transformation and Identity - The Face and Plastic Surgery*, Quadrangle/New York Times, New York.

MacGregor, F. (1990), 'Facial Disfigurement: Problems and Management of Social Interaction and Implications For Mental Health', *Aesthetic Plastic Surgery*, 14 (4), 249-257.

MacGregor, F.C., Abel, T.M., Bryt, A., Lauer, E. and Weissmann, S. (1953), *Facial Deformity and Plastic Surgery*, C.C. Thomas, Springfield, Illinois.

McGuire, D.E. (1990), 'An Evaluation of A Social Skills Program For Adolescents With Facial Disfigurement', *unpublished Doctoral Dissertation*, University of Illinois at Chicago.

MacMahon, B. and McKeown, T. (1953), 'The Incidence of Harelip and Cleft Palate Related To Birth Rank and Maternal Age', *Am. J. Hum. Genet.*, 5, 176-183.

McWilliams, B.J. (1974), 'Clinical Use of The Peabody Picture Vocabulary Test With Cleft Palate Pre-Schoolers', *Cleft Palate Jour.*, 11, 439-442.

McWilliams, B.J. (1982), 'Social and Psychological Problems Associated With Cleft Palate. Symposium On Social and Psychological Considerations In Plastic Surgery', *Clinics in Plastic Surgery*, vol. 9, no. 3, July, 317-326.

McWilliams, B., Bluestone, C. and Musgrave, R. (1969), 'Diagnostic Implication of Vocal Cord Nodules In Children With Cleft Palate', *Laryngoscope*, 79, 1972,-1980.

McWilliams, B.J. and Musgrave, R. (1972), 'Psychological Implications of Articulation Disorders In Cleft Palate Children', *Cleft Palate Jour.*, 9,

294-303.

McWilliams, B.J. and Paradise, L.P. (1973), 'Education, Occupational and Marital Status of Cleft Palate Adults', *Cleft Palate Jour.,* 10, 223-229.

McWilliams, B., Lavorato, A. and Bluestone, C. (1973), 'Vocal Cord Abnormalities In Children With Velopharyngeal Valving Problems', *Laryngoscope,* 83, 1745-1753.

McWilliams, B.J. and Matthews, H.P. (1979), 'A Comparison of Intelligence and Social Maturity In Children With Unilateral Complete Clefts and Those With Isolated Cleft Palates', *Cleft Palate Journal,* vol. 16, no. 4, October, 363-372.

McWilliams, B.J., Morris, H.L. and Shelton, R.L. (1984), *Cleft Palate Speech,* B.C. Decker Inc., The C.V. Mosby Company, Saint Louis.

Maw, A.R. (1986), 'Ear Disease' in Albery, E.H., Hathorn, I.S. and Pigott, R.W. (eds), *Cleft Lip and Palate: A Team Approach,* Wright, Bristol, 63-67.

Means, B. and Irwin, J. (1954), 'An Analysis of Certain Measures of Intelligence and Hearing In A Sample of The Wisconsin Cleft Palate Population', *Cleft Palate Newsletter,* 4, 2-4.

Meyerson, L. (1955), 'Somatopsychology of Physical Disability' in W.M. Cruickshank, W.M. (ed.), *Psychol. Except. Children and Youth,* Prentice-Hall, Englewood Cliffs, N.J..

Miller, G.A. (1969), 'Presidential Address', American Psychological Association, (1969), in D. Larson, D. (ed.), (1984), *Teaching Psychological Skills: Models For Giving Psychology Away,* Brooks / Cole Publishing Company, P.V (Preface).

Moll, K. (1968), 'Speech Characteristics of Individuals With Cleft Lip and Palate', in Spriestersbach, D. and Sherman, D. (eds), *Cleft Palate and Communication,* Academic Press, New York, 61-118.

Moore, P., Blakeney, P., Broemeling, L., Portman, S., Herndon, D. and Robson, M. (1993), 'Psychological Adjustment After Childhood Burn Injuries As Predicted By Personality Traits', *Jour. Burn Care and Rehabilitation,* 14, (1), 80-82.

Mordecai, R.M. (1984), 'The Orthodontic Management of Cleft Lip and Palate Patients', *Dent. Update,* 11, 567-583.

Morley, M.E. (1965), *The Development and Disorders of Speech In Children,* 2nd Edition, Livingstone, Edinburgh and London.

Morley, M.E. (1966), *Cleft Palate and Speech,* 6th Edition,Churchill Livingstone, Edinburgh.

Morley, M.E. (1970), *Cleft Palate and Speech,* 7th Edition, Churchill Livingstone, Edinburgh.

Morris, H.L. (1962), 'Communication Skills of Children With Cleft Lips and Palates', *Jour. Speech and Hearing Research,* 5, 79-90.

Morris, H. (1973), 'Velopharyngeal Competence and Primary Cleft Palate Surgery, (1960),-(1971),: A Critical Review', *Cleft Palate Jour.,* 10, 62-70.

Morris, H.L. (1979), 'Evaluation of Abnormal Articulation Patterns' in Bzoch, K.R. (ed.), *Communicative Disorders Related To Cleft Lip and Palate*, Little, Brown and Company, Boston.

Mousset, M.R. and Trichet, C. (1985), 'Babbling and Phonetic Acquisitions After Early Complete Surgical Repair of Cleft Lip and Palate', *Paper presented at the Fifth international Congress On Cleft Palate and Related Craniofacial Abnormalities*, MonteCarlo.

Munson, S. and May, A. (1955), 'Are Cleft Palate Persons of Subnormal Intelligence?', *Educ. Res. Jour.*, 48, 617-622.

Musgrave, R., McWilliams, B.J. and Matthews, H. (1975), 'A Review of The Results of Two Different Surgical Procedures For The Repair of Clefts of The Soft Palate Only', *Cleft Palate Jour.*, 12, 281-290.

Nash, P.R. (1993), 'Psychosocial Implications of Being Born With A Cleft Palate (With Instances of Additional Cleft Lip)', *Unpublished Doctoral Thesis*, University of Southampton.

Nation, J.E. (1970), 'Vocabulary Comprehension and Usage of Preschool Cleft Palate and Normal Children', *Cleft Palate Journal*, 7, 639-644.

Nation, J.E. and Aram, D.M. (1977), *Diagnosis of Speech and Language Disorders*, C.V. Mosby, St. Louis.

Nation, J.E. and Wetherbee, M.A. (1985), 'Cognitive-Communicative Development of Identical Triplets, One With Unilateral Cleft Lip and Palate', *Cleft Palate Jour.*, 22, 38-50.

Natsume, N., Suzuki, T., and Kawai, T. (1987), 'Maternal Reactions To The Birth of A Child With Cleft Lip and/or Palate',*Correspondence and Brief Communications, Plastic and Reconstr. Surgery*, June, 1003-1004.

Noar, J.H. (1988), 'Cleft Patients, Parents and The Cleft Palate Team', MSc. *Thesis in Orthodontics*, University of London.

Noar, J.H. (1991), 'Questionnaire Survey of Attitudes and Concerns of Patients With Cleft Lip and Palate and Their Parents', *Cleft Palate-Craniofacial Journal*, vol. 28, no. 3, July, 279-284.

Noar, J.H. (1992), 'A Questionnaire Survey of Attitudes and Concerns of Three Professional Groups Involved In The Cleft Palate Team', *Cleft Palate-Craniofacial Jour.*, vol. 29, no. 1 , 92-95.

Offer, D., Ostrov, E. and Howard, K.I. (1984), 'Patterns of Adolescent Self-Image' in Lamb, H.R. (ed.), *New Directions For Mental Health Services.*, Jossey-Bass, San Francisco.

O'Gara, M.M., and Logemann, J.A. (1988), 'Phonetic Analyses of The Speech Development of Babies With Cleft Palate', *Cleft Palate Journal*, vol. 25, no. 2, April, 122-134.

Oldfield, M. and Tate, G.T. (1964), 'Cleft Lip and Palate: Some Ideas On Prevention and Treatment, Based On 1,166 Cases', *Brit. Jour. Plastic Surgery*, 17, 1-9.

Oppenheim, A.N. (1966), *Questionnaire Design and Attitude Measurement*, Heinemann, London.

O'Riain, S. and Hammond, B.N. (1972), 'Speech Results In Cleft Palate Surgery, A Survey of 249 Patients', *Brit. Jour. Plastic Surgery*, 25, 380-387.

Orr, D., Reznikoff, M. and Smith, G. (1989), 'Body Image, Self-Esteem and Depression In Burn-Injured Adolescents and Young Adults', *Jour. Burn Care and Rehabilitation*, 10, (5), 454-461.

Osborne, J. (1986), 'Genetic Counselling' in Albery, E.H., Hathorn, I.S. and Pigott, R.W. (eds), *Cleft Lip and Palate: A Team Approach*, Wright, Bristol, 75-77.

Owen, D.R. (1970), 'Behavioral Concomitants of A Psychometric Scale of Inhibition Developed From Mothers' Reports' in Pauker, J.D. (Chm.), *Age, Sex, Response Communality, and Behavioral Descriptive Categories As The Basis For Psychometric Dimensions of Children's Personality*, Symposium presented at the Midwestern Psychological Association, Cincinnati, April.

Owens, J.R., Jones, J.W. and Harris, F. (1985), 'Epidemiology of Facial Clefting', *Arch. Dis. Child*, 60, 521-529.

Palkes, H.S., Marsh, J.L. and Talent, B.K. (1986), 'Pediatric Craniofacial Surgery and Parental Attitudes', *Cleft Palate Journal*, vol. 23, no. 2, April, 137-143.

Palmer, G. (1988), *The Politics of Breastfeeding*, Pandora Press, London.

Palmer, J. and Adams, M. (1962), 'The Oral Image of Children With Cleft Lip and Palate', *Cleft Palate Bull.*, 12, 72-76.

Pannbacker, M. (1975), 'Oral Language Skills of Adult Cleft Palate Speakers', *Cleft Palate Jour.*, 12, 95.

Pannbacker, M. (1988), 'Prevention of Communication Problems Associated With Cleft Palate', *Jour. Commun. Disord.*, 21, 401-408.

Paradise, J.L. (1975), 'Middle Ear Problems Associated With Cleft Palate', *Cleft Palate Jour.*, 12, 17.

Parkes, C.M. (1972), *Bereavement: Studies in Grief in Adult Life*, Int. Univ. Press, Inc., New York.

Partridge, J., (1992), 'Workshops and Advice For The Facially Disfigured', *'Changing Faces'* Literature, 'Changing Faces' Charity, London.

Partridge, J., Coutinho, W., Robinson, E. and Rumsey, N. (1994), 'Changing Faces: Two Years On', *Nursing Standard*, 8 May, (34), 54-58.

Patterson, D., Everett, J., Bombardier, C., Questad, K., Lee, V. and Marvin, J. (1993), 'Psychological Effects of Severe Burn Injuries', *Psychological Bulletin*, 113, (2), 362-378.

Patzer, G.L. (1984), *The Physical Attractiveness Phenomena*, Plenum Press, New York.

Pecyna, P.M., Feeney-Giacoma, M.E. and Neiman, G.S. (1987), 'Development of The Object Permanence Concept In Cleft Lip and Palate and Noncleft Lip and Palate Infants', *Journal Commun. Disord.*, 20, 233-243.

Pertschuk, M.J. and Whitaker, L.A. (1985), 'Psychosocial Adjustment and Craniofacial Malformations In Childhood', *Plastic and Reconstr. Surgery*, vol. 75, no. 2, February, 177-184.

Peter, J.P. and Chinsky, R.R. (1974), 'Sociological Aspects of Cleft Palate Adults: I. Marriage', *Cleft Palate Jour.*, 11, 295-309.

Peter, J.P., Chinsky, R.R. and Fisher, M.H. (1975), 'Sociological Aspects of Cleft Palate Adults: IV. Social Integration', *Cleft Palate Jour.*, 12, 304-310.

Philips, B.J. and Harrison, R.J. (1969), 'Language Skills of Preschool Cleft Palate Children', *Cleft Palate Jour.*, 6, 108-119.

Phillips, J.L. Jr. (1975), *The Origins of Intellect: Piaget's Theory*, 2nd Edition, W.H. Freeman and Company, San Francisco.

Phillips, P. (1975), *Speech and Hearing Problems In The Classroom*, Cliff Notes, Inc., Lincoln, Nebraska.

Phillips, P. and Stengelhofen, J. (1989), 'Towards Partnership With Parents' in Stengelhofen, J. (ed.), *Cleft Palate, The Nature and Remediation of Communication Problems*, Churchill Livingstone, Edinburgh, 165-185.

Philp, M. and Duckworth, D. (1982), *Children With Disabilities and Their Families: A Review of Research*, NFER-Nelson, Windsor.

Piaget, J. (1950), *The Psychology of Intelligence*, Routledge and Kegan Paul, London.

Piers, E.V. (1984), *Manual For The Piers-Harris Children's Self-Concept Scale*, The Western Psychologial Services, Acklen, T.N..

Piers, E.V. and Harris, D.B. (1964), 'Age and Other Correlates of Self-Concept', *Jour. Educ. Psych.*, 55, 91-95.

Pigott, R.W. (1986), 'Primary Repair of The Cleft Lip and Palate' in Albery, E.H., Hathorn, I.S. and Pigott, R.W. (eds), *Cleft Lip and Palate: A Team Approach*, Wright, Bristol, 20-30.

Pigott, R.W. (1986), 'Secondary Surgery' in Albery, E.H., Hathorn, I.S. and Pigott, R.W. (eds), *Cleft Lip and Palate: A Team Approach*, Wright, Bristol, 31-41.

Pillemer, F.G. and Cook, K.V. (1989), 'The PsychosocialAdjustment of Pediatric Craniofacial Patients After Surgery', *Cleft Palate Jour.*, vol. 26, no. 3, July, 201-208.

Pinkerton, P. (1970), 'Parental Acceptance of The Handicapped Child', *Devel. Med. Child Neurol.*, 12, 207.

Podeanu-Czehofsky, I. (1975), 'It Is Only The Child's Guilt? Some Aspects of Family Life of Cerebral Palsied Children', *Rehabilitation Literature*, 36, 308-311.

Police Sergeant, Henley Training Centre, (1988), 'Quotation' in Jones, P., *Lipservice: The Story of Talk In Schools*, Open University Press, Milton Keynes, p.111.

Porter, J., Beuf, A., Lerner, A. and Norlund, J. (1986), 'Psychosocial Effect of Vitiligo: A Comparison of Vitiligo Patients With 'Normal' Control

Subjects, With Psoriasis Patients, and With Patients With Other Pigmentary Disorders', *Jour. American Academy of Dermatology*, 15, (2), 220-224.

Porter, J., Beuf, A., Lerner, A. and Norlund, J. (1990), 'The Effect of Vitiligo On Sexual Relationships', *Jour. American Academy of Dermatology*, 22, 221-222.

Prugh, D.G. (1956), 'Psychological and Psychophysiological Aspects of Oral Activities In Childhood', *Pediat. Clin. N. Am.*, 3, 1049-1072.

Pruzinsky, T. and Edgerton, M. (1990), 'Body-Image Change In Cosmetic Plastic Surgery' in Pruzinsky, T. and Cash, T. (eds), *Body Images: Development, Deviance and Change*, Guilford Press, New York, 217-236

Pugh, G. (1985), 'Parents and Professionals In Partnership. Issues and Implications In Parent Involvement', *Partnership Paper 2.*, National Children's Bureau, London.

Quinn, P.O. and Rapoport, J.L. (1974), 'Minor Physical Anomalies and Neurologic Status In Hyperactive Boys', *Pediatrics*, 53, 742-747.

Rapoport, J.L. and Quinn, P.O. (1975), 'Minor Physical Anomalies (Stigmata), and Early Developmental Deviation: A Major Biologic Subgroups of 'Hyperactive Children'', *Int. J. Ment. Health*, 4, 29-44.

Reich, J. (1969), 'The Surgery of Appearance', *Medical Jour. of Australia*, 2, 5-13.

Richards, I.D.G. and Lowe, C.R. (1971), 'Incidence of Congenital Defects In South Wales 1964-6', *Br. J. Prev. Soc. Med.*, 25, 59-64.

Richards, I.D.G. and McIntosh, H.T. (1973), 'Spina Bifida Survivors and Their Parents - A Study of Problems and Services', *Development Medicine and Child Neurology*, 15, 292-304.

Richardson, S. (1970), 'Age and Sex Differences In Values Towards Physical Handicaps', *Jour. Health and Social Behaviour*, 11, 207-214.

Richardson, S. (1971), 'Handicap, Appearance and Stigma', *Social Science and Medicine*, 5, 621-628.

Richardson, S.A., Goodman, N., Hastorf, A.H. and Dornbusch, S.M. (1961), 'Cultural Uniformity In Reaction To Physical Disabilities', *Am. Sociol. Rev.*, 26, 241-247.

Richardson, S.A., Hastorf, A.H., and Dornsbuch, M. (1964), 'Effects of A Physical Disability On A Child's Description of Himself',*Child Development*, 35, 893-907.

Richman, L.C. (1976), 'Behavior and Achievement of The Cleft Palate Child', *Cleft Palate Jour.*, 13, 4-10.

Richman, L.C. (1978a), 'The Effects of Facial Disfigurement On Teachers Perception of Ability In Cleft Palate Children', *Cleft Palate Jour.*, 15, 155-160.

Richman, L.C. (1978b), 'Parents and Teachers: Differing Views of Behavior of Cleft Palate Children', *Cleft Palate Jour.*, 15, 360-364.

Richman, L.C. (1979), 'Language Variables Related To Reading Ability of

Children With Verbal Deficits', *Psych. in The Schools*, 16, 299-305.

Richman, L.C. (1980), 'Cognitive Patterns and Learning Disabilities In Cleft Palate Children With Verbal Deficits', *Jour. Speech and Hearing Research*, 23, June, 447-456.

Richman, L.C. (1983), 'Self-Reported Social, Speech, and Facial Concerns and Personality Adjustment of Adolescents With Cleft Lip and Palate', *Cleft Palate Journal*, vol. 20, no. 2, April, 108-112.

Richman, L.C. (1989), 'Editorial Commentary' on Broder and Strauss, (1989), *op cit.*

Richman, L.C. and Harper, D.C. (1978), 'School Adjustment of Children With Observable Disabilities', *Jour. Abnormal Child Psychology*, vol. 6, no. 1, 11-18.

Richman, L.C. and Harper, D.C. (1979), 'Self-Identified Personality Patterns of Children With Facial or Orthopedic Disfigurement', *Cleft Palate Journal*, vol. 16, no. 3, 257-261.

Richman, L.C. and Eliason, M. (1982), 'Psychological Characteristics of Children With Cleft Lip and Palate: Intellectual, Achievement, Behavioral and Personality Variables', *Cleft Palate Jour.*, vol. 19, no. 4, October, 249-257.

Richman, L.C. and Eliason, M. (1984), 'Type of Reading Disability Related To Cleft Type and Neuropsychological Patterns', *Cleft Palate Journal*, vol. 21, no. 1, 1-6.

Richman, L.C., Holmes, C.S. and Eliason, M.J. (1985), 'Adolescents With Cleft Lip and Palate: Self-Perceptions of Appearance and Behavior Related To Personality Adjustment', *Cleft Palate Journal*, vol. 22, no. 2, April, 93-96.

Richman, L.C., Eliason, M. and Lindgren, S.D. (1988), 'Reading Disability In Children With Clefts', *Cleft Palate Jour.*, vol. 25, no. 1, 21-25.

Roberts, J., Prince, R., Gold, G. Et Al. (1970), 'Social and Mental Health Survey', *Montreal, Summary Report, Poverty and Social Policy In Canada*, edited by Mann, W.E., Copp Clark Publishing Company, 85, Toronto.

Roger, D. (1992), 'The Development and Evaluation of A Work Skills and Stress Management Training Programme', *Paper presented at the Annual Conference of The British Psychological Society*, April, Scarborough.

Rosenberg, M. (1965), *Society and The Adolescent Self-Image*, Princeton University Press, Princeton, N.J..

Rosenberg, L., Mitchell, A.A., Parsells, J.L., Pashayan, H., Louick, C. and Sapiro, S. (1983), 'Lack of Relation of Oral Clefts To Diazepam During Pregnancy', *N. Engl. J. Med.*, 309, 1282-1285.

Rotter, J.B. (1966), 'Generalised Expectancies For Internal Versus External Control of Reinforcement', *Psychological Monographs*, 80, 1, (entire issue).

The Royal College of Physicians, (1990), *Report-Research involving Patients*, January, The Royal College of Physicians of London.

The Royal College of Physicians, (1990), *Report - Guidelines On The Practice of Ethics Committees in Medical Research involving Human Subjects*, January, The Royal College of Physicians of London.

Rubinow, D., Peck, G., Squillace, K. and Gnatt, G. (1987), 'Reduced Anxiety and Depression In Cystic Acne Patients After Successful Treatment With Oral Isotretinoin', *Jour. American Academy of Dermatology*, 17, (1), 25-32.

Ruess, A.L. (1965), 'A Comparative Study of Cleft Palate Children and Their Siblings', *Journal Clinical Psychology*, vol. 21, 354-360.

Rumsey, N., Bull, R. and Gahagen, D. (1986), 'A Preliminary Study of The Potential of Social Skills Training For Improving The Quality of Social Interaction For The Facially Disfigured', *Soc. Beh.*, 1, 143-145.

Russell, J. (1989), 'Early Intervention' in Stengelhofen, J. (ed.), *Cleft Palate, The Nature and Remediation of Communication Problems*, Churchill Livingstone, Edinburgh, 31-63.

Russel, L.B. and Russel, W.L. (1952), 'Radiation Hazards To The Embryo and Foetus', *Radiol.*, 58, 376-396.

Rutter, M. (1972), *Maternal Deprivation Reassessed*, Penguin, London

Rutter, M., Tizard, J. and Whitmore, K. (1970b), *Education, Health and Behaviour*, Longmans, London.

Safra, M.J. and Oakly, G.P. (1975), 'Association Between Cleft Lip With or Without Cleft Palate and Prenatal Exposure To Diazepam', *Lancet*, 2 478-480.

Salvia, J. and Ysseldyke, J. (1978), *Assessment In Special and Remedial Education*, Houghton Miflin, Boston, Mass..

Salvia, J., Algozzine, R. and Sheare, J. (1977), 'Attractiveness and School Achievement', *Jour. School Psychology*, 15, 60-67.

Sandstrom, C.I. (1968), *The Psychology of Childhood and Adolescence*, Pelican.

Saxman, J. and Bless, D. (1973), 'Patterns of Language In Cleft Palate Children Aged 3 To 8 Years', *Paper presented at the Annual Meeting of The American Cleft Palate Association*, Oklahoma City.

Schade, G.L. (1974), 'Induction of Cleft Palate By Amniotic Sac Puncture', *Acta Morphol Neerl Scand.*, 12, 159-166.

Schaffer, R. (1977), *Mothering*, Fontana Press, London.

Scheper-Hughes, N.M. (1987b), 'The Cultural Politics of Child Survival' in Scheper-Hughes, N.M. (ed.), *Child Survival: Anthropological Approaches To The Treatment and Maltreatment of Children*, D. Reidel Publishing Company, Dordrecht, 1-32.

Scheper-Hughes, N.M. (1990), 'Difference and Danger: The Cultural Dynamics of Childhood Stigma, Rejection and Rescue', *Cleft Palate Jour.*, vol. 27, no. 3, July, 301-307.

Schonfeld, W.A. (1969), 'The Body and The Body-Image In Adolescents' in

Caplan, G. and Lebovici, S. (eds), *Adolescence: Psychological Perspectives*, Basic Books, New York, 50-78.

Schontz, F.C. (1975), *The Psychological Aspects of Physical Illness and Disability*, The Macmillan Publishing Company, Inc., New York.

Schneider, D.J., Hastorf, A.H. and Ellsworth, P.C. (1979), *Person Perception*, Addison-Wesley, Reading, Ma..

Schneiderman, C.R. and Auer, K.E. (1984), 'The Behavior of The Child With Cleft Lip and Palate As Perceived By Parents and Teachers', *Cleft Palate Jour.*, vol. 21, no. 3, July, 224-228.

Schneiderman, C.R. and Harding, J.B. (1984), 'Social Ratings of Children With Cleft Lip By School Peers', *Cleft Palate Journal*, vol. 21, No. 3, July, 219-223.

Schutt, W.H. (1977), 'Handicapped Children' in Mitchell, R.G. (ed.), *Child Health in The Community: A Handbook of Social and Community Paediatrics*, Churchill Livingstone, Edinburgh.

Scott, C. (1961), 'Research On Mail Surveys', *Jour. Roy. Stat. Soc.*, 24, Series A, 143-195.

Secord, P. and Jourard, S. (1953), 'The Appraisal of Body-Cathexis: Body Cathexis and The Self', *Jour. Consult. Psychol.*, 17, 343-347.

Seidman, S., Allen, R., and Wasserman, G. (1986), 'Productive Language of Premature and Physically Handicapped Two-Year-Olds', *Jour. Commun. Disord.*, (19, 61-73.

Seligman, M.E. (1975), *Helplessness*, W.H. Freeman, Reading.

Semin, G.R. and Manstead, A.S.R. (1983), *The Accountability of Conduct: A Social Psychological Analysis*, Academic Press, New York.

Shafer, W.G., Hine, M.K. and Levy, B.M. (1974), *A Textbook of Oral Pathology*, 3rd Edition, Saunders.

Shaw, W.C. (1981), 'Folklore Surrounding Facial Deformity and The Origins of Facial Prejudice', *Brit. Jour. Plastic Surgery*, 34, 237-246.

Shaw, W.C., Meek, S. and Jones, D. (1980), 'Nicknames, Teasing, Harassment and The Salience of Dental Features Among School Children', *Br. Jour. Orthodont.*, 7, 75-80.

Shaw, W.C. and Humphreys, S. (1982), 'Influence of Children's Dentofacial Appearance On Teacher Expectations', *Community Dent. Oral Epidemiol.*, 10 (6),, December, 313-319.

Sigelman, C.K. and Singleton, L.C. (1986), 'Stigmatization In Childhood: A Survey of Developmental Trends and Issues' in Ainlay, S.C., Becker, G. and Coleman, L.M. (eds), *The Dilemma of Difference: A Mutidisciplinary View of Stigma*, Plenum Press, New York.

Sigelman, C.K., Miller, T.E. and Whitworth, L.A. (1986), 'The Early Stigmatizing Reactions To Physical Differences', *Jour. Appl. Dev. Psych.*, 7, 17-32.

Simmonds, J.F. and Heimburger, R.E. (1978), 'Psychiatric Evaluation of Youth With Cleft Lip-Palate Matched With A Control Group', *Cleft Palate Jour.*, 15, 193.

Sinclair De Zwart, H. (1973), 'Language Acquisition and Cognitive Development' in Moore, T. (ed.), *Cognitive Development and The Acquisition of Language*, Academic, New York.

Sinicrope, P.E. and Clifford, E. (1973), 'Effects of Cleft Lip and Palate On Body Satisfaction', *Paper presented at the American Cleft Palate Association Annual Meeting*, Oklahoma City, Oklahoma.

Slutsky, H. (1969), 'Maternal Reaction and Adjustment To Birth and Care of Cleft Palate Child', *Cleft Palate Jour.*, 6, 425-429.

Smith, R.M. and McWilliams, B.J. (1968), 'Psycholinguistic Considerations In The Management of Children With Cleft Palate', *Jour. Speech and Hearing Disorders*, 33, 1, 26-33.

Smith, B., Skef, Z., Cohen, M. and Dorf, D. (1986), 'Aerodynamic Assessment In The Results of Pharyngeal Flap Surgery: A Preliminary Investigation', *Plast. Reconstr. Surg.*,76, 402-410.

Snyder, L. (1975), 'Pragmatics In Language Disabled Children: Their Prelinguistic and Early Verbal Performative and Presuppositions', *Doctoral Dissertation*, University of Colorado.

Social Trends 22 (1992), *A Publication of The Government Statistical Service*, 1992 Edition, Central Statistical Office, HMSO.

Spiedel, B.D. and Medow, S.R. (1972), 'Maternal Epilepsy and Abnormalities of The Foetus and Newborn', *Lancet*, 2, 839-843.

Spriestersbach, (1961a), 'Counseling Parents of Children With Cleft Lips and Palates', *Jour. Chron. Diseases*, 13, 244-252.

Spriestersbach, D.C. (1973), *Psychological Aspects of The 'Cleft Palate Problem'*, Vols. 1 and 2, University of Iowa Press, Iowa.

Spriestersbach, D.C. and Sherman, D. (1968), (eds), *Cleft Palate and Communication*, Academic Press, New York.

Spriestersbach, D.C., Darley, F.L. and Morris, H.L. (1958), 'Language Skills In Children With Cleft Palates', *Jour. Speech Hearing Research.*, 1, 279-285.

Starr, P. and Heiserman, K. (1977), 'Acceptance of Disability By Teenagers With Oral Facial Clefts', *Rehab. Couns. Bull.*, 28, 198.

Starr, P., Chinsky, R., Canter, H. and Meier, J. (1977), 'Mental, Motor and Social Behaviour of Infants With Cleft Lip and/or Cleft Palate', *Cleft Palate Jour.*, 14, 140.

Steinhausen, H-C. (1981), 'Chronically Ill and Handicapped Children and Adolescents: Personality Studies In Relation To Disease', *Jour. Abnormal Child Psychology*, vol. 9, no. 2, 291-297.

Stengelhofen, J. (1989), 'The Nature and Causes of Communication Problems In Cleft Palate' in Stengelhofen, J. (ed.), *Cleft Palate, The Nature and Remediation of Communication Problems*, Churchill Livingstone, Edinburgh, 1-30.

Stengelhofen, J. (1990), *Working With Cleft Palate*, Winslow Press, Bicester.

Stengelhofen, J. and Foster, T.D. (1979), 'An Investigation Into The

Effects of Residual Oro-Nasal Fistula In Repaired Cleft Palate', *Proceedings of The 8th National Conference of The College of Speech Therapists*, London.

Strauss, R. and Broder, H. (1991), 'Directions and Issues In Psychosocial Research and Methods As Applied To Cleft Lip and Palate and Craniofacial Anomalies', *Cleft Palate-Craniofacial Jour.*, vol.28, No.2, April, 50-156.

Strauss, R.P., Broder, H. and Helms, R.W. (1988), 'Perceptions of Appearance and Speech By Adolescent Patients With Cleft Lip and Palate and By Their Parents', *Cleft Palate Journal*, vol. 25, no. 4, October, 335-342.

Strean, L.P. and Peer, L.A. (1956), 'Stress As An Etiologic Factor In The Development of Cleft Palate', *Plastic Reconstr. Surg.*, 18, 1-8.

Stricker, G., Clifford, E., Cohen, L.K., Giddon, D.B., Meskin, L.H., and Evans, C.A. (1979), 'Psychosocial Aspects of Craniofacial Disfigurement: A 'State of The Art' Assessment Conducted By The Craniofacial Anomalies Program Branch', The National Institute of Dental Research, *Am. J. Orthod.*, vol. 76, no. 4, October, 410-422.

Sudman, S. and Bradburn, N. (1984), 'Improving Mailed Questionnaire Design' in Lockhart, D.C. (ed.), *Making Effective Use Of Mailed Questionnaires*, New Directions For Program Evaluation, no.21, Jossey-Bass, San Francisco.

Tagiuri, R. (1969), 'Person Perception' in Lindzey, G. and Aronson, E. (eds), *Handbook of Social Psychology*, Addison-Wesley, Reading, M.A..

Tattum, D. and Herbert, G. (1990), *Bullying: A Positive Response-Advice For Parents, Governors and Staff in Schools*, Cardiff Institute of Higher Education Learning Resources Centre, Cardiff.

Tavormina, J.B., Kastner, L.S., Slater, P.M. and Watt, S.L. (1976), 'Chronically Ill Children. A Psychologically and Emotionally Deviant Population?', *Jour. Abnormal Child Psychology*, 4, 99-110.

Tedesco, L.A., Albino, J.E., Cunat, J.J, Green, L.J., Lewis, E.A. and Slakter, M.J. (1983a), 'A Dento-Facial Attractiveness Scale. Part I: Reliability and Validity', *Am. Jour. Orthod.*, 83, 38-43.

Tempest, M.N. (1958), 'Some Observations On Blood Loss In Harelip and Cleft Palate Surgery', *Brit. Jour. P lastic Surgery*, 11, 34-44.

Tisza, V.B., Silverstone, B., Rosenblum, G. and Hanlon, N. (1958), 'Psychiatric Observations of Children With Cleft Palate', *Am. Jour. Orthopsychiat.*, 28, 416-423.

Tisza, V.B. and Gumpertz, E. (1962), 'The Parents' Reaction To The Birth and Early Care of Children With Cleft Palate', *Paediatrics*, 30, 86-90.

Tobiasen, J.M. (1984), 'Psychosocial Correlates of Congenital Facial Clefts: A Conceptualization and Model', *Cleft Palate Journal*, vol. 21, no. 3, July, 131-139.

Tobiasen, J.M. (1987), 'Social Judgements of Facial Deformity', *Cleft Palate Journal*, vol. 24, no. 4, October, 323-327.

Tobiasen, J.M. (1989), 'Scaling Facial Impairment', *Cleft Palate Journal*, vol. 26, no. 3, July, 249-254.

Tobiasen, J.M. (1991), 'Editorial Commentary' on Eliason, M. et al., (1991), *op cit.*

Tobiasen, J.M. and Hiebert, J.M. (1988), 'Reliability of Esthetic Ratings of Cleft Impairment', *Cleft Palate Journal*, vol. 25, no. 3, 313-317.

Trower, P., Bryant, B. and Argyle, M. (1978), *Social Skills and Mental Health*, Methuen.

Van Demark, D. and Harden, M. (1990), 'Speech Therapy For The Child With Cleft Lip and Palate' in Bardach, J. and Morris, H.L. (eds), *Multidisciplinary Management of Cleft Lip and Palate*, W.B. Saunders, Philadelphia, 99-805.

Van Demark, D. and Olin, W. (1986), 'The Iowa Approach' in Hotz, M., Gnoinski, W., Perko, M., Nussbaumer, H., Hoff, E. and Haubensak, R. (eds), *Early Treatment of Cleft Lip and Palate*, Hans Huber Publishers, Toronto, 20-23.

Van Demark, D. and Van Demark, A. (1970), 'Speech and Socio-Vocational Aspects of Individuals With Cleft Palate', *Cleft Palate Jour.*, 7, 284-299.

Varni, J., Wilcox, K.T., and Hanson, V. (1988), 'Mediating Effects of Family Social Support On Child Psychological Adjustment In Juvenile Rheumatoid Arthritis', *Health Psychol.*, 7, 421-432.

Varni, J., Rubenfeld, L., Talbot, D. and Setoguchi, Y. (1989a), 'Determinants of Self-Esteem In Children With Congenital/Acquired Limb Deficiencies', *Jour. Dev. Behav. Pediatr.*, 10, 13-16.

Varni, J., Rubenfeld, L., Talbot, D. and Setoguchi, Y. (1989b), 'Stress, Social Support, and Depressive Symptomatology In Children With Congenital/Acquired Limb Deficiencies', *Jour. Pediatr. Psychol.*, 14, 515-530.

Varni, J. and Setoguchi, Y. (1991), 'Correlates of Perceived Physical Appearance In Children With Congenital/Acquired Limb Deficiencies', *Jour. Dev. Behav. Pediatr.*, 12, 171-176.

Veau, V. (1931), *Division Palatine; Anatomie, Chirurgie, Phonetique*, Paris Masson et Cie.

Verma, G.K. and Beard, R.M. (1981), *What Is Educational Research? Perspectives On Techniques of Research*, Gower, Aldershot.

Videbeck, R. (1960), 'Self-Conception and The Reaction of Others', *Sociometry*, 23, 231-239.

Waldrop, M.F. and Halverson, C.F. (1971), 'Minor Physical Anomalies and Hyperactive Behavior In Young Children' in Hellmuth, J. (ed.), *Exceptional Infant: Studies In Abnormalities*, vol. 2, Brunner/Mazel, Inc., New York.

Walker, B.E. and Crain, B.Jr. (1960), 'Effects of Hypervitaminosis A On Palate Development In Two Strains of Mice', *Am. J. Anat.*, 107, 49-58.

Wall, A. (1989), *Ethics and The Health Services Manager*, King Edward's

Hospital Fund For London.

Wallander, J. and Varni, J. (1989), 'Social Support and Adjustment In Chronically Ill and Handicapped Children', *Am. Jour. Commun. Psychol.*, 17, 185-201.

Wallander, J., Feldman, W. and Varni, J. (1989), 'Physical Status and Psychosocial Adjustment In Children With Spina Bifida', *Jour. Pediatr. Psychol.*, 14, 89-102.

Warren, D.W. and Devereux, J.L. (1966), 'An Analog Study of Cleft Palate Speech', *Cleft Palate Jour.*, 3, 103.

Wasserman, G.A., Green, A. and Solomon, C.R. (1985), 'At-Risk Toddlers and Their Mothers: The Special Case of Physical Handicap', *Child Dev.*, 56, 363-389.

Wasserman, G.A., Shilansky, M. and Hahn, H. (1986), 'A Matter of Degree: Maternal Interaction With Infants of Varying Levels of Retardation',*Child Study Jour.*, 16, 241-253.

Wasserman, G.A., Allen, R. and Linares, L.O. (1988), 'Maternal Interaction and Language Development In Children With and Without Speech-Related Anomalies', *Jour. Commun. Disord.*, 21, 319-331.

Watson, C.G. (1964), 'Personality Maladjustment In Boys With Cleft Lip and Palate', *Cleft Palate Jour.*, 1, 130-138.

Weachter, E.H. (1959), 'Concerns of Parents Related To The Birth of A Child With A Cleft of The Lip and Palate With Implications For Nurses', *M.A. Thesis*, University of Chicago, Chicago, Illinois.

Westlake, H. and Rutherford, D. (1966), *Cleft Palate*, Prentice Hall, Englewood Cliffs, N.J..

White, A. (1982), 'Psychiatric Study of Patients With Severe Burn Injuries', *British Medical Journal*, 284, 465-467.

White, M. (1989), 'Magic Circle', *Times Educ. Supplement*, 30.6.89

Whitfield, R. (1988), 'Quotation' in Jones, P. *Lipservice: The Story of Talk In Schools*, Open University Press, Milton Keynes, p.xi.

Williams, E. and Griffiths, T. (1991), 'Psychological Consequences of Burn Injury', *Burns*, 17, (6), 478-480.

Wirls, C.J. (1971), 'Psychosocial Aspects of Cleft Lip and Palate' in Graff, W. Rosenstein, S. and Bzoch, K. (eds), *Cleft Lip and Palate Surgical, Dental and Speech Aspects*, Little, Brown and Company, Boston, chapter viii.

Wirls, C.J. and Plotkin, R.R. (1971), 'A Comparison of Children With Cleft Palate and Their Siblings On Projective Test Personality Factors', *Cleft Palate Jour.*, 8, 399-408.

Wolff, S. (1969), *Children Under Stress*, Allen Lane, Penguin Press.

Wood, P.H.N. (1975), 'Classification of Impairments and Handicaps', *Document WHO / ICDO / REV / CONF / 75.15*, World Health Organization, Geneva.

Wood, P.H.N. and Badley, E.M. (1978), 'An Epidemiological Appraisal of Disablement' in Bennett, A.E. (ed.), *Recent Advances In Community*

Medicine, Churchill Livingstone, Edinburgh.

Woodburn, M.F. (1973), *The Social Implications of Spina Bifida,* Scottish Spina Bifida Association (Eastern Branch), subsequently NFER Publishing Company, Windsor.

WHO, (1980b), *International Classification of Impairments, Disabilities and Handicaps,* World Health Organization, Geneva.

Wright, B.A. (1964), 'Spread In Adjustment To Disability', *Bulletin, Menninger Clinic,* 28, 198-208.

Wylie, R., Miller, P., Cowles, S. and Wilson, A. (1979), *The Self-Concept,* Theory and Research On Selected Topics, vol.2, Revised Edition, University of Nebraska Press, Lincoln, N.E..